OXFORD SPECIALTY TRAINING

Clinical Medicine for the MRCP PACES
Volume 2

History-taking, communication and ethics

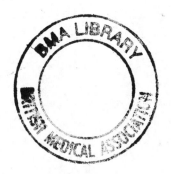

OXFORD SPECIALTY TRAINING

Clinical Medicine for the MRCP PACES Volume 2

History-taking, communication and ethics

Edited by

Gautam Mehta
Specialist Registrar in Gastroenterology
Wellcome Trust Research Fellow
Institute of Hepatology
University College London

Bilal Iqbal
Specialist Registrar in Cardiology
Hammersmith Hospital
Imperial College London

Deborah Bowman
Senior Lecturer in Medical Ethics and Law
Centre for Medical and Healthcare Education
St. George's, University of London
London

Forewords by
Professor Sir Kenneth Calman
Chief Medical Officer (1991–8)

Professor Sir Graeme Catto
President, General Medical Council (2002–9)

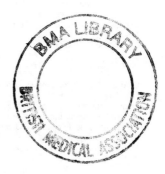

OXFORD
UNIVERSITY PRESS

Great Clarendon Street, Oxford OX2 6DP

Oxford University Press is a department of the University of Oxford.
It furthers the University's objective of excellence in research, scholarship,
and education by publishing worldwide in

Oxford New York

Auckland Cape Town Dar es Salaam Hong Kong Karachi
Kuala Lumpur Madrid Melbourne Mexico City Nairobi
New Delhi Shanghai Taipei Toronto

With offices in

Argentina Austria Brazil Chile Czech Republic France Greece
Guatemala Hungary Italy Japan Poland Portugal Singapore
South Korea Switzerland Thailand Turkey Ukraine Vietnam

Oxford is a registered trade mark of Oxford University Press
in the UK and in certain other countries

Published in the United States
by Oxford University Press Inc., New York

British Library Cataloguing in Publication Data
Data available

Library of Congress Cataloguing in Publication Data
Data available

Typeset by Glyph International, Bangalore, India
Printed in Great Britain
by Ashford Colour Press Ltd., Gosport, Hampshire

ISBN 978–0–19–955749–3

10 9 8

Foreword

Ask any patient what matters about their care, and communication is likely to be near the top of their agenda. The communication they need is not just about the language used, and the depth of the explanation, but about the way in which the process is conducted. Communication allows the transmission of empathy, compassion, and care as well as facts about the illness and possible treatment. It is also about listening, not just hearing, what the patient says.

One of the privileges of being a doctor is to be allowed to share the stories of patients. These allow the doctor to become involved and by listening enabled to interpret the story, understand it and make some sense of it. That is a very particular skill and is at the heart of the consultation. Add to this the need to consider a wide variety of ethical issues and the task becomes even more complex. Discussions on consent, or on whether to proceed with treatment, are not easy. But it is what doctors do, and the newer methods of learning to communicate, and not just to be dropped in at the deep end, can make a difference. This is what this book is about.

Patients have huge experience of their illness and their symptoms and what they mean to them. The privilege is being allowed to share that and to have an opportunity of changing things for the better. Two lessons have been important for me. First, the mantra of not getting involved with patients, was one that was taught to me as an undergraduate. I don't think it works. Empathy, kindness, and compassion require involvement and professionalism does not mean that one cannot feel concern for a patient or a family and want to make a difference. I read somewhere of the patient who asked, 'my story is broken, can you help me fix it?' To do that effectively does require active listening and participation.

The second is that patients are highly sophisticated and can teach doctors a lot about how to behave. As an oncologist many years ago, I set up a series of cancer support groups. I like to think that they made contribution to helping patients and their families. However what I am sure of is that they helped the clinical staff understand better what the problems really were. We benefited as least as much as the patients did, if not more, and I have always been grateful for all that they taught me.

Finally, a word on equanimity. This was the subject of one of Sir William Osler's great essays. It means the ability to be able to keep a clear head, provide a way forward and give confidence and calmness when things get difficult. It too is part of the communication which is so important between patient and doctor.

Kenneth C Calman

Foreword

The message is loud and clear. Patients, the public and the medical profession itself expect doctors to practise safe and high quality medicine. Of course, how we perform in practice is inevitably influenced by the knowledge, skills, and behaviours we acquire—and that in turn depends on appropriate assessment procedures. Over the last few years, the Royal Colleges of Physicians have revised the way they assess candidates for the MRCP (UK), an almost essential prerequisite to becoming a consultant physician in the UK. The new PACES examinations remain clinically relevant while ensuring greater objectivity in marking.

These two volumes adopt an innovative approach to help the postgraduate student prepare for these new assessments. Based on a selection of clinical cases from the various systems of the body, the authors emphasize the importance of communication skills and ethical considerations. What make these books different, however, are the *clinical notes* sections which not only guide the candidate through the technique of clinical examination but also integrate investigative results and consider relevant differential diagnoses. Each section also includes a number of questions commonly asked by examiners.

The authors are senior registrars and medical educators with experience of preparing candidates for the MRCP PACES examination. They have produced two volumes packed with the information needed to pass PACES and to practise high quality medicine. While written specifically for those aspiring to be physicians, these volumes deserve to be widely read by all with an interest in clinical medicine. Candidates in particular and patients have good reason to welcome these volumes.

Professor Sir Graeme Catto

Preface

'The single biggest problem with communication is the illusion it has taken place.'

George Bernard Shaw

Clinical medicine is evolving. The public's perception of safety and quality in healthcare is evolving. Moreover, the MRCP PACES examination continues to evolve to establish the benchmark for professional medical practice in a modern healthcare system. Effective communication skills, whether giving or receiving information, are the foundation of good medical practice. Although often neglected by undergraduate and postgraduate teaching programmes, the abilities to establish professional relationships, to communicate effectively, and to work within a sound ethical framework, represent the peak of professional performance. Eliciting a history from a vulnerable patient requires not only knowledge and technique, but also complex skills of rapport, empathy, and sensitivity. At the same time, medical professionals must be able to synthesize the facts presented before them, develop a safe, effective, and ethical management plan, and be able to communicate these facts to colleagues.

Hence, the pressures on the candidate for the MRCP (PACES) examination are considerable and varied. On the one hand, the candidate is faced with the task of learning the endless factual knowledge presented in medical texts, and mastering the various clinical examination techniques essential to pass Stations 1, 3, and 5 of the MRCP (PACES) examination. However, the College recognizes that the qualities of a medical professional represent more than just the sum of history and examination skills. To that end, the MRCP (PACES) examination has evolved to assess the higher-order skills that embody the contemporary physician, such as empathy, rapport, problem-solving abilities, professionalism, and ethical practice.

Many candidates assume that communication skills cannot be taught, and are 'innate' characteristics of the person. Although communication is closely bound to self-perception, self-esteem, and personal style, knowing how to converse with friends is not the same as interviewing a patient. Because we all have some experience of communicating with peers and patients, most candidates prepare for these stations by clinical 'experience'. Unfortunately, experience is a poor teacher of effective communication, since good and bad habits are reinforced equally. Effective patient interviewing requires a series of learned skills, which when performed correctly have been demonstrated to improve the accuracy of patient diagnoses, increase patient satisfaction, improve patient compliance with treatment, decrease patient stress and anxiety, as well as increase doctor well-being and provide cost-savings. However, most candidates still neglect to systematically prepare these skills for the PACES examination or for their medical practice. Indeed, Stations 2 and 4 are the stations most frequently failed by candidates sitting the MRCP (PACES) examination.

This volume is intended to be a comprehensive guide, not only to the history-taking and ethico-legal curriculum required for the MRCP (PACES) examination, but also to clinical practice. Successful learning requires the understanding of conceptual building blocks, which are then applied to a range of clinical contexts. This book applies experimental and constructivist learning theory to clinical practice, with key conceptual themes that underpin the succeeding clinical scenarios.

Following this introduction, the history-taking section begins with a review of the key concepts of effective patient interviewing. The subsequent clinical scenarios are a comprehensive selection of the cases that the candidate can expect to encounter in the PACES examination, and in clinical practice.

In a similar fashion to Volume 1, an evidence-based approach is taken to patient interviewing, followed by examiner's questions, which further promote an evidence-based review of the medical problem. The reader is provided with a strategy for sensitive and empathic interviewing, and a resource to promote evidence-based practice. The section covering communication skills and medical ethics also begins with an overview of the main principles of ethico-legal practice. The subsequent four sections are structured around core themes. In each section key concepts are introduced, and are translated to a range of scenarios.

The first of these sections is concerned with capacity. The reason for beginning with capacity is that it is fundamental to how doctors facilitate choices and decisions about care. Capacity provides the freedom for self-determination and raises the ethical bar when it is absent. Before seeking consent, doctors must consider capacity thoroughly. Of the four criteria for valid consent, capacity is the first to be considered and in its absence, the other three criteria are redundant. For that reason, capacity is discussed before all else in this volume.

Consent is discussed in detail, with the aim of deconstructing its elements and application in diverse clinical scenarios, thereby enabling readers to become familiar with, and confident in applying, the core concepts to varied situations. In seeking to prepare for PACES or any other examination, deep and effective learning should be the aim. Such an approach means that learners are able to discern key principles, core concepts, and relevant frameworks whilst adapting to diverse or even novel situations. In this section, consent is presented as much more than a series of ethico-legal rules. Rather the clinical scenarios presented demonstrate the therapeutic value of seeking meaningful consent, the importance of, and limits to, patient choice, the virtue of a flexible of approach, and the need to respect difference.

The section discussing confidentiality and information sharing is divided into two subsections dealing separately with the basic principles of, and qualifications to, confidentiality, and then with the sharing or provision of healthcare information. The practical business of working with other agencies and third parties is covered throughout this section of the book with an emphasis on demonstrating how to balance both the legal framework and professional discretion that are particular to handling confidential information in medicine.

Finally, professionalism is discussed, in relation to probity and accountability. Once again, core themes are considered in relation to a range of situations that may challenge the ways in which an individual doctor interacts both with, and on behalf of, the National Health Service. This section discusses what it means to be 'professional' when dealing with conflict, responding to complaints, recording critical incidents, defining standards of care, maintaining professional competence, and working with others. It is a section that encompasses what might be described as 'pure bioethics' and is informed by the law, but the discussion also extends beyond disciplinary boundaries to reflect the complexity of skills, values, and behaviour that a 'good' doctor should bring to his or her practice.

To close, this volume represents the synthesis of the authors' perceptions of professionalism within a modern healthcare system. The cardinal feature of a professional is the ability to recognize similar attributes in his or her peers. The new MRCP (PACES) examination applies this principle, by assessing clinical performance as well as simply knowledge or technique. The new Station 5 is the best example of this development in learning and assessment, whereby candidates are measured by their overall performance and professionalism. The concepts of this book are designed to prepare candidates for the demands of the (PACES) examination, and their ongoing development as physicians and professionals.

Acknowledgements

First, I would like to thank my co-authors Bilal and Deborah for their never-ending patience and effort. Without their spirit and enthusiasm, this project would have been filed along with most of my other great ideas! Many thanks also to the other contributors—Fatima, Paul, and Rimona for their sterling work.

No work of this magnitude is possible without mentorship, and I am particularly indebted to Andrew Thillainayagam for his unwavering support and guidance. It was those memorable first words from my first post-take ward round, 'Gautam, are you sure you want to be a physician?' that inspired me to pursue excellence in my chosen field. I also owe a debt of gratitude to Ian Curran, and my medical education colleagues at the London Deanery and Barts & Royal London, for introducing me to the concepts of learning and teaching that underpin this book.

I am grateful to all those at Oxford University Press for making this idea a reality—Fiona Goodgame, Christopher Reid, Stephanie Ireland, and Joanna Hardern to name but a few.

Whatever the weaknesses of these books, they would have been far greater without the help of my friends Mathena and Samer, who reviewed the manuscript more times than they care to remember. Special thanks also to Alex for never-ending support and inspiration.

Finally, these books are dedicated to my parents, to whom I owe so much. My mother for her love and affection, and my father for being my role-model in medicine and in life.

Gautam Mehta

First, I would like to thank my co-authors Gautam and Deborah for all their hard work, time and patience, without which this venture would never have been completed. I would like to thank Fatima, Paul, and Rimona for their contributions and feedback.

I am forever indebted to Chris Wathen for his invaluable advice, support, and guidance in orientating this project, especially at such a time of unprecedented change to the curriculum and structure of the MRCP (PACES) examination.

If it were not for Oxford University Press, our concepts for novel MRCP (PACES) textbooks would have remained as such, and would never have become a reality. I would particularly like to thank our colleagues, Fiona, Stephanie, Chris, and Joanna at Oxford University Press for their friendly advice, support, and patience throughout every stage of this project.

I cannot be grateful enough to Nabila and Adam for their everlasting support, resilience and patience at home, without which, I would never have been able to complete this, for what once felt like a never-ending project.

Finally, I would like to dedicate these books to my parents, as it if were not for their affection and inspiration at every stage of my life and career, I would not be where I am today.

Bilal Iqbal

Deborah Bowman is grateful to the staff and students at St George's who provide such a stimulating environment in which to develop ideas, and to those clinicians who, having passed MRCP, applied their skills and knowledge so kindly when a period of illness threatened to derail the project.

Deborah Bowman

Contributor details

Fatima Jaffer

CTI Core Medical Training

National Hospital for Neurology and Neurosurgery

Queen Square

London, UK

Structure of the MRCP (PACES) examination

Structure of the examination

The 5 stations comprising the MRCP (PACES) examinations are set up, such that at any one time, 5 candidates can be examined. The duration of each station is 20 minutes. Stations 2 and 4 are designated 20 minutes each, whereas stations 1, 3, and 5 are further split into two 10-minute clinical encounters. Each station is preceded by a 5-minute interval. This is particularly useful for stations 2, 4, and 5, where the initial candidate information that outlines the scenario(s) can be used to gather your thoughts, organize your history-taking approach and develop preliminary differential diagnoses.

Skills tested in the examination

From October 2009, the marking scheme for the MRCP (PACES) examination has changed. There are now seven clinical skills tested in the examination. The Clinical Skills tested are:

A. Physical Examination
B. Identifying Physical Signs
C. Clinical Communication
D. Differential Diagnosis
E. Clinical Judgement
F. Managing Patients' Concerns
G. Maintaining Patient Welfare

The marking scheme

Each skill is designated a mark: 0 (unsatisfactory), 1 (borderline), and 2 (satisfactory).

			Skills tested							
Station	**Encounter**	**Time (min)**	**A**	**B**	**C**	**D**	**E**	**F**	**G**	**Maximum marks (per examiner)**
1	Abdomen	10	•	•		•	•		•	10
1	Respiratory	10	•	•		•	•		•	10
2	History	20			•	•	•	•	•	10
3	Cardiovascular	10	•	•		•	•		•	10
3	Nervous system	10	•	•		•	•		•	10
4	Communication	20			•		•	•	•	8
5	Brief Clinical Consultation (1)	10	•	•	•	•	•	•	•	14
5	Brief Clinical Consultation (2)	10	•	•	•	•	•	•	•	14

Examiners are no longer required to award an overall judgement mark for each encounter. Given that 2 examiners will each score the candidate, the total marks are 172. Station 5 now constitutes 56 marks—that's almost a third of the total marks.

For specific mark sheets and further information about the MRCP (PACES) structure, please visit

(a) www.mrcpuk.org/PACES/Pages/PacesMarkSheets.aspx

(b) www.mrcpuk.org/PACES/Pages/PacesFormat.aspx

Contents

List of Abbreviations

↑	raised
↓	lowered
A&E	Accident and Emergency Department
AAFB	acid-alcohol fast bacilli
ABCD$_2$	Age, Blood pressure, Clinical features, Duration of symptoms and Diabetes mellitus
A&E	Accident and Emergency Department
ABPA	allergic bronchopulmonary aspergillosis
ABVD	adriamycin, bleomycin, vinblastine, dacrabazine
AC	air conduction
ACC	American College of Cardiology
ACE	angiotensin converting enzyme
ACR	American College of Rheumatology
ACTH	adrenocorticotrophic hormone
ADA	Adenosine deaminase activity
ADH	antidiuretic hormone
ADPKD	autosomal dominant polycystic kidney disease
AF	atrial fibrillation
AFLP	acute fatty liver of pregnancy
AFP	alph-fetoprotein
AHA	American Heart Association
AICA	anterior inferior cerebellar artery infarction
AIDP	acute inflammatory demyelinating polyradiculoneuropathy
AIDS	aquired immunodeficiency syndrome
AIP	acute interstitial pneumonia
ALP	alkaline phosphatase
ALT	alanine aminotransferase
AML	acute myeloid leukaemia
AMPA	α-amino-hydroxy-5-methylisoxasole-4 propionic acid
AMTS	abbreviated mental test score
ANA	antinuclear autoantibody
ANCA	anti-neutrophil cytoplasmic antibody
anti-CCP	Anti-cyclic citrullinated peptide
anti-GBM	anti-glomerular basement membrane antibody
anti-RNP	anti-ribonucleoprotein antibody
AP	antero-posterior
APC	adenomatous polyposis coli
APTT	activated partial thromboplastin time
APUD	amine precursor uptake and decarboxylation
ARDS	acute respiratory distress syndrome
A-R-P	Accommodation Reflex Preserved
ARPKD	Autosomal recessive polycystic kidney disease
ASA	atrial septal aneurysm
ASD	atrial septal defect
ATS	American Thoracic Society
AVM	arteriovenous malformations
AVNRT	atrioventricular nodal re-entry tachycardia

AVRT	atrioventricular re-entry tachycardia
BC	bone conduction
BCC	basal cell carcinoma
BEACOPP	bleomycin, etoposide, doxorubicin, cyclophosphamide, Oncovin (vincristine), prednisolone, procarabazine
BMD	Becker's muscular dystrophy
BMI	body mass index
BNF	British National Formulary
BNP	brain natriuretic peptide
BP	blood pressure
bpm	beats per minute
BPPV	benign paroxysmal positional vertigo
CAB	Citizens Advice Bureau
CABG	coronary artery bypass graft
CADASIL	cerebral autosomal dominant arteriopathy with subcortical infarcts and leucoencephalopathy
CAM	Confusion Assessment Method
cAMP	cyclic adenosine monophosphate
c-ANCA	cytoplasmic anti-neutrophil cytoplasmic antibody
CAT	computerized axial tomography
CHD	coronary heart disease
CIDP	chronic inflammatory demyelinating polyneuropathy
CINCA	Chronic Infantile, Neurologic, Cutaneous, and Articular
CJD	Creutzfeldt-Jakob disease
CK	creatine kinase
CML	chronic myeloid leukaemia
CMV	cytomegalovirus
CNS	central nervous system
COMT	catechol-O-methyl transferase
COP	cryptogenic organizing pneumonia
COPD	chronic obstructive pulmonary disease
COPP	cyclophosphamide, Oncovin (vincristine), prednisolone, procarbazine
CPA	cerebellopontine angle
CPEO	chronic progressive external ophthalmoplegia
CPR	cardiopulmonary resuscitation
CRC	colorectal carcinoma
CRH	corticotrophin releasing hormone
CRP	C-reactive protein
CSF	cerebrospinal fluid
CT	computed tomography
CT KUB	CT— kidneys, ureters, bladder
CXR	chest X-ray
D-AB	Dorsal-ABduct
DAFNE	Dose Adjustment for Normal Eating programme
DCCT	Diabetes Control and Complications Trial
DDAVP	desmopressin acetate (synthetic analogue of vasopressin)
DHS	Drug Hypersensitivity Syndrome
DI	diabetes insipidus
DIC	disseminated intravascular coagulation
DIP	desquamative interstitial pneumonia
DIP	distal interphalangeal

DKA	diabetic ketoacidosis
DMARDs	disease modifying anti-rheumatic drugs
DMD	Duchenne's muscular dystrophy
DNAR	do not attempt resuscitation
DNCB	dinitrochlorobenzene
DPA	Data Protection Act (1998)
DPCP	diphenylcypropenone
DPP-IV	dipeptidyl peptidase IV
DRESS	Drug Reaction with Eosinophilia and Systemic Symptoms
DVLA	Driver and Vehicle Licensing Agency
DVT	deep vein thrombosis
EAA	extrinsic allergic alveolitis
EBV	Epstein-Barr virus
ECCE	extracapsular cataract extraction
ECG	electrocardiogram
EDIC	Epidemiology of Diabetes Interventions and Complications trial
EDTA	ethylenediaminetetraacetic acid
EEG	electroencephalogram
EIA	enzyme immunoassay
EMG	electromyography
ENA	extractable nuclear antigen
ENT	ear, nose, and throat
EPS	electrophysiological studies
ERCP	endoscopic retrograde cholangiopancreatography
ERG	electroretinogram
ERS	European Respiratory Society
ESR	erythrocyte sedimentation rate
FAP	familial adenomatous polyposis
FBC	full blood count
FDA	Food and Drug Administration
FDR	first-degree relative
FET	forced expiratory time
FEV	forced expiratory volume
FH	family history
FNA	fine-needle aspiration
FOB	faecal occult blood
FRC	functional residual capacity
FSH	follicle stimulating hormone
FTA	fluorescent treponemal antibody
FVC	forced vital capacity
GALS	gait, arms, legs, spine
GBS	Guillain-Barré syndrome
GFR	glomerular filtration rate
GGT	gamma glutamyl transpeptidase
GH	growth hormone
GHRH	growth hormone-releasing hormone
GI	gastrointestinal
GIST	gastrointestinal stromal tumour
GLP-1	Glucagon-like peptide 1
GMC	General Medical Council

GN	glomerulonephritis
GORD	gastrooesophageal reflux disease
GTN	glyceryl trinitrate
HAART	highly active anti-retroviral therapy
Hb	haemoglobin
HCC	hepatocellular carcinoma
hCG	human chorionic gonadotrophin
HCV	hepatitis C virus
HDL	high density lipoprotein
HELLP	Haemolysis, Elevated Liver enzymes, Low Platelets
HHT	hereditary haemorrhagic telangiectasia
HHV-6	human herpesvirus 6
HIV	human immunodeficiency virus
HL	Hodgkin's lymphoma
HMSN	hereditary motor and sensory neuropathy
HNPCC	hereditary nonpolyposis colorectal cancer
HNPP	hereditary neuropathy with pressure palsy
HONK	hyperosmolar hyperglycaemic non-ketotic
HR	heart rate
HRA	Human Rights Act (1998)
HRCT	high resolution CT (scan)
HSV	herpes simplex virus
HTLV-1	human T-lymphotropic virus-1
IBD	inflammatory bowel disease
IBS	irritable bowel syndrome
ICAS	Independent Complaints Advocacy Service
ICD	implantable cardioverter defibrillator
ICCE	intracapsular cataract extraction
ICU	Intensive Care Unit
IDA	iron-deficiency anaemia
IGF-1	insulin-like growth factor-I
IH	immunohistochemistry
IM	intramuscular
IMCA	independent mental capacity advocates
INO	internuclear ophthalmoplegia
INR	international normalized ratio
IPV	inactivated polio virus
IV	intravenous
IVC	inferior vena cava
IVIG	intravenous immunoglobulin
IVTA	Intravitreal triamcinolone acetonide
JVP	jugular venous pressure
LA	left atrium
LABA	long acting β_2 agonist
LACI	lacunar circulation infarct
LADA	latent autoimmune disease of the adult
LDH	lactate dehydrogenase
LDL	low density lipoprotein
LEMS	Lambert-Eaton myasthenic syndrome
LFT	liver function tests

LH	luteinising hormone
LIP	lymphoid interstitial pneumonia
LMN	lower motor neurone
LP	lumbar puncture
LPHs	lipotropins
LV	left ventricle
MALT	mucosal-associated lymphoid tissue
MCA	middle cerebral artery
MCP	metacarpophalangeal
MDR TB	multi-drug resistant tuberculosis
MEN	mulitple endocrine neoplasia
MGUS	Monoclonal gammopathy of undetermined significance
MI	myocardial infarction
MMSE	Mini Mental State Examination
MND	motor neurone disease
MPTP	1-methyl-4-phenyl-1,2,3,6-tetrahydropridine
MPZ	myelin protein zero gene
MRA	magnetic resonance angiogram
MRCP	magnetic resonance cholangiopancreatography
MRI	magnetic resonance imaging
MRSA	Methycillin resistant staphylococcus aureus
MRV	magnetic resonance venography
MSA	multiple systems atrophy
MSH	melanocyte-stimulating hormone
MSI	microsatellite instability
MSM	men who sleep with men
MuSK	muscle-specific kinase
NAAT	nucleic acid amplification test
nAChR	nicotinic acetylcholine receptors
NAFLD	non-alcoholic fatty liver disease
NCS	nerve conduction study
NHL	non-Hodgkin's lymphoma
NICE	National Institute for Health and Clinical Excellence
NMDA	N-methyl-D-aspartic acid
NO	nitric oxide
NSAID	nonsteroidal anti-inflammatory drug
NSCLC	non-small cell carcinoma
NSIP	non-specific interstitial pneumonia
NSTEMI	non-ST segment elevation myocardial infarction
NYHA	New York Heart Association
OA	osteoarthritis
OIs	opportunistic infections
OGD	oesophago-gastro-duodenoscopy
OPV	oral live attenuated polio virus
PA	pulmonary artery
PACI	partial anterior circulation infarct
P-AD	Palmar-ADduct
p-ANCA	perinuclear anti-neutrophil cytoplasmic antibody
PALS	Patient Advocacy and Liaison
PAN	polyarteritis nodosa

PBC	primary biliary cirrhosis
PCI	percutaneous coronary intervention
PCP	pneumocystis carinii pneumonia
PCR	polymerase chain reaction
PCWP	pulmonary capillary wedge pressure
PDA	patent ductus arteriosus
PE	pulmonary embolism
PEFR	peat expiratory flow rate
PEG	percutaneous gastronomy
PFO	patent foramen ovale
PFT	pulmonary function test
PI	protease inhibitor
PICA	posterior inferior cerebellar artery
PIP	proximal interphalangeal
PJS	Peutz-Jehgers syndrome
PMF	pulmonary massive fibrosis
PMP22	peripheral myelin protein-22 gene
POCI	posterior circulation infarct
POEMS	Polyneuropathy, Organomegaly, Endocrinopathy, Monoclonal gammopathy, and Skin changes
POMC	proopiomelanocortin
PPD	purified protein derivative
PR	per rectum
PSA	Prostate Specific Antigen
PSC	primary sclerosing cholangitis
PSP	progressive supranuclear palsy
PTH	parathyroid hormone
PTU	propylthiouracil
PVS	persistent vegetative state
QALYS	Quality Adjusted Life Years
RA	rheumatoid arthritis
RA	right atrium
RAPD	relative afferent pupillary defects
RBC	red blood cell
RB-ILD	respiratory bronchiolitis-interstitial lung disease
REM	rapid eye movement
RhF	Rheumatoid factor
RNA	ribonucleic acid
RNP	ribonuclear protein
RPGN	Rapidly Progressive Glomerulonephritis
RPR	Rapid Plasmin Reagin
RV	right ventricle
SADBE	squaric acid dinitryl ester
SAH	subarachnoid haemorrhage
SCC	squamous cell carcinoma
SCLC	small cell lung carcinoma
SHBG	sex hormone-binding globulin
SHO	Senior House Officer
SIADH	syndrome of inappropriate anti-diuretic hormone
SLE	systemic lupus erythematosus

SPECT	Single Photon Emission Computed Tomography
SSRI	selective serotonin reuptake inhibitor
STEMI	ST segment elevation myocardial infarction
STI	sexually transmitted infection
SUDEP	Sudden Unexpected Death in Epilepsy
SVC	superior vena cava
SVTs	supraventricular tachycardias
TACI	total anterior circulation infarct
TB	tuberculosis
TED	thrombo-embolus deterrent
TGF	transforming growth factor
TIA	transient ischaemic attack
TIPS	transjugular intrahepatic portosystemic shunt
TLC	total lung capacity
TNF	tumour necrosis factor
TNM	classification system: spread of primary tumour (T); extent of lymph node involvment (N); and presence or absence of metastases (M)
TPHA	*T pallidum* haemagglutination
TTP	thrombotic thrombocytopenic purpura
TSH	thyroid stimulating hormone
TSI	thyroid stimulating immunoglobulin
TVO	transient visual obscuration
U&E	urea and electrolytes
UC	ulcerative colitis
UIP	usual interstitial pneumonia
UKPDS	UK Prospective Diabetes Study
UMN	upper motor neurone
USA	unstable angina
VDRL	Venereal Disease Reference Laboratory
VEGF	vascular endothelial growth factor
VF	ventricular fibrillation
VHFs	viral haemorrhagic fevers
V-Q	ventilation-perfusion
VSD	ventricular septal defect
VT	ventricular tachychardia
VZV	varicella zoster virus
WBC	white blood cell
WCC	white cell count
WHO	World Health Organization
WPW	Wolff-Parkinson-White syndrome

Station 2 ◆ **History Taking Skills**

Core Concepts and Overview

Core concepts and overview

Recent years have seen a shift in the perception of communication skills from being considered subjective personal traits, to an objective, evidence-based curriculum of skills and techniques. This development was founded on the recognition that core communication skills are identifiable, can be taught, and form the basis of the majority of professional encounters.

The core skills required for the patient interview in the MRCP (PACES) examination can be broadly divided into three areas: *content* skills, *process* skills, and *perceptual* skills. The *content* of the medical interview refers to the information the candidate is attempting to gather, or to give, during the course of the interview. The detail of this content is covered in the subsequent case histories of this book. However, the ability of the candidate to communicate or acquire this content depends largely on the *process* of the interview, and their *perceptual* skills.

The *process* of the interview refers to the manner in which the candidate communicates with the patient. Although the candidate's agenda may be to establish the content of the interview, this will not be successful unless the patient's agenda in considered. In Stations 2 and 4 of the PACES examination, the candidate is provided with clear written instructions (such as a GP letter), followed by 14 minutes for patient interaction. The candidate then has 1 minute for reflection, followed by 5 minutes of discussion with the examiners. Despite the limited time available in the PACES Stations 2 and 4, the examiners will expect the candidate to develop rapport, show empahty, appropriately use silencce during the interview, and interpret non-verbal cues. Indeed, these processes are the key to obtaining the content of the interview, not just for the examination but also for clinical practice.

Perceptual skills refer to the candidate's decision making, problem solving, and clinical reasoning skills. These are complex, higher-order skills, which reflect the individual's attitudes, beliefs, and self-perception. Indeed, if the content of the interview reflects the candidate's 'knowledge', and the process of the interview is a reflection of 'technique', then these perceptual skills are a demonstration of appropriate 'behaviour' or 'performance'.

Nevertheless, the distinction between these skills is artificial since they are inextricably linked, and the MRCP candidate must employ all three areas to be considered a professional—the summation of knowledge, technique, and behaviour. The purpose of this section of the book is to provide the candidate with a framework to develop the necessary techniques for successful medical interviewing.

The most commonly used framework for acquiring a medical history is the traditional model, whcih reflects the 'content' of the interview (Box 2.1). Whilst this model is the established order of case presentation, and the 'currency' of communicating salient facts to colleagues, this model has also become embedded in the *process* of the interview. This linear model is based around the clinician's agenda of acquiring information, and promotes a closed questioning style to fulfil this agenda. Moreover, in the examination setting, candidates use the history-taking station to demonstrate their knowledge by saying it out loud in the form of the questions they ask. Inevitably, this involves closed questions, which neglect the patient's agenda and the doctor–patient relationship.

Box 2.1 Traditional history-taking model

- Presenting complaint
- History of presenting complaint
- Past medical history
- Drug history
- Allergy history
- Family history
- Social history
- Systems review

Instead, the art of patient-centred communication lies in using the process of the interview to establish the patient's perspective of the consultation, and *translating* that information into the traditional history structure when presenting to colleagues or documenting written notes. Time constraints, whether in the PACES examination or in clinical practice, often compel candidates to adopt an interrogative interview technique in an attempt to be more time efficient. However, this approach will isolate the patient and dismay examiners, even if it satisifies the candidate's agenda.

The Calgary-Cambridge guide by Kurtz and colleagues[1] is a useful framework to the process of effective medical interviewing, and is one of the most widely used tools in patient communication. Although there is only a window of 14 minutes to acquire the history in the PACES examination, application of the abridged framework presented below will allow the candidate to target the consultation to the patient's agenda, and thus establish the content of the consultaion in the most efficient manner.

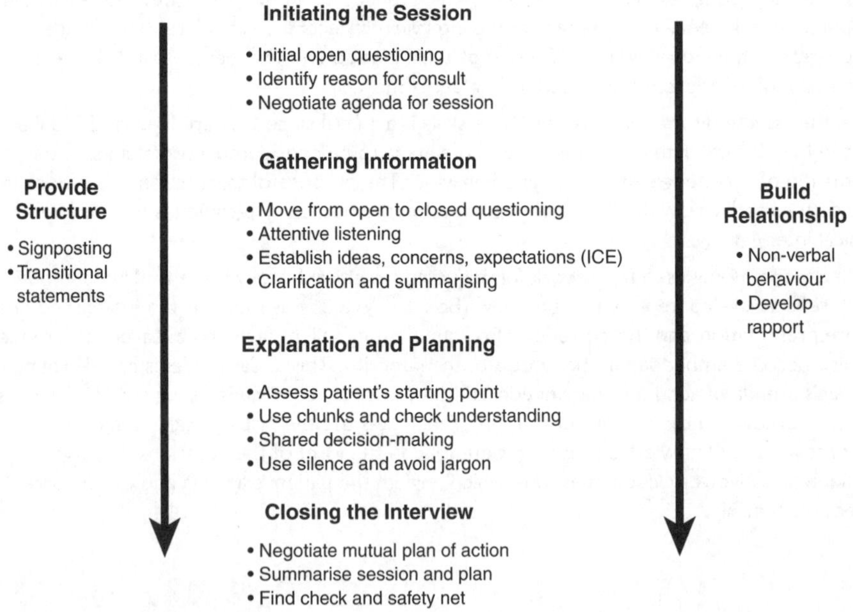

Initiating the Session

- Initial open questioning
- Identify reason for consult
- Negotiate agenda for session

Gathering Information

Provide Structure

- Signposting
- Transitional statements

- Move from open to closed questioning
- Attentive listening
- Establish ideas, concerns, expectations (ICE)
- Clarification and summarising

Build Relationship

- Non-verbal behaviour
- Develop rapport

Explanation and Planning

- Assess patient's starting point
- Use chunks and check understanding
- Shared decision-making
- Use silence and avoid jargon

Closing the Interview

- Negotiate mutual plan of action
- Summarise session and plan
- Find check and safety net

Figure 1 Calgary-Cambridge framework.
Modified from Kurtz and Silverman[1]

Initiating the session

Begin by greeting the patient and obtaining their name. Introduce yourself, your role, and the nature of the interview. If appropriate, obtain verbal consent for the interview: *'Is it alright if we discuss the reason why you are here today?'* Identify the reason for the consult by asking appropriate open questions, e.g. *'What would you like to discuss today?'*, or *'What questions were you hoping to ask me today?'*

Use *attentive listening* to hear the patient's initial response without interruption or direction. This may feel like a long time in the examination scenario, but allowing the patient to make an uninterrupted opening statement minimizes the risk that 'hidden agendas' will arise later in the interview. Once the patient has finished speaking, use *summarizing* and *checking* to maintain a structure to the interview, and screen for other problems: *'So that's abdominal pain and vomiting, anything else?'*

If the list of problems is unrealistic for a single consultation, it may be necessary to negotiate the agenda with the patient: *'Since the pain and the vomiting are new, shall we concentrate on those today and talk about your eye drops at the next appointment?'* However, even though the scenario in the PACES examination will give a background to the patient's problem, they may still have a hidden agenda and it is important not to dismiss the patient's issues just because they are not listed in the introduction to the scenario.

Gathering information

Encourage the patient to tell the story in their own words, from beginning to end. Use open questioning initially; *'Tell me how your symptoms started?'* Move on to use closed questions for details and to establish dates and times: *'What prompted you to finally go to the doctor?'*, *'How long was it before you came to hospital?'*

Use *clarification* if the patient uses statements that are unclear: *'Could you explain what you mean by sick? Do you mean vomiting or unwell?'* Avoid the use of *jargon*, e.g gastrostomy, echocardiogram.

Actively try to determine:

I   the patient's *ideas* about their illness; 'What do you think may be causing your symptoms?'
C   their *concerns*, 'Is the anything you are worried this may be?'
E   their *expectations*: 'What do you see happening to yourself after treatment?', 'I see you are keen to start treatment "quickly— is there anything specific that you are trying to get better for?'

During the process of acquiring the content of the interview, use *signposting* to direct the interview and maintain structure, *'I'm now going to ask you some questions about your bowel habits'*. Sharing thinking with the patient, if done sensitively and cautiously, also encourages patient involvement and develops rapport, *'What I'm thinking now is this may be a problem with your digestion. Have you had these symptoms before?'*

Explanation and planning

Begin by assessing the patient's starting point, by asking how much they understand about their problems or the process so far. Use small chunks of information when explaining a plan, and check for understanding at each stage. Use the patient's responses and non-verbal cues as a guide to how to proceed. Use visual aids or diagrams if possible.

The goal is to achieve a shared understanding of the medical problem. This involves relating the issues to the patient's perspective, and to their ideas, concerns, and expectations that were previously discussed. This phase of the interview is built upon the relationship that has been established by the candidate's techniques, behaviour, and professionalism. Sharing the interviewer's thoughts and dilemmas during the course of the interview is an important way of empowering the patient to engage in shared decision making. *'I can see that you are concerned about the thought of having a biopsy. Let me explain the issues from my perspective so we can make this decision together.' 'Whilst there is a lot of research in this area, we still don't know the best treatment. Let me explain why I think we should avoid antibiotics.'*

Finally, summarize the session and check with the patient that their concerns have been addressed. A safety net must also be mentioned—what to do if the plan is not working, e.g. call the secretary, attend the emergency department. Finish by asking for final questions and check agreement with the plan of action.

Whilst this framework provides a structure for the candidate to fall back on in the PACES examination, it must be remembered that allowing the patient to determine the content of the interview facilitates patient-centred interviewing. The art of the skilled interviewer is to use the techniques mentioned above to provide structure to the interview, without encroaching on the patient's agenda. If the candidate can apply these techniques on the background of the evidence-base presented in the forthcoming case histories, they will have the foundation for effective communication in the PACES examination and their professional practice.

References

1. Kurtz SM, Silverman JD. The Calgary-Cambridge Referenced Observation Guides: an aid to defining the curriculum and organizing the teaching in communication training programmes. Medical Education 1986; 30:83–9.

History-Taking Skills

Case 1 ◆ Hypertension

INFORMATION FOR THE CANDIDATE

Dear Doctor,

Thank you for seeing this 52-year old gentleman with an elevated blood pressure. He has been found to have three successive blood pressure readings of 158/98 mmHg, 160/95 mmHg, and 156/96 mmHg. He has been taking bendroflumethiazide 2.5mg daily for the last 4 months, with little effect. There is no history of stroke or ischaemic heart disease. He is a smoker of 20 cigarettes per day, and drinks up to 12 pints of lager at weekends. He is currently a self-employed electrician.

Many thanks for your opinion.

Acquiring the history

A. History of presenting complaint:

- Are there symptoms of uncontrolled hypertension—headache, visual disturbance?
- Are there symptoms of end-organ damage—chest pain, palpitations, dyspnoea, ankle oedema, neurological symptoms?
    - ◆ MACROVASCULAR DISEASE
        Coronary artery disease: chest pain, breathlessness, orthopnoea, paroxysmal nocturnal dyspnoea, ankle oedema
        Peripheral vascular disease: cold extremities, claudication
        Cerebrovascular disease: visual disturbances, neurological deficit
    - ◆ MICROVASCULAR DISEASE
        Retinal disease: visual disturbance
        Renal disease: nausea, lethargy, ankle swelling
- Are there symptoms of an underlying medical disorder causing secondary hypertension (see question 1).
    - ◆ Enquire about symptoms of endocrine disease:
        Hyperthyroidism: anxiety, sweating, palpitations, tremor, weight loss, diarrhoea
        Acromegaly: headaches, change in appearance, glove and shoe size, visual field disturbance
        Cushing's syndrome: steroid use, striae, purpura, centripetal fat deposition, proximal myopathy
        Conn's syndrome: weakness, lethargy, muscle cramps (hypokalaemia)
        Phaeochromocytoma: palpitations, sweating and weight loss.
    - ◆ Enquire about symptoms of renal disease. Are there any urinary symptoms, obstructive symptoms, or symptoms of uraemia, i.e. lethargy, nausea, pruritis?
- Are there symptoms of an underlying anxiety disorder, or of 'white-coat hypertension'? Has the patient had their blood pressure measured outside a hospital or clinic?

B. Relevant medical and family history:

- ◆ Ask about conditions which predispose to secondary hypertension (see question 1)
- ◆ The major complications of hypertension are coronary heart disease (CHD), stroke, renal disease, heart failure and peripheral vascular disease. Ask specifically about these conditions.
- ◆ A family history of hypertension makes essential hypertension more likely. However, a family history of endocrine disease (*specifically MEN 2*), CHD and risk factors such as dyslipidaemia should be sought.

C. Medications and interactions:

- Remember, most hypertensive patients will use over the counter or prescribed medications which alter blood pressure, or interact with common antihypertensive medications:
  - ◆ Nonsteroidal anti-inflammatory drugs (NSAIDs) can cause sodium retention, and resistance to hypertension treatment.
  - ◆ Over the counter nasal sprays and decongestants may contain vasoactive agents such as ephedrine and pseudoephedrine, which can induce hypertension.
- Oral contraceptive agents frequently cause a mild elevation in blood pressure, although oestrogen containing compounds may induce overt hypertension.
- Corticosteroids (topical and systemic) cause sodium retention and hypertension. Ask specifically about symptoms of Cushing's syndrome.
- Ciclosporin may also cause progressive hypertension.
- Illicit drug use, such as cocaine, MDMA (ecstasy) and amphetamines, must not be overlooked in patients with resistant hypertension.
- Ask about anabolic steroid use in young patients, especially atheletic male patients.
- Ask about compliance with prescribed medications. If compliance is poor, ask about common adverse reactions to therapy (e.g. bendroflumethiazide—impotence, gout; calcium-channel blockers—ankle swelling, constipation; angiotensin converting enzyme (ACE) inhibitors—cough).

D. Social issues:

- Alcohol excess and obesity are the most common causes of reversible hypertension. Ask about lifestyle, diet (caffeine and salt intake) and alcohol use.
- Cigarette smoking is also a major contributor to CHD risk.
- Enquire about illicit drug use (see above).
- Ask about occupation, and how the patient is supporting himself financially.
- If any risk factors for impotence are present, such as diabetes mellitus, peripheral vascular disease, or bendroflumethiazide or beta blocker use, ask sensitively about marital problems.

Formulating a plan of action

- Explain that the diagnosis of hypertension is not in itself serious, but control of blood pressure is necessary to prevent serious complications like heart disease and stroke, and that causes are primary (essential hypertension) and secondary. If 'white coat hypertension' is likely, then an ambulatory 24-hour BP monitor may be necessary.
- Tell the patient that you would like to request routine blood tests (to exclude possible secondary causes of hypertension) and an ECG (electrocardiogram) (to look for evidence of left ventricular hypertrophy).
- Advise about lifestyle factors and modifications.
- Tell the patient that a follow-up appointment will be given to discuss the results of above tests.

Questions commonly asked by examiners

What are the causes of secondary hypertension, and how common is it?

Secondary hypertension accounts for 5% of the prevalence of hypertension in primary care. The causes are:

- **Renal**
  - Renal parenchymal disease
  - Renovascular disease
  - Chronic renal disease of any aetiology
- **Endocrine**
  - Cushing's syndrome
  - Hyperaldosteronism
  - Adrenal hyperplasia
  - Phaechromocytoma
  - Acromegaly
  - Thyroid disease
- **Cardiorespiratory**
  - Coarctation of the aorta
  - Obstructive sleep apnoea
- **Drug-induced**

Which patients with hypertension should receive treatment?

The National Institute for Health and Clinical Excellence (NICE) guidelines[1] (2006) recommend that all hypertensive patients with an estimated 10-year CHD risk of greater than 20%, or a persistent blood pressure over 160/100mmHg, should receive pharmacological treatment. All patients with diabetes mellitus or pre-existing cardiovascular disease should also be treated, as guided by the National Service Frameworks for these diseases.

How is cardiovascular risk assessed in a hypertensive patient?

The 10-year CHD risk is estimated using Coronary Risk Prediction Charts,[2] derived from data acquired from the Framingham Heart Study. These charts provide an estimate of CHD risk based on gender, age, systolic blood pressure, smoking status, total cholesterol, and HDL cholesterol. However, these charts are only suitable for primary prevention. These charts cannot be used for patients with established cardiovascular disease, familial hypercholesterolaemia or other inherited dyslipidaemias, chronic renal disease or diabetes mellitus.

How would you manage this patient?

- **Confirm diagnosis** – hypertension should be diagnosed with an appropriate sized blood pressure cuff, with an elevated blood pressure found on three separate occasions.
- **Lifestyle interventions** – advice should be provided regarding reducing salt intake, decreasing alcohol consumption, smoking cessation, and regular exercise.
- **Manage cardiovascular risk** – modifiable risk factors such as obesity, hyperlipidaemia, diabetes mellitus and smoking must be identified and treated. All patients with a 10-year CHD risk greater than 30% should receive lipid lowering therapy.
- **Drug treatment** – patients aged over 55 should be treated according to the NICE guidelines (Figure 1.1).

What blood pressure would you be aiming for with treatment?

For patients without diabetes mellitus, the aim of treatment should be a systolic pressure <140mmHg, and a diastolic pressure <85mmHg.

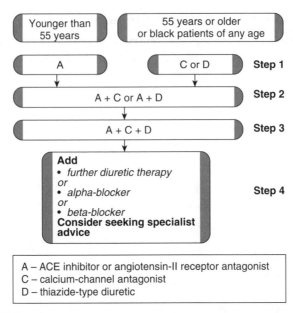

Figure 1.1 BHS/NICE flow chart.

In patients with diabetes mellitus, chronic renal disease, or established cardiovascular disease, the optimal treatment goals are systolic pressure <130mmHg, and diastolic pressure <80mmHg.

What is the role of beta blockers in the management of hypertension?

Beta blockers are no longer considered first-line antihypertensives for patients over the age of 55 in the most recent NICE guidance.[1] This is following a series of studies suggesting decreased efficacy in reducing stroke risk, including the ASCOT[3] and LIFE[4] trials. A meta-analysis of these trials demonstrated a 16% higher incidence of stroke among patients treated with beta blockers, primarily atenolol, than those treated with other antihypertensive medications.[5]

Beta blockers may still be useful in younger patients, or those with associated CHD.

What about elderly patients?

Until recently, there was no data to support the treatment of hypertension in patients over the age of 80. However, the recent HYVET study was stopped early due to a lower rate of fatal or non-fatal stroke in elderly patients receiving indapamide, with or without perindopril, over placebo.[6]

References

1. National Institute for Health and Clinical Excellence Hypertension: management of hypertension in adults in primary care. London: NICE, June 2006.

2. Jackson R, Lawes CM, Bennett DA, et al. Treatment with drugs to lower blood pressure and blood cholesterol based on an individual's absolute cardiovascular risk. Lancet 2005; 365:434–41.

3. Dahlof B, Sever PS, Poulter NR, et al. Prevention of cardiovascular events with an antihypertensive regimen of amlodipine adding perindopril as required versus atenolol adding bendroflumethiazide as required, in the Anglo-Scandinavian Cardiac Outcomes Trial – Blood Pressure Lowering Arm (ASCOT-BPLA): a multicentre randomised control trial. Lancet 2005; 366:895–906.

4. Reihms HM, Oparil S, Kjeldsen SE et al. Losartan benefits over atenolol in non-smoking hypertensive patients with left ventricular hypertrophy—the LIFE study. Blood pressure 2004; 13:376-84.

5. Lindholm LH, Carlberg B, Samuelsson O. Should beta blockers remain first choice in the treatment of primary hypertension? A meta-analysis. Lancet 2005; 366:1545–53.

6. Beckett NS, Peters R, Fletcher AE, et al. Treatment of hypertension in patients 80 years of age or older. New Engl J Med. 2008; 358:1887–98.

Case 2 ◆ **Dyspepsia**

INFORMATION FOR THE CANDIDATE

Dear Doctor,

Thank you for seeing this 42-year old lady with a three month history of bloating and epigastric pain. She feels she may also have lost some weight, however her bowel habit is regular. She has been taking lansoprazole 15mg daily with some benefit, but is still symptomatic. She smokes 30 cigarettes per day. There is no other significant past medical history.

Many thanks for your opinion.

Acquiring the history

A. History of presenting complaint:

- Characterize the abdominal pain—site, type, radiation, intensity, duration, onset, frequency, previous episodes?
- Is there associated nausea or vomiting?
- Are there associated reflux symptoms—retrosternal burning, acid brash, regurgitation, worse on lying flat?
- Is the pain relieved by, or precipitated by, meals?
- Is the pain pancreatic in origin—radiates to back, precipitated by eating, relieved by leaning forward?
- Is the pain biliary in origin—right sided abdominal pain, precipitated by eating, with associated nausea?
- Is the pain colonic in origin—lower abdominal pain, colicky in nature, partially relieved by defaecation?
- Could the pain be cardiac in origin—exertional chest pain, dyspnoea?
- Are there any alarm features, suggesting gastrointestinal malignancy?
    - Dysphagia?
    - Weight loss?
    - Early satiety?
    - Jaundice?
    - Anaemia?
    - Progressive vomiting?
    - Previous gastric ulcer?
    - Previous gastric surgery?
- Nocturnal symptoms? Posture during sleep (number of pillows, etc.)?
- Is the patient eating late in the day, precipitating nocturnal symptoms?
- Are the symptoms affecting the patient's quality of life?

B. Relevant medical and family history:

- Previous gastric ulcer or gastric surgery?
- Previous pancreatitis?
- Previous gall stone disease or cholesystectomy?
- Haemoglobinopathy (pigment gall stones)?
- Iron deficiency anaemia (except premenopausal women)?
- Any previous endoscopic or radiological investigations?
- Family history of gastrointestinal malignancy?
- Hyperlipidaemia (markedly elevated triglycerides are a risk factor for pancreatitis)?

C. Medications and interactions:

- Ask about proton pump inhibitor use, or other antacid compounds?
- Ask about compliance with current drug regimen?
- Any drugs which may cause gastric ulceration—NSAIDs, corticosteroids, bisphosphonates?
- Any drugs which may precipitate gastro-oesphageal reflux—nitrates, calcium antagonists, theophyllines, bisphosphonates?
- Any drugs which may cause pancreatitis—azathioprine, antiretroviral drugs, loop and thiazide diuretics?

D. Social issues:

- Alcohol excess and obesity are common precipitants of abdominal pain. Ask about lifestyle, diet, and alcohol use.
- Cigarette smoking is also a major contributor to dyspepsia, and gastrointestinal cancer risk.
- Ask about occupation, and how the patient is supporting himself financially.

Formulating a plan of action

- Explain that there are several possible diagnoses of abdominal pain and dyspepsia, but a trial of therapy may be the best initial strategy prior to investigation.
- Explain that endoscopy would be an initial test if alarm symptoms are present, or if the patient is aged over 55.[1]
- If endoscopy is not indicated initially, tell the patient that the initial management would be a trial of proton pump inhibitor for four weeks, followed by Helicobacter pylori testing if the patient is still symptomatic.
- Suggest an abdominal ultrasound if biliary or pancreatic pain is a feature.
- If reflux symptoms are present, advise the patient to elevate the head of their bed, and avoid eating late in the day, to prevent nocturnal symptoms.
- Provide general advice about weight loss, smoking cessation, limiting alcohol intake, and avoiding dietary precipitants of dyspepsia—although avoid the concept of 'food allergy'.
- Tell the patient that a follow-up appointment will be given to discuss the results of above tests.

Questions commonly asked by examiners

What are the major risk factors for gastric cancer?

- *Helicobacter pylori* infection—causes atrophic gastritis, progressing to metaplasia, dysplasia and cancer
- Previous gastric surgery—due to hypochlorhydria, or bile reflux
- Cigarette smoking—associated with a 1.5 fold increase in risk
- Blood group A—may be in linkage dysequilibrium with other genes close to blood group antigens
- Gastric cancer has been described in association with certain cancer syndromes, including hereditary non-polyposis colorectal cancer, familial adenomatous polyposis, and Peutz-Jehger's syndrome.

Tell me about methods of diagnosing Helicobacter pylori infection?

Non-invasive methods of diagnosis include ^{13}C-urea breath testing, and Helicobacter stool antigen detection. The sensitivity and specificity of both these tests exceeds 95%, although the use of proton pump inhibitors may lead to false negative results.

Rapid urease testing from endoscopic biopsies has a sensitivity and specificity of 90–95%. Helicobacter can also be diagnosed on routine histology from the gastric antrum and body. It can also provide information about intestinal metaplasia and mucosal-associated lymphoid tissue (MALT), both of which are associated with Helicobacter infection.

Bacterial culture and sensitivity testing is not routinely recommended, but may provide information in refractory disease.

What is role of Helicobacter pylori infection in peptic ulcer disease?

Epidemiologically, Helicobacter is associated with up to 95% of patients with duodenal ulcers. Furthermore, treatment of Helicobacter reduces the incidence of ulcer recurrence.

Helicobacter is also found in 65–95% of patients with gastric ulcers, and 70–90% of patients with gastric cancer. However, Helicobacter eradication has not been proven to reduce gastric adenocarcinoma risk, although MALT-type lymphomas may achieve remission following Helicobacter eradication.

The mechanism of disease is thought to be due to bacterial effects on gastric acid secretion, gastric metaplasia, immune responses to infection, and mucosal defence mechanisms.

What is the role of Helicobacter pylori infection in non-ulcerative dyspepsia?

Helicobacter infection has also been reported in 20–60% of patients with non-ulcerative dyspepsia, although the prevalence in asymptomatic individuals is 20–45%. The effect of treating Helicobacter in these patients has been studied several times, although the studies have provided mixed results, with only a small benefit on symptoms demonstrated on meta-analysis.

References

1. Dyspepsia: Managing dyspepsia in adults in primary care. National Institute of Health and Clinical Excellence, August 2004.

Case 3 ♦ **Weight Loss**

INFORMATION FOR THE CANDIDATE

Dear Doctor,

Thank you for seeing this 82-year old gentleman who has lost 3 stone in the last 2 months. His appetite is poor, although there are no other symptoms of note. He is an ex-smoker and has also has chronic obstructive pulmonary disease (COPD) and hypertension which are managed with inhalers and antihypertensives.

Many thanks for your opinion.

Acquiring the history

Weight loss is a common but worrying symptom for patients, particularly the elderly. The aim of the history is detect features of serious physical and psychological illness, and to establish the need for further invasive investigation.

The focus of much of the history is to screen for underlying causes of weight loss, hence many of the questions are 'closed'. Therefore, initially establish that weight loss is the patients' only complaint, and ask openly if the patient has any other concerns or is worried about anything in particular; *'Before we discuss your weight loss, may I ask if there is anything else bothering you? Is there anything in particular you are worried may be causing the weight loss?'*.

A. History of presenting complaint:

- **Determine nature of weight loss:**
  - Quantify degree of weight loss: Clinically significant weight loss may be defined as greater than 5% of body weight over a period of up to 12 months, and is associated with increased mortality. However, patients may under-estimate or over-estimate the degree of weight loss. Up to one-third of patients complaining of weight loss have not actually lost weight. Attempt to quantify the amount and duration of weight loss. *'How much weight have you lost?'*, *'Over how long?'*. If possible, calculate the Body Mass Index—weight(kg)/height(m)^2. Additionally, corroborate the weight loss by asking family members for an opinion and asking about changes in clothing size, *'Have you noticed your clothes becoming looser or hanging off you?'*.
  - Is the weight loss voluntary or involuntary?
  - Does the weight loss coincide with a change in diet, physical activity or lifestyle?
  - Establish if the patient has lost their appetite, *'Do you still feel hungry?'*, *'Are you enjoying your food?'*, *'How is your appetite?'*.

Involuntary weight loss with *preserved* appetite	Involuntary weight loss with *loss* of appetite
Uncontrolled diabetes mellitius	Malignancy
Hyperthyroidism	Severe cardiac or respiratory failure
Malabsorption	Advanced chronic renal disease
Phaeochromocytoma	Oesophageal disease (causing dysphagia or odynophagia)
	Gastroduodenal disease (causing vomiting or abdominal pain)
	Depression
	HIV
	Chronic inflammatory disease of any cause

- **Screen for alarm symptoms:**
  - Dysphagia: *'Do you have problems swallowing, or does the food ever get stuck?'* See Case 6, Dysphagia for subsidiary questions.
  - Early satiety: *'Are you able to manage a meal, or have you been getting full quickly?'*
  - Abdominal pain: *'Do you ever experience any pain in your stomach or abdomen?'*. Ask about post-prandial pain (suggesting gastroduodenal disease or mesenteric ischaemia) and pancreatic pain in particular. *'Does the pain come on after meals? Does it go through to your back?'* See Case 8, Abdominal pain.
  - Change in bowel habit: *'Have you noticed a change in your bowels? Any diarrhoea or constipation? What colour are the stools?'* This is often a difficult question for patients to answer accurately, so a closed question may help *'Are they pale, like this?'* whilst pointing to a pale yellow object (often the colour of casenotes folders!).

- ♦ Melaena/haematochezia: *'Have you passed any blood in your motions? Is the blood red or dark? Is it bright red—like a letterbox?'*
- ♦ Respiratory symptoms: *'Have you noticed a change in your breathing or cough? Have you coughed up any blood?'*
- ♦ Bone pain: *'Have you had any pain in your back or your joints?'*. Bone pain or night pain may suggest metastatic malignancy.
- ♦ Endocrine symptoms: hyperthyroidism—*'Have you had sweats recently, or been unusually warm or nervous?'*, diabetes—*'Have you been unusually thirsty or passing a lot of urine?'*, adrenal insufficiency—*'Have you had any nausea or dizziness recently?'*.
- ♦ Other constitutional symptoms: night sweats, fatigue.

- • **Establish the patient's nutritional intake:**

An assessment of nutritional intake should be made, along with an assessment of the patient's nutritional requirements which are influenced by co-morbid conditions and functional status. Ask about:

(i) the number of meals and snacks consumed during a typical 24-hour period
(ii) the consumption of meat and dairy produce
(iii) who prepares the food, and whether the patient finishes the portions
(iv) the use of nutritional and vitamin supplements
(v) previous dietetic consults

Also ask about any other problems with eating meals, such as problems with dentition or painful swallowing (odynophagia).

Remember that the physiological energy requirements will be higher for patients who have chronic illnesses and those that are particularly mobile.

- • **Screen for psychological causes of weight loss:**

Psychiatric disease is a common cause of weight loss, particularly in young females or in the elderly.

(i) *'Have you ever tried to lose weight deliberately?'*
(ii) *'Does your weight fluctuate a lot?'*
(iii) *'How many diets have you been on in the past year?'*
(iv) *'How has your mood been over recent weeks?'*

B. Relevant medical and family history:

- • Several chronic medical conditions can cause weight loss: COPD, cardiac failure, diabetes, chronic renal disease.
- • Ask about gastrointestinal (GI) conditions such as peptic ulcer disease, pancreatic disease, or Crohn's disease.
- • Ask about previous GI surgery which may predispose to malabsorption, such as small bowel resection or pancreatic surgery.
- • Patients with peripheral vascular disease, and/or vascular risk factors are prone to mesenteric ischaemia.
- • Ask about a family history of malignancy, particularly colorectal, breast, and ovarian cancer.

C. Medications and interactions:

- • Some medications may directly contribute to weight loss by affecting appetite: selective serotonin reuptake inhibitors (SSRIs), levodopa, metformin, theophylline, and digoxin.
- • GI side effects may also contribute to weight loss:
  - ♦ Dry mouth: anticholinergics, diuretics
  - ♦ Dysphagia: bisphosphonates, NSAIDs, theophylline
  - ♦ Nausea: antibiotics, digoxin, metformin, iron

- Pancreatitis may be caused by azathioprine, HIV anti-retrovirals, loop diuretics, thiazide diuretics and metronidazole. Ensure that patients with chronic pancreatitis on pancreatic enzyme replacements are also on acid-suppression, since gastric acid may denature the enzyme supplements.
- Illicit drug use, such as cocaine and amphetamines, must not be overlooked in young patients with weight loss.

D. Social issues:

- Alcohol excess is a common cause of chronic pancreatitis.
- Cigarette smoking is a risk factor for several malignancies.
- Ask about HIV risk factors, since HIV is a cause of unexplained weight loss.
- Document travel history as a risk factor for chronic infection (eg. Giardia, Campylobacter, Cryptosporidium)

Formulating a plan of action

- Reassure the patient that whilst weight loss is a serious symptom, a cause is usually found (in 75% of cases).
- Tell the patient that you would like to perform a full examination and request routine blood tests. Explain that a dietetic consultation may also be helpful.
- Initial tests to consider include:
  - Full blood count (FBC), electrolytes, liver function tests (LFTs), albumin (not a sensitive marker of nutritional status, since it varies with severe co-morbidity), C-reactive protein (CRP), iron studies.
  - Thyroid function tests, glucose, 9am cortisol or synacthen test.
  - Serum B12, calcium, vitamin D, prothrombin time (markers of vitamin malabsorption).
  - Tumor markers: CEA, Ca19-9, Ca-125, αFP, PSA.
  - Faecal sudan stain (qualitative marker of fat malabsorption), faecal elastase (low in chronic pancreatitis).
  - Coeliac antibodies
- Tell the patient that a follow-up appointment will be given to discuss the results of above tests, and establish the need for further investigations (such as imaging or endoscopy).

Questions commonly asked by examiners

How would you assess a patient's nutritional status?

The Subjective Global Assessment[1] is a validated dietetic tool to assess nutritional status. It is based on six features, which are assessed by history and examination:

(i)   Change in weight
(ii) Dietary intake
(iii) Functional capacity
(iv) Gastrointestinal symptoms with nutritional impact (e.g. diarrhoea)
(v)   Metabolic stress of current disease
(vi) Examination findings of poor nutrition

The patient's nutritional requirements are affected by functional capacity and co-morbidity, but can be estimated:

$$1000 + (10 \times \text{body weight}) = \text{approximate energy requirement (kcal)}$$

An assessment must also include an approximation of the patient's fluid requirements, which will be influenced by fluid losses due to fever, malabsorption, stoma output, etc.

Clinical examination will help to determine fluid balance status, however the degree of fat and muscle stores can also be estimated:

(i)   fat stores: triceps skinfold thickness
(ii) muscle stores: arm muscle circumference, temporalis muscle wasting
(iii) muscle function: hand grip dynometry

Biochemistry is also used to assist nutritional assessment, however no single test directly reflects nutritional state. In particular, the serum albumin is inversely correlated with the CRP, and may therefore reflect inflammation rather the nutritional state. Moreover, the albumin only falls in severe malnutrition, hence patients may have significant undernutrition with a normal albumin.

Measurement of electrolytes, in particular the sodium, potassium, calcium, magnesium, and phosphate, is important when commencing feeding for early detection of re-feeding syndrome (see below).

What are the principles of management of malnutrition?

1.   Eliminate sepsis—since nutritional support is ineffective in the presence of active sepsis, infection must be detected and treated. Malnourished patients may not exhibit the classical signs of sepsis, so a high degree of suspicion is required.
2.   Diagnose and treat GI disease—malabsorption may be a consequence of coeliac disease, Crohn's disease, bacterial overgrowth, pancreatic insufficiency, lactose deficiency or short bowel syndrome. This must be treated alongside nutritional supplementation.
3.   Treat micronutrient deficiencies—all patients should have thiamine supplementation before feeding is commenced, since re-feeding may precipitate Wernicke's encephalopathy in malnourished patients with thiamine deficiency.
4.   Attempt nutritional support enterally—if the GI tract is intact and functioning then this is the preferred route of supplementation, since enteral feeding prevents gram-negative bacterial translocation across the gut lumen, and is not associated with the complications of parenteral line-feeding.
5.   Monitor and replace electrolytes to prevent re-feeding syndrome—in malnourished patients who are undergoing gluconeogenesis, the sudden introduction of nutrition causes a surge in insulin to facilitate glucose uptake. However, this insulin also causes an intracellular shift in potassium, phosphate, and magnesium, resulting in very low serum levels. This may cause clinical consequences including arrhythmias, rhabdomyolysis, and death. Therefore, these electrolytes must be measured and replaced daily until feeding is established and there are no further electrolyte shifts.
6.   Parenteral nutrition—this is administered through a tunnelled intravenous catheter (Broviac catheter). The short-term complications include those from line placement (bleeding, pneumothorax, line sepsis, and thrombosis), hyperglycaemia, re-feeding syndrome, and abnormal LFTs. If excess nutrition is provided, greater than 500kcal over energy requirements, then acute fatty liver, jaundice, and liver failure may occur. The long-term complications include line sepsis, line thrombosis, gallstones, renal stones, and bone disease.

How would you approach weight loss in elderly patients?

Weight loss in elderly patients may not be due to medical conditions, but may be consequence of dementia or social factors. Elderly patients also have impaired smell and taste, and altered GI function, which affect appetite and intake. Furthermore, polypharmacy is common in this group and medications may contribute to weight loss directly (see above) or indirectly by causing GI side effects (e.g. altered taste, nausea).

All elderly patients with weight loss should undergo screening for depression and dementia. Furthermore, elderly patients with weight loss and iron-deficiency anaemia should undergo evaluation of the upper and lower GI tract. The causes of weight loss in the elderly are listed in Box 1.

Box 1 Unintentional weight loss in the elderly: 'Meals on Wheels'	
M	Medication effects
E	Emotional problems (eg. depression)
A	Anorexia, alcoholism
L	Late-life paranoia
S	Swallowing disorders
O	Oral health (e.g. poorly fitting dentures)
N	No money
W	Wandering and dementia behaviour
H	Hyper/hypothyroidism, hypercalcaemia, hypoadrenalism
E	Enteric problems (eg. malabsorption)
E	Eating problems (eg. inability to feed oneself)
L	Low salt, low cholesterol diets
S	Social problems (e.g. isolation, difficulty shopping)
Source: Adapted from Morley and Silver[2]	

References

1. Detsky AS, McLaughlin JR, Baker JP, et al. What is subjective global assessment of nutritional status? JPEN J Parenter Enteral Nutr 1987; 11:8–13.

2. Morley JE, Silver AJ. Nutritional issues in nursing home care. Ann Intern Med 1995;123(11):850–9.

Case 4 ◆ Change in Bowel Habit

INFORMATION FOR THE CANDIDATE

Dear Doctor,

Thank you for seeing this 48-year old lady with a 3-month history of altered bowel habit. She has lost a stone in weight over this time, but has not had any rectal bleeding. She has a history of longstanding type 1 diabetes, for which she takes insulin. She is concerned because she has a cousin with ulcerative colitis and her uncle recently died from colon cancer. I wonder if she needs a colonoscopy?

Many thanks for your opinion.

Acquiring the history

Altered bowel habit is a common symptom, and the challenge for the candidate is not only to consider the broad list of differential diagnoses, but also to determine which patients require further invasive investigation. Moreover, distinguishing between the many causes of diarrhoea and constipation requires questioning about other GI and systemic symptoms. Therefore, sensitive and open questioning is essential to detect symptoms that the patient may regard as trivial or embarrassing, but which may be highly relevant to their investigation and management.

A. History of presenting complaint:

• **Determine what the patient means by a change in bowel habit.**

'What has been the trouble with your bowels recently?'; 'Can you tell me exactly what you mean by constipation/diarrhoea/loose stool?'; 'How is this different from your normal bowel habit?'.

◆ **Constipation:** Determine what the patient means by 'constipation'. The classic definition is of fewer than 3 bowel movements per week, however patients use the term to describe a broad range of symptoms. Determine the patient's 'normal' bowel habit, and how things have changed.

Ask about stool frequency, consistency, associated straining, and the sensation of incomplete evacuation. *'How often do you open your bowels in an average week?'; 'What do you pass?', 'Is the stool hard or soft? Does it hurt or do you strain when you pass stool?'; 'Have you noticed any blood in the toilet or in your stool?'; 'When you finish, do you ever have the feeling that you still need to open your bowels?'*

Ask about onset, duration, and progression of symptoms. Acute or recent-onset constipation is more likely to represent colon cancer or intestinal obstruction. *'Are you still passing wind?'*—failure to pass flatus suggests complete intestinal obstruction.

Defecatory disorders are the cause in a significant proportion of patients with constipation (20–25%). These are caused by pelvic floor dysfunction, where the puborectalis muscle and external anal sphincter fail to relax during defecation, possibly due to incorrect learned behaviour earlier in life. In fact, this syndrome is associated with psychological symptoms such as depression and anxiety, and a large proportion of patients (40%) have a history of sexual abuse. Sensitive and open questioning is therefore essential, particularly once initial questioning is complete and rapport has been established (see below). More focused questions include, *'Do you ever have difficulty passing soft stools as well as hard stools?', 'Do you ever find it difficult to relax or let go in order to pass stool', 'Do you ever need to push around, or put your finger into, your vagina/rectum to help you pass stool?'.* Also ask about incontinence; *'Do you ever lose control of your bowels?'.* In the presence of urgency this suggests proctitis (see below), although 'overflow diarrhoea' due to faecal impaction typically presents with incontinence in the absence of urgency.

◆ **Diarrhoea:** Again, confirm what the patient means by 'diarrhoea'. Patients may use the term 'diarrhoea' to describe faecal incontinence, an increased frequency of normal stool or an acute diarrhoeal illness. Several definitions of diarrhoea exist—increased stool weight (>200g/day) or a general change increase in liquidity of stool.

There are several patterns of presentation of 'diarrhoea' which may give a clue to diagnosis:

(i) Large volumes of watery stool, unaffected by fasting, suggesting a secretory process
(ii) Moderate volume of loose stool, which improves on fasting, suggesting an osmotic process
(iii) Bloody diarrhoea and abdominal pain, suggesting an inflammatory process
(iv) Steatorrhoea, the passage of pale, greasy stools suggesting malabsorption (see Case 3 Weight Loss).
(v) Urgency suggests proctitis, or inflammation of the rectum.
(vi) Nocturnal diarrhoea, or waking from sleep to pass stool, suggests organic disease such as inflammatory bowel disease (IBD) or autonomic neuropathy due to diabetes mellitus

Therefore, ask specifically whether the diarrhoea improves at night or if the patient fasts for a while. Ask about pale stools and the presence of blood (melaena and haematochezia). Urgency or incontinence can be extremely disabling for patients: for example, they may be unable to use public transport. Appreciation of this through the use of empathy may help with rapport; *'I can see that must make your life very difficult, particularly if you have to travel to work'.* Ask sensitively how the patient is coping with their symptoms—how do they travel, do they use incontinence pads?

- **Associated GI symptoms:** Screen with focused questions for:
  - Upper GI symptoms: nausea, vomiting, dysphagia, reflux, dyspepsia, early satiety (see Case 2 Dyspepsia)
  - Abdominal pain: in particular, pain that is relieved by defaecation suggesting irritable bowel syndrome (IBS), or pancreatic pain suggesting chronic pancreatitis. (see Case8 Abdominal Pain)
  - Weight loss (see Case 3 Weight Loss)
- **Associated systemic symptoms:**
  - Fever, tachycardia: systemic upset suggests IBD or infectious colitis (see below).
  - Extraintestinal symptoms: joint pains, oral ulceration, rash, red or painful eyes. These may be features of IBD or may occur following GI infection (reactive arthritis or Reiter's syndrome; see Case 23 Joint Pains).
- **Associated risk factors:**

If the diarrhoea is of recent onset:

  - *'Have you recently started any new medications?'*; (see below).
  - *'Have you noticed any foods that make your symptoms better or worse? How about dairy products?'*. Patients often attribute their symptoms to diet, although genuine food allergy/intolerance is rare as ide from lactose intolerance and coeliac disease. True lactase deficiency causing lactose intolerance is common in African and Asian populations, and is diagnosed using a lactose-hydrogen breath test. In the remaining patients this symptom should not be ignored, since a systematic food elimination approach under the supervision of a dietitian may be indicated.
  - *'Have you recently had any antibiotics? Have you been hospitalized or attended hospital in the last 2 months?'* Clostridium difficile infection is an increasing cause of acute diarrhoea in both hospitals and the community. These patients may have systemic symptoms such as fever. Viral infections may also be acquired from healthcare settings.
  - *'Have you ever had surgery on your abdomen? In particular, have you had surgery to your gall bladder, surgery for ulcers, or removal of a segment of intestine?'* GI surgery may cause abdominal pain and intestinal obstruction due to adhesions. Bile acid malabsorption is also a cause of chronic watery diarrhoea—this occurs following terminal ileal resection or following cholecystectomy or vagotomy.
  - *'Have you been in contact with anyone with similar symptoms?' 'Have you eaten anything unusual over recent days?' 'How long after eating did the symptoms start?'*
    - <6 hours following ingestion—*Staphylococcus aureus* infection (mayonnaise, poultry); *Bacillus cereus*
    - 8–14 hours—*Clostridium perfringens* infection (re-heated meat or poultry).
    - >14 hours—viral infection

B. Relevant medical and family history:

- Ask about a past personal and family history of IBD and colorectal carcinoma (CRC).
- Other conditions associated with constipation include:
  - Hypothyroidism
  - Hypercalcaemia—due to malignancy, hyperparathyroidism, sarcoidosis, etc.
  - Previous spinal cord injury or spinal surgery
  - Diverticular disease
- Other conditions associated with diarrhoea include:
  - Diabetes mellitus (see below)
  - Chronic pancreatitis

- Hyperthyroidism
- Antibody mediated autoimmune disease (eg. vitiligo, Grave's disease)—associated with coeliac disease
- Systemic sclerosis—associated with small bowel bacterial overgrowth
- Carcinoid syndrome—patients may have diarrhoea associated with flushing, wheeze, and rash (pellagra)

C. Medications and interactions:

- Several medications (including alcohol) can cause diarrhoea:
  - Antibiotics
  - ACE inhibitors
  - Digoxin
  - SSRIs
  - Statins
  - Proton pump inhibitors – particularly lansoprazole.
  - Laxatives
  - Magnesium in antacid preparations

D. Social issues:

- Alcohol excess is a cause of diarrhoea and of chronic pancreatitis.
- Cigarette smoking is a common cause of exacerbation of Crohn's disease, and a risk factor for colorectal cancer.
- Dietary habits, such as the use of laxatives, should also be enquired about. This may be related to underlying psychological disease such as an eating disorder, and should therefore be approached sensitively. Excessive use of sugar-free gum may also cause diarrhoea, since sorbitol may be an inadvertent source of laxative.
- Ask sensitively about HIV risk factors (see Case 17 Sexually Transmitted Infection). Diarrhoea in HIV is common, and may be due to infection in an immunocompromized host, or due to other complications such as small intestinal lymphoma. Infectious agents include *Cryptosporidium*, *Microsporidium*, *Isospora*, *Cytomegalovirus* (CMV), and *Mycobacterium avium complex*.
- Anal intercourse also predisposes to infectious proctitis, in the absence of HIV, by agents such as *Neisseria gonorrhoea* and *Chlamydia trachomatis* (causing lymphogranuloma venereum). These infections are often mistaken for proctitis due to ulcerative colitis.

Formulating a plan of action

- Use the technique of summarizing to demonstrate to the patient that you have heard their concerns, and to clarify what may be a complicated history. At this point, it may be helpful to ask openly, 'What do you think may be causing your symptoms?'. A significant proportion of patients have functional, non-organic symptoms, although this is difficult to accept for many. Further sensitive questioning regarding other aspects of the patient's life may be helpful, 'Has there been a particular change in your life during the time you have had these symptoms?', 'Did the symptoms come on during a particular time of stress?'.
- If there is considerable anxiety, the patient may insist on further investigation even if not indicated. In such cases, conflict resolution is a key communication skill that the candidate must demonstrate (see Case 5 Family History of Cancer).
- Explain to the patient that initial investigations will involve blood tests, and possibly stool samples if the diarrhoea is of recent onset (see below). Initial tests to consider include:
  - FBC, electrolytes, LFTs, albumin, CRP.
  - Thyroid function tests.

- ◆ Iron studies, serum B12, calcium, vitamin D, prothrombin time (markers of iron-deficiency anaemia (IDA) or malabsorption).
- ◆ Coeliac antibodies.
- ◆ Stool microscopy, culture and sensitivity including *Clostridium difficile* toxin
- ◆ Faecal elastase (low in chronic pancreatitis), faecal sudan stain (qualitative marker of fat malabsorption).
- Some patients may merit further investigations (see below). The reasons for this, along with the risks and benefits, should be clearly explained to the patient. Tell the patient that a follow-up appointment will be given to discuss the results of the above tests, and establish the need for further investigations (such as imaging or endoscopy).

Questions commonly asked by examiners

How do you treat a patient with a flare of IBD colitis?

The principles of treatment of IBD-related colitis are similar, regardless of whether the aetiology is Crohn's disease or ulcerative colitis (UC). The differences relate to the decreased efficacy of 5-ASA drugs in Crohn's disease, and whether anti-TNF (tumour necrosis factor) therapy is of benefit in acute UC.

All patients with a flare of IBD should have infection excluded by stool cultures for community-acquired bacterial pathogens and *C.Difficile*.

- *Proctitis*: First-line treatment is topical 5-ASA suppositories used once-daily, with steroid foams used once-daily as a second-line addition.
- *Mild/moderate left-sided colitis*: In the absence of systemic symptoms, patients can be treated with 5-ASA enemas, with steroid foam enemas as a second-line addition. High-dose oral 5-ASA tablets can be added to topical 5-ASA therapy, in a 'top-down, bottom-up regimen'. For example, 2g twice-daily mesalazine may be added to a 1g daily mesalazine enema.[1] If rectal bleeding persists beyond 10–14 days, oral steroids should be added.[2]
- *Extensive colitis*: Patients with severe colitis, as determined by the Truelove and Witt criteria (see below) require hospitalization and should receive intravenous steroids and subcutaneous low molecular weight heparin for thromboprophylaxis. Patients should have a daily abdominal X-ray to rule out progression to toxic megacolon (colonic diameter >6cm), and GI surgeons should be involved early in the patient's management. For patients with ulcerative colitis, if the patient's CRP is >45mg/L after 72 hours of intravenous steroids along with greater than 3 stools in 24 hours, the risk of colectomy on that admission is 85%.[3] Therefore, these patients should be considered for colectomy after 3 days of medical therapy. Alternatives include intravenous ciclosporin, or for UC a single dose of infliximab. These decisions should be made by a specialist IBD team, including physicians, surgeons, and nurses.

Box 2 Truelove and Witt Criteria for Severe Colitis
Bowel frequency >6 times per 24 hours *and* one or more of the systemic manifestations: • Haemoglobin <10.5g/dL   • erythrocyte sedimentation rate (ESR) >30mm/hr   • Pulse rate >90 beats per min   • Temperature >37.5°C

What are the causes of diarrhoea in diabetes mellitus?

Potential causes of diarrhoea in the diabetic patient include:

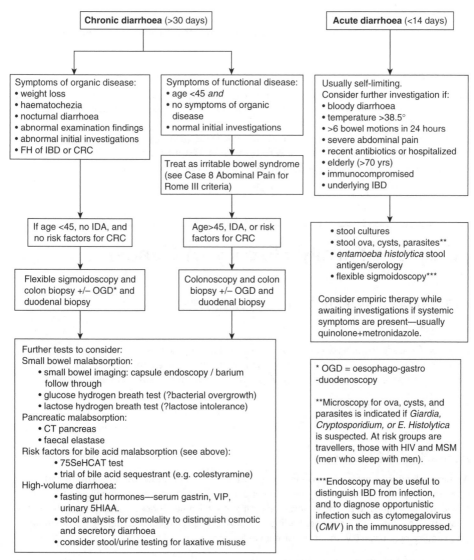

Figure 4.1
Source: Modified from Thomas, et al. Guidelines for the investigation of chronic diarrhoea, 2nd edn. Gut. 2003; 52 Suppl 5:v1–15.

- Diabetic autonomic neuropathy of the enteric nervous system. This may cause delayed or increased small bowel motility. The diarrhoea is typically painless and watery, and occurs at night. Anorectal dysfunction may also occur causing faecal incontinence.

- Small bowel bacterial overgrowth, causing chronic diarrhoea, may occur in patients with decreased small bowel mobility.

- Coeliac disease is associated with type 1 diabetes mellitus, since both are antibody-mediated autoimmune diseases. The prevalence of coeliac disease in type 1 diabetic adults is around 5%.

- Metformin causes GI side effects, including diarrhoea, in 30% of patients.
- Sorbitol in artificial sweeteners, frequently used by diabetic patients, may cause osmotic diarrhoea.

References

1. Marteau P, et al., Combined oral and enema treatment with Pentasa (mesalazine) is superior to oral therapy alone in patients with extensive mild/moderate active ulcerative colitis: a randomised, double blind, placebo controlled study. Gut. 2005; 54(7):960–65.

2. Hanauer SB, et al., Delayed-release oral mesalamine at 4.8 g/day (800 mg tablet) for the treatment of moderately active ulcerative colitis: the ASCEND II trial. Am J Gastroenterol. 2005; 100(11):2478–85.

3. Travis SP, et al., Predicting outcome in severe ulcerative colitis. Gut. 1996; 38(6):905–10.

Case 5 ◆ Family History of Cancer

INFORMATION FOR THE CANDIDATE

Dear Doctor,

Thank you for seeing this 53-year old lady, whose son was recently diagnosed with metastatic colon cancer. She has a past history of endometrial cancer, for which she underwent hysterectomy and oophrectomy. I am concerned that she may need a colonoscopy. Please could you see and advise.

Many thanks for your opinion.

Acquiring the history

Acquiring the family history is a routine part of clinical practice. However, an accurate and detailed family history has gained renewed importance with the advent of sophisticated molecular techniques to diagnose hereditary cancer syndromes. Indeed, a detailed family history is essential to differentiate asymptomatic patients who require further screening from patients who require reassurance without invasive investigation.

A. History of presenting complaint:

Since the patient may be concerned although asymptomatic, initial open questioning is vital to identify symptoms which the patient may perceive as trivial yet may be clinically relevant: *'How have you been feeling recently? Have there been any recent changes to your health or your lifestyle?'*.

Remember that patients with a recent bereavement or illness in their family are likely to be anxious or still grieving. In these situations, *empathic* responses are usually the most effective ways of developing a rapport with the patient, rather than using a *sympathetic* response or ignoring the patient's anxieties altogether (see introduction for further detail on empathic and sympathetic responses). An example of an empathic response may be *'I can see things have been difficult for you during your son's illness. Tell me how you have been feeling?'*. By contrast, a sympathetic response would invoke 'pity' as a means of dealing with the patient's anxieties and proceeding with the history according to the 'physician's agenda'—*'I'm so sorry to hear about your son's illness. Have you had any health problems recently?'*.

Even in the time-pressured situation of the MRCP (PACES) examination, examiners will look favourably on candidates who persevere with *active listening* and *empathy* rather than pursue their own agenda or turn the history into an 'interrogation'.

More focused questioning should cover symptoms relevant to the common inherited cancer syndromes:

- Lynch syndrome (Hereditary Non-Polyposis Colorectal Cancer)
1. Colonic symptoms:
    - change in bowel habit?
    - rectal bleeding?
    - weight loss?
    - previous colonoscopy / colonic polyps?
2. Extra-colonic symptoms:
    - post-menopausal vaginal bleeding (endometrial cancer)?
    - abdominal or pelvic pain (ovarian cancer)?
    - jaundice or epigastric pain (hepatobiliary / pancreatic cancer)?
    - early satiety or dyspepsia (gastric cancer)?
    - any unusual skin lesions or moles (sebaceous adenomas, carcinomas, and keratocanthomas)?
- Multiple endocrine neoplasia:
    - history of thyroid / parathyroid disease?
    - symptoms of hypercalcaemia (musculoskeletal pain, constipation)?
    - history of pituitary disease?
    - visual disturbance—particularly loss of peripheral vision?
- *BRCA1* and *BRCA2* mutations:
    - Past history of breast lumps / lumpectomy?

B. Family history:

Determine the family history of the patient, going back three generations. For each cancer, attempt to document:

- Age of *diagnosis* (rather than treatment or death)?
- Site/type of cancer?
- At which medical unit was the patient treated?
- Type of treatment (surgical/adjuvant/neo-adjuvant)

Differentiate first-degree relatives (parent, sibling, child) from second-degree relatives (grandparent, cousin, niece, nephew). Also ask about a family history of colonic polyps, for which the patient's relative may have had colonoscopy and polypectomy.

For the patient referral above, the Amsterdam II criteria* may be used to determine the risk of Lynch syndrome:

- Three or more relatives with Lynch syndrome-associated cancers (colorectal cancer, endometrial cancer, small-intestine tumours, or renal cell cancer), one of whom is a first-degree relative of the other two and in whom FAP has been excluded.
- Lynch syndrome-associated cancers involving at least two generations.
- One or more cancers diagnosed before the age of 50.

---

* These criteria can be remembered by the '3–2–1 rule': 3 affected members over 2 generations, of whom 1 is under age 50.

However, these criteria only have a sensitivity of 50% for Lynch syndrome as defined by genetic testing. Therefore, if suspicion of Lynch syndrome remains high but the family does not meet Amsterdam II criteria, then they should not be falsely reassured but should be referred for genetic counselling and genetic testing for Lynch syndrome (see below). In some cases, tumour specimens from the affected relative may be obtained and tested for genetic markers of Lynch syndrome, so asking where the patient's relative underwent treatment is an important question.

Even if genetic testing for Lynch syndrome is negative, these patients remain at increased risk due to their significant family history and require a higher level of colon surveillance (see below).

C. Relevant past medical history:

- Other risk factors for colorectal cancer: adenomatous polyps, inflammatory bowel disease, diabetes mellitus, cigarette smoking.
- Other risk factors for breast cancer: benign breast disease, early menarche, later menopause, use of HRT. High parity and oophrectomy before the age of 40 are protective.

E. Relevant social history:

As with other cases, the social history should include questioning about lifestyle, occupation and disability. Additionally, as mentioned above, the patient may still be grieving about a recent bereavement. Although the focus of this history is not the patient's stage of bereavement, a brief open question about the patient's loss will be appreciated by the examiners: *'How have you been coping since the death of your son?'*. The phases of grief have been described as: denial and isolation, anger, bargaining, depression, and finally acceptance.[1] Whilst there is not time to counsel the patient fully in the MRCP (PACES) examination, the good candidate will be able to make an assessment of the patient's progress through these stages of grief.

Formulating a plan of action

- Reassure the patient that in the absence of symptoms, significant pathology is unlikely. However, in view of the family history, it is sensible to investigate further to determine the risk of cancer and treat any 'small growths (polyps) that may turn into cancer over years'.
- If the patient's family history fulfils the Amsterdam II criteria, or if the patient has colonic symptoms, then explain that colon investigation will be necessary. This may be either colonoscopy (optical colonoscopy) or CT (computed tomography) colonography (virtual colonoscopy). Both require bowel preparation, although optical colonoscopy is the preferred modality (see below).

However, a definitive diagnosis of Lynch syndrome requires genetic testing, initially on tumour tissue from the affected relative: microsatellite instability (MSI), and immunohistochemistry (IH). This is because tumours from Lynch kindreds typically have high MSI, and they also do not possess the Lynch syndrome gene product, which can be demonstrated by IH. The next step is gene testing of the patient for mismatch-repair gene mutations (see below). Since this diagnosis carries implications for the whole family, testing is only done following genetic counselling, and if there is a strong suspicion of Lynch syndrome.

- Finally, even if the patient does not fulfil the Amsterdam II criteria, it may be that the patient requires colon screening at an earlier age than usual (before the age of 50). There is a marginal benefit in colon screening for people with one affected first-degree relative (FDR) aged under 45 years or two affected FDRs. Patients with a lesser family history do not require surveillance over and above that of the general population, and should be reassured as such.
- If the patient's anxiety persists over a risk of cancer, despite no clinical features to mandate colon surveillance, then the initial response should be empathic; *'Since your son's illness was*

such a shock, I can see that you must be worried about your own health'. It may be necessary to explore the reasons for the patients' anxiety, most likely due to not completing the grieving process (above), although this should be done sensitively without engaging in conflict about further tests.

If the patient is adamant about the need for a colonoscopy, then the role of the physician is to share their agenda with the patient at the same time as facilitating patient autonomy (see Calgary–Cambridge model in introduction). Conflict resolution is a key communication skill and frequently arises in the MRCP (PACES) examination, especially in the setting of a patient demanding a test/treatment. In general, conflict can be minimized by developing rapport with the patient and using empathic responses. Reassurance should only be provided once the patient's agenda has been established—premature reassurance may sound false and be counter-productive. Facilitating autonomy involves explanation about the risks/benefits of colonoscopy in this setting, and fully explaining other options including routine blood tests and giving the patient time to consider their options. Ideally, the consultation should finish with a shared plan made jointly between physician and patient.

Questions commonly asked by examiners

What do you know about the hereditary colorectal cancer syndromes?

(i) Lynch syndrome

This is the most common of the hereditary colon cancer syndromes, accounting for 2–3% of all CRC and 2% of uterine cancer. It is an autosomal dominant disorder caused by a germline mutation in one of several DNA mismatch repair genes:

- hMSH2 (human MutS homolog 2)—chromosome 2p16
- hMLH1 (human MutL homolog 1)—chromosome 3p21
- hPMS1 (human postmeiotic segregation 1)—chromosome 2q31
- hPMS2 (human postmeiotic segregation 2)—chromosome 7p22
- hMSH6 (human MutS homolog 6)—chromosome 2p16

Patients with Lynch syndrome have a markedly increased risk of CRC, as well as other cancers including gynaecological, urological, gastric, small intestine, biliary, pancreatic, skin, and brain. The overall cancer risk is 80%, and for CRC is 50–70%. CRC presents typically 10–20 years earlier than sporadic CRC. Cancers are thought to develop from adenomas in similar fashion to sporadic CRC, although the polyps have a 'flat' morphology, the cancers occur more proximally in the colon and are usually less differentiated.

Two variants of Lynch syndrome are Muir-Torre (Lynch syndrome with associated sebaceous tumors, cutaneous keratoacanthomas, and visceral carcinomas) and Turcot syndrome (Lynch syndrome with associated brain tumors, typically gliomas). These are likely to be types of Lynch syndrome rather than distinct disease entities.

The genetic hallmark of Lynch syndrome is MSI. This refers to the expansion or contraction of short repetitive DNA sequences due to defective DNA repair. MSI can be tested for in tumours using the polymerase chain reaction (PCR) to amplify a DNA sequence. The presence of MSI is highly sensitive for Lynch syndrome, although not specific, hence further genetic tests are required to confirm the diagnosis.

Surveillance for patients from Lynch families involves annual/biannual colonoscopy for patients beginning at age 20–25. Patients also undergo annual ultrasound screening for ovarian and endometrial cancer from age 30–35, annual urinalysis and urine cytology from age 25–35, annual skin surveillance and periodic upper GI endoscopy.

Although regular drug treatment with aspirin has been shown to decrease the incidence of sporadic colonic adenomas and CRC, no benefit was found in a recent large study of patients with Lynch syndrome.[2]

(ii) Familial adenomatous polyposis

Familial adenomatous polyposis (FAP) is also an autosomal dominant disorder, characterized by the presence of more than 100 (often hundreds) of colorectal adenomas. The disease is caused by mutations in the adenomatous polyposis coli (APC) gene. FAP accounts for less than 1% of the burden of CRC. However, FAP is also associated with an increased risk of duodenal ampullary carcinoma, follicular or papillary thyroid cancer, and gastric carcinoma.

Gardner's syndrome is a variant of FAP with additional extra-intestinal features, such as desmoid tumours, sebaceous or epidermoid cysts, lipomas, osteomas, supernumerary teeth, and gastric polyps. Turcot's syndrome is a further variant of FAP associated with central nervous system (CNS) medulloblastomas.

The risk of CRC in classical FAP is almost 100% by age 45. For this reason, most patients undergo colectomy after adolescence—this may be a complete proctocolectomy with ileo-anal anastomosis or a subtotal colectomy with ongoing surveillance of the rectum. Patients should also have upper GI endoscopy for surveillance of gastroduodenal polyps. Cox-2 inhibitors have also been shown to reduce GI polyps in FAP,[3] unlike in Lynch syndrome, although they should be used in additon to colectomy rather than as a replacement for surgery.

(iii)Peutz-Jehgers Syndrome

Peutz-Jehgers syndrome (PJS) is also an autosomal dominant syndrome. It is characterized by the presence of pigmented lesions on the lips and buccal mucosa, and multiple GI harmatomatous polyps (see Volume 1, Case136 Peutz-Jeghers Syndrome). Hamartomas occur most frequently in the small intestine (65–95%), although they may also occur in the colon (60%) and stomach (50%).

The cancer risk is markedly elevated in PJS, for sites including the colon, small intestine, stomach, pancreas, and breast. The lifetime risk of CRC is 39%. Genetic testing is not widely available, hence FDRs are screened with upper and lower GI endoscopy and small intestine imaging. Affected individuals also require surveillance for GI, pancreatic, and breast tumours.

What do you know about colorectal cancer screening in the United Kingdom?

CRC screening using faecal occult blood (FOB) testing, annually or biannually, has been shown to reduce cumulative CRC mortality over an 18-year follow-up.[4] On the basis of this evidence and pilot studies, a CRC screening programme was introduced in the UK in 2009. This involves offering biannual FOB testing for all individuals aged 60–69. Abnormal tests are found in 2% of the population, and these are followed up with a screening colonoscopy. The major disadvantage of the FOB test is the high false positive rate.

Aside from population screening, which other patients require surveillance for colorectal cancer?

What is the role of CT in screening for colorectal cancer?

CT colonography (virtual colonoscopy) is performed following bowel preparation with laxatives in a similar fashion to optical colonoscopy. Subsequently, the colon is inflated with air, passed via rectal tube, and CT images are acquired. Sophisticated software is then used to reconstruct an image of the colon which is viewed in a similar way to conventional optical colonoscopy. The sensitivity of CT for polyps greater than 1cm in size and for CRC is similar to colonoscopy.

The advantages of CT are a lower risk of perforation, lack of sedation, and the possible benefit of detecting other extra-colonic lesions on the images. However, patients with polyps will need a

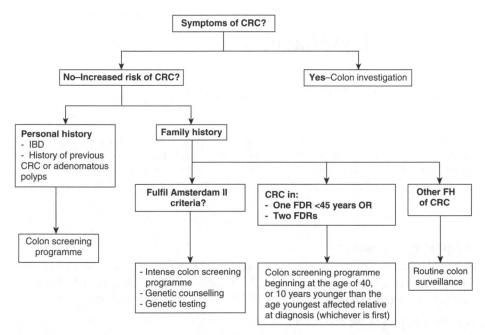

Figure 5.1

subsequent colonoscopy to remove them, thus leading to an extra procedure with cumulative cost and risk. A further disadvantage is the radiation dose—less than a barium enema, but the long-term effects of repeated screening ae unknown. Moreover, the trials of CT screening of CRC have been mainly performed in younger adults, so the efficacy of CT screening the elderly has not been proven.[5]

CT is currently used for patients unable (for example cannot lie on their side or cannot receive sedation) or unwilling to undergo colonoscopy. It may play a wider role in screening if future studies confirm safety and effectiveness in older populations.

References

1. Kubler-Ross, E. On Grief and Grieving: Finding the Meaning of Grief Through the Five Stages of Loss, New York: Simon & Schuster Ltd.; 2005.

2. Burn J, Bishop DT, Mecklin JP et al. Effect of aspirin or resistant starch on colorectal neoplasia in the Lynch syndrome. N Engl J Med. 2008; 359:2567–78.

3. Phillips RK, Wallace MH, Lynch PM et al. A randomised, double blind, placebo controlled study of celecoxib, a selective cyclooxygenase 2 inhibitor, on duodenal polyposis in familial adenomatous polyposis. Gut 2002; 50:857–60.

4. Mandel JS, Bond JH, Church TR et al. Reducing mortality from colorectal cancer by screening for fecal occult blood. Minnesota Colon Cancer Control Study. N Engl J Med. 1993; 328:1365–71.

5. Dhruva S, Phurrough SE, Salive ME et al. CMS's Landmark Decision on CT Colonography—Examining the Relevant Data. N Engl J Med. 2009; 360:2699–701.

Case 6 ◆ **Dysphagia**

INFORMATION FOR THE CANDIDATE

Dear Doctor,

This 78-year-old lady has had difficulty swallowing for the last two months. She is struggling with solids and liquids, and has lost a stone in weight. Her past medical history is of arthritis and hypertension, for which she takes amlodipine, bendroflumethiazide, and diclofenac. I wonder if she needs an endoscopy?

Many thanks for your opinion.

Acquiring the history

The history is a vital part of the assessment of patients with dysphagia, since the history can distuinguish oropharyngeal from oesophageal dysphagia in over 80% of cases. For this reason, dysphagia is a relatively common case in the MRCP (PACES) history-taking station.

A. History of presenting complaint:

Begin with an open question to allow the patient to describe their symptoms. *'I gather from your doctor that you have had difficulty swallowing. Could you tell me about it?'*; *'Describe to me what happens when you swallow.'*

The aim of this part of the history is to elicit the features that differentiate oropharyngeal and oesophageal dysphagia, using focused questions for clarification only after the patient has finished describing their symptoms.

Oropharyngeal dysphagia	Oesophageal dysphagia
Difficulty *initiating* swallowing	No difficulty in initiation, but food 'sticks' soon after swallowing
Associated nasal *regurgitation*	
Associated *coughing, choking*	Worse with solids than liquids
Worse with liquids than solids	May be associated *reflux* and *dyspepsia*
History of aspiration pneumonia	Symptoms may be *progressive*
History of neurological disease, including stroke	May be associated with *alarm symptoms*
Associated with other neurological symptoms (e.g. dysarthria, weakness)	

Consider the following areas:

- Age of onset—older age, male sex, and the presence of heartburn or weight loss predict mechanical (obstructive) causes of dysphagia.
- Characteristics
  - ◆ Initiation – *'Do you have trouble starting your swallow?'*; *'Do you need to turn your head or change position to swallow?'*. Patients with oropharyngeal dysphagia, who have difficulty transferring food from the mouth to the pharynx, may reposition their body or use their fingers to move food into the pharynx.

- ◆ Associated features of regurgitation and aspiration. *'Do you cough or choke after you swallow?'*; *'Does food ever come back up your nose when you swallow?'*.
- ◆ Type of food: *'Do you have difficulty with liquids, solids, or both?'*. If mainly solids, *'Is it worse with tough foods like bread and meat? What food have you been eating?'*. If mainly liquids, *'Have you tried anything to make liquids easier to swallow? Is it easier with thicker liquids?'*.

Dysphagia that is worse with solids is likely to be a mechanical cause of dysphagia. Symptoms that are worse with liquids suggests an oropharyngeal cause. Dysphagia that affects solids and liquids equally may be an oesophageal motility disorder.

- Progression—*'Are your symptoms getting worse, or do they come and go? Have you lost weight?'*. Rapidly progessive symptoms raise the possibility of malignancy. Intermittent, non-progressive symptoms suggest an oesophageal web or ring.
- Location—*'Where exactly does the food get stuck?'* Patients with oropharyngeal dysphagia may point to their pharynx, whereas those with oesophageal dysphagia are more likely to point to their sternum.

Associated symptoms:

- **Gastrointestinal**
  - ◆ Odynophagia—*'Is it painful to swallow?'* This suggests an inflammatory cause, such as oesophagitis or oesophageal infection.
  - ◆ Chest pain—*'Does it hurt anywhere in your chest when you swallow?'* Associated with motor disorders of the oesophagus (e.g. diffuse oesophageal spasm, achalasia, systemic sclerosis).
  - ◆ Heartburn / dysphagia—*'Have you had any heartburn during the time you have been unwell? What about during the night?'* Acid reflux predisposes to oesophagitis, oesophageal strictures, and oesophageal adenocarcinoma.
  - ◆ Acid brash / regurgitation—*'Do you ever wake up with an acidic taste in your mouth in the mornings?'*; *'Do you ever bring up food you have just eaten?'* Acid brash is associated with acid reflux. Passive regurgitation may occur with benign oesophageal lesions, such as an oesophageal diverticulum or achalasia.
- **Neurological**
  - ◆ Tremor—Parkinson's disease is associated with neuromuscular dysphagia.
  - ◆ Ptosis or intermittent weakness—Myasthenia gravis is also a cause of neuromuscular dysphagia.
  - ◆ Weakness, dysarthria—Stroke is the most common cause of oropharyngeal dysphagia—45% of all stroke patients experience dysphagia at 3 months.

B. Relevant medical history:

Past medical history:

- Neurological disease: Stroke, Parkinson's disease, multiple sclerosis, myasthenia gravis, amyotrophic lateral sclerosis, cerebral palsy.
- Sjögren's disease—ask about dry eyes and a dry mouth.
- Systemic sclerosis.
- Osteoarthritis—cervical spondylosis may cause oesophageal compression.
- Previous radiotherapy to the thorax—radiation oesophagitis.
- Valvular heart disease—an enlarged left atrium may also compress the oesophagus.
- HIV / immunosuppressive treatment—predispose to oesophageal infection.
- Atopy / hayfever—associated with eosinophilic oesophagitis.

C. Medications:

Drugs causing oesophageal injury

Several drugs are corrosive to the oesophageal mucosa, and can cause 'pill-oesophagitis':

- Doxycycline
- Bisphosphonates
- NSAIDs
- Iron sulphate

Drugs affecting lower oesophageal sphincter pressure

- Nitrates
- Calcium antagonists

D. Social issues:

- Take a careful smoking and alcohol history. Both cigarette smoking and alcohol use are associated with oropharyngeal, laryngeal, and oesophageal squamous cell carcinomas. Cigarette smoking is also a risk factor for oesophageal adenocarcinoma.
- Ask how the patient has been feeding themselves, and maintaining their nutritional intake.
- Sensitively enquire about psychological symptoms—*globus pharyngeus* is the sensation of a lump or foreign body in the throat, in the absence of dysphagia, odynophagia, and evidence of gastro-oesophageal reflux. Symptoms are thought to be a form of somatization. *'How have things been in your life generally over recent months? What was going on in your life at the time the symptoms came on? Do you have any particular stresses or worries in your life at the moment?'.*

Formulating a plan of action

Explain to the patient that further investigation will be needed to determine the cause of dysphagia. The most likely initial test is upper GI endoscopy for almost all cases of dysphagia (see Case 2 Dyspepsia, for alarm symptoms for endoscopy) even if a neuromuscular cause is suspected—to rule out a concomitant oesophageal lesion. An alternative approach is to arrange a barium study first if an oropharyngeal lesion or oesophageal diverticulum is suspected. This is because intubation of the upper oesophagus is not well visualized at endoscopy, so there is a small risk of perforation if there is upper oesophageal pathology.

Explain that the endoscopy may be done with or without a sedative, and is a very quick day-case procedure. The initial results will be available on the day of the test, but a follow-up appointment will be arranged to discuss the results of biopsies and blood tests.

Questions commonly asked by examiners

What is the differential diagnosis of oesophageal dysphagia?

- *Peptic stricture*—this is complication of acid reflux, affecting 10% of patients who seek medical attention for reflux. Symptoms are of gradually progressive dysphagia to solids. Endoscopic biopsy is used to confirm that the stricture is benign, following which the stricture can be endoscopically dilated.
- *Oesophageal carcinoma*—squamous cell carcinoma is associated with smoking and alcohol use, and is common in South East Asia. Adenocarcinoma is associated with acid reflux and Barrett's oesophagus, and the incidence is one of the most rapidly increasing amongst cancers in the Western world. Symptoms are of rapidly progressive dysphagia and weight loss.

- *Achalasia*—is a characterized by loss of peristalsis in the distal oesophagus, and failure of the lower oesophageal sphincter to relax. Almost complete dysphagia may occur to both solids and liquids. Oesophageal manometry studies will diagnose elevated lower oesophageal pressure. However, endoscopy is required to rule out 'pseudo-achalasia', due to gastric cancer causing malignant infiltration of the myenteric plexus. Treatment may be endoscopic botulinum injection, endoscopic dilatation, or surgery.

- *Diffuse oesophageal spasm*—is a motility disorder characterized by simultaneous, uncoordinated oesophageal contractions. Symptoms are of intermittent chest pain and dysphagia, which may be triggered by acid reflux or hot and cold food. Calcium antagonists are used for therapy.

- *Systemic sclerosis*—is associated with low amplitude oesophageal contractions and acid reflux. Peptic strictures are also common. Patients may also experience delayed gastric emptying, leading to recurrent vomiting, and are also at risk of small-bowel bacterial overgrowth causing chronic diarrhoea and malabsorption.

- *Eosinophilic oesophagitis*—is a condition associated with atopy and food allergies. It presents in younger patients with food bolus impaction.

- *Radiation injury*—radiation oesophagitis and subsequent fibrosis and stricturing may occur following radiotherapy to the trunk.

- *Extrinsic compression*—an enlarged left atrium, thoracic aortic aneurysm, or mediastinal lymph nodes may cause oesophageal compression.

- *Oesophageal infection*—i.e. fungal or CMV infection, may cause dysphagia and odynophagia in immunocompromised patients

Tell me about surveillance for Barrett's oesophagitis?

Barrett's oesophagitis develops as a consequence of chronic gastrooesophageal reflux disease (GORD), and predisposes to the development of adenocarcinoma of the oesophagus. The stratified squamous epithelium that normally lines the distal oesophagus is replaced by columnar epithelium.

The prevalence of Barrett's oesophagitis is between 1 and 4%. The rate of transformation to adenocarcinoma is 0.2–2% per year. Endoscopy has been used as a surveillance tool, on the basis that curable dysplasia may be detected earlier, although this approach has not yet been proven to reduce mortality. The British Society of Gastroenterology, and American Society for Gastrointestinal Endoscopy, recommend endoscopic surveillance every 2–3 years for patients who would be candidates for oesophagectomy.

What is the approach to the diagnosis of oropharyngeal dysphagia?

After upper GI endoscopy, and possibly oesophageal manometry, to rule out an oesophageal lesion, most patients are investigated under the supervision of speech therapists and ear, nose, and throat (ENT) surgeons. Video fluoroscopy is an X-ray study using barium, which is filmed during real-time from both anterior–posterior and lateral directions, to closely study the mechanisms of swallowing. The elevation of the hyoid bone and larynx, relaxation of the upper oesophageal sphincter and contraction of the pharynx can be examined.

If neuromuscular abnormalities are found, by features such aspiration or pooling of barium, or muscle paralysis, treatment can be introduced. This may involve thickening of fluids, or manoeuvres during swallowing which reduce dysphagia and aspiration (e.g. head tilting, forced valsalva manoeuvre).

Case 7 ◆ Jaundice

INFORMATION FOR THE CANDIDATE

Dear Doctor,

Thank you for seeing this 49-year old man with a 5-day history of jaundice. He tells me his urine has also been dark in colour, but he is otherwise well with no pale stools or fevers.

Many thanks for your help.

Acquiring the history

Patients rarely complain of 'jaundice' themselves—they, or someone else, may have noticed a change in the colour of their eyes or skin, but more commonly they will complain of associated symptoms. Since jaundice usually is a sign of a serious illness, it is vital to allow the patient time to disclose their other symptoms before proceeding to closed questioning.

A. Presenting complaint:
Begin with an open question, without focusing on the jaundice referred to in the referral letter. *'I understand from your doctor that you haven't been feeling so well over recent weeks—when did you last feel your health was normal?'*; *How have you been feeling since?'*; *'Can you tell me a little more about that…?'*.

B. History of presenting complaint:
Now focus on the onset and duration of the jaundice. *'When did you notice that your eyes/skin had changed colour?'*; *'How have things progressed since then?'*.

- Acute onset (days):
    - Gall stone disease (choledocholithiasis, cholangitis)
    - acute hepatitis
    - Acute Budd-Chiari syndrome
    - Haemolysis
- Subacute onset (weeks–months):
    - Pancreatic and hepatobiliary malignancy
    - Intrahepatic cholestasis (eg. drug-induced, autoimmune, infiltrative liver disease)
    - Right-sided heart failure
- Recurrent episodes:
    - Gallstone disease (choledocholithiasis, cholangitis)
    - Disorder of bile transport (e.g. Gilbert's syndrome)

Ask about these associated symptoms:
- *Fever:* may occur in cholangitis, viral hepatitis, or rare causes of cholecystitis causing jaundice (e.g. Mirizzi's syndrome—compression of the hepatic duct by chronic inflammation in Hartmann's pouch of the gallbladder). Fever is also a feature of alcoholic hepatitis.
- *Right upper quadrant pain:* this suggests cholangitis or acute hepatitis in the context of jaundice. Other causes are Budd-Chiari syndrome causing acute liver failure, or Mirizzi's syndrome (as above). Right upper quadrant pain in the absence of jaundice has a wider

differential diagnosis (see Case 8 Abdominal Pain). Gradual-onset 'painless' cholestatic jaundice classically suggests pancreatic or bile duct malignancy, but drug-related or autoimmune cholestasis are also usually painless.

- *Confusion*: the presence of altered mental status strongly suggests a serious underlying cause, such as sepsis due to cholangitis, or hepatic encephalopathy due to acute or chronic liver failure. Other causes include intracranial haemorrhage as a consequence of coagulopathy caused by liver failure, hypoglycaemia due to liver failure, or a post-ictal state following a seizure due to alcohol or substance withdrawal.
- *Mucosal bleeding / bruising*: ask specifically about gum bleeding, nosebleeds, and easy bruising. Aside from coagulopathy caused by liver failure, other causes of mucosal bleeding and jaundice include disseminated intravascular coagulation (DIC) due to cholangitis and sepsis, thrombocytopenia due to portal hypertension (hypersplenism), thrombotic thrombocytopenic purpura (TTP), or severe malaria.
- *Back pain*: is a feature of viral hepatitis (along with right upper quadrant pain) and severe haemolysis.
- *Dark urine / pale stools*: these are classically symptoms of 'obstructive' jaundice, which causes excess conjugated bile to appear in the urine. Additionally, the lack of conjugated bile secreted into the intestines leads to a lack of stool pigment—'pale' stools. However, severe haemolysis may cause dark urine due to haemoglobinuria. Therefore, these questions may be better at following the progress of jaundice once the diagnosis is known, rather than distinguishing obstructive jaundice from haemolysis.
- *Pruritus*: is a feature of all cholestatic processes, including bile duct obstruction, drug-induced and autoimmune. Other systemic diseases causing pruritus include chronic renal disease, haematological malignancy, and thyrotoxicosis.
- *Weight loss*: involuntary weight loss is associated with pancreatic or hepatobiliary malignancy. Patients with advanced chronic liver disease are also usually malnourished, although their weight loss may be balanced by the development of ascites.

C. Associated risk factors:

Risk factors for viral hepatitis:

- Needle and blood exposure—shared needles, tattoos, piercings, dental, or medical care abroad?
- Sexual history—ask sensitively about sexual contacts, type of encounter (heterosexual, homosexual), number of partners and the use of barrier protection (see Case 17 Sexually Transmitted Infection).
- Exposure to hepatitis A—exposure to individuals with viral illness or history of eating shellfish? Document travel history in last 6 weeks.
- Recent immunosuppression—patients who may be asymptomatic carriers of hepatitis B may develop liver failure due to viral reactivation after starting immunosuppressant therapy (e.g. steroids, chemotherapy).

Risk factors for alcoholic hepatitis and acute liver failure

- Alcohol intake—ask openly and non-judgementally about alcohol intake. Many patients may under-report the amount of alcohol they consume. After an open question, such as *'How much alcohol do you drink in an average weekend?'*, it may help to provide the patient with a choice of answers, to allow them to acknowledge their alcohol intake without fear of judgement. For example, *'Would you say you drink more like one to two beers/whiskies a night, or eight to ten beers/whiskies a night?'*. It may also help to provide the patient with a social 'excuse' for drinking, *'A lot of people find that a drink helps them sleep at night—do you ever do the same?'*.

- Medications—*'Do you take painkillers or cold remedies containing paracetamol?'*; *'Have you recently started any new medications or over-the-counter remedies?'*; *'Do you drink herbal teas or herbal remedies?'*. Several drugs are associated with acute liver failure, including paracetamol, antituberculous medications and antiepileptics. Herbal teas containing pyrrolizidine alkaloids may also cause hepatic veno-occlusive disease and liver failure.

- Vascular risk factors for Budd-Chiari syndrome—*'Have you, or anyone in your family, ever had a blood clot?'*; *'Have you ever been diagnosed with a blood disorder?'*. Up to half of cases of Budd-Chiari syndrome may be due to an underlying myeloproliferative disorder, such as poly-cythaemia vera or essential thrombocythaemia. In women of reproductive age, also ask about use of the contraceptive pill.

Risk factors for cholestatic jaundice

- Gallstones—ask about a history of gallstones, and a past history of post-prandial right upper quadrant pain. Also ask about risk factors for gallstones, such as a haemolytic anaemia (pigment stones), previous parenteral nutrition, gastric bypass surgery, or use of somatosta-tin analogues such as Lanreotide for carcinoid syndrome or acromegaly.

- Previous hepatic or biliary surgery—risk of biliary strictures.

- Previous pancreatitis may result in pancreatic pseudocyst formation, which can compress the biliary tree.

- History of sickle cell anaemia—associated with haemolysis and biliary disease due to pigment gallstones, but also ischaemic cholangiopathy caused by sickling in the end arteries supplying the biliary tree.

- History of ulcerative colitis—associated with primary sclerosing cholangitis in 1–4% of cases (67% of patients with primary sclerosising cholangitis have ulcerative colitis).

D. Travel history:

The incubation period of hepatitis A virus infection is 4–6 weeks. Therefore, document all areas visited in the preceding 2 months. Hepatitis B virus infection is also common (prevalence up to 20%) in South East Asia, Eastern Europe, and sub-Saharan Africa—ask specifically about travel to these areas. Additionally, liver fluke infection (Clonorchiasis and Opisthorchiasis) may be acquired in South East Asia. These infections may cause biliary strictures, resulting in jaundice and recurrent cholangitis.

E. Relevant family history:

Ask about a family history of liver disease, hepatitis, or blood disorders. Haemachromatosis, Wilson's disease, and Gilbert's syndrome are familial, as are several haemolytic anaemias such as sickle cell anaemia and G6PD deficiency. Hepatitis B may also be vertically transmitted.

F. Medications and vaccines:

- Ask about all prescription, over-the-counter, and herbal medications. Document starting date and compliance for each drug.

- Ask specifically about vaccinations for hepatitis B (see above) and hepatitis A.

G. Gynaecological and obstetric history:

- In women of child-bearing age, ask about last menstrual period and chances of pregnancy. (see below - liver disease in pregnancy)

- In pregnant women, ask about a history of pre-eclampsia and liver abnormalities in previous pregnancies (see below).

Formulating a plan of action

- Use the technique of summarizing to ensure that you have covered all of the patient's concerns. This is especially likely if the patient was unaware of the jaundice prior to the consultation. *'Is there anything that we haven't discussed that you are worried about?'*.

- Explain that a full examination, blood tests, and an ultrasound scan of the liver will be necessary to determine the diagnosis.
- Aside from routine blood tests and a screen for causes of hepatitis and chronic liver disease (see below), the most important test is an ultrasound scan which will differentiate 'obstructive' from 'non-obstructive' jaundice. The normal diameter of the common bile duct on ultrasound in adults is 7mm. This may increase in the very elderly or following cholecystectomy, but in general if the common bile duct is greater than 7mm in diameter this suggests biliary obstruction.

Blood tests in patients presenting with jaundice:

- FBC
- LFTs (AST, ALT, γGT, ALP)*
- Urea, creatinine, electrolytes
- Bilirubin
- Albumin, prothrombin time*
- Viral hepatitis serology (Hepatitis A IgM, Hepatitis B sAg, Hepatitis C Ab, EBV IgM).
- Liver autoantibodies (Anti- smooth muscle/mitochondrial/LKS antibodies)
- Serum iron, transferrin, ferritin, ceruloplasmin, and α1 anti trypsin levels

Consider:

- Tumor markers (including Ca19-9, αFP, CEA, PSA, Ca125)—if malignancy is suspected.
- Proportion of unconjugated/conjugated bilirubin—to differentiate 'pre-hepatic' from 'hepatic' and 'post-hepatic' jaundice. Unconjugated jaundice due to pre-hepatic causes is rarely greater than 100μmol/L. Deep jaundice is usually conjugated. Urine dipstick testing for urobilinogen is unreliable.
- Haemolysis screen (blood film, LDH, haptoglobin, reticulocyte count)
- Hepatitis E IgM—if a history of travel to endemic area or in pregnant women
- Thrombophilia screen (including antiphospholipid antibodies, Protein C, Protein S, and Antithrombin levels, Factor V Leiden genotype, JAK2 genotype)—if evidence of Budd-Chiari syndrome.
- Bile acid concentration in pregnancy—elevated cholic acid and chenodeoxycholic acid may be the only abnormalities in obstetric cholestasis. In pregnancy, the alkaline phosphatase is raised due to placental production, and thus is not useful for cholestasis.
- HIV test in high risk patients.

Questions commonly asked by examiners

Could you briefly outline the pathophysiology of jaundice?

Unconjugated bilirubin is formed from haemoglobin degradation in the reticuloendothelial system (spleen, liver, bone marrow). The unconjugated bilirubin is not soluble in water, and is transported to the liver bound to albumin so that it is not excreted in the urine. In the liver, it is conjugated to glucuronic acid within hepatocytes to form conjugated bilirubin which is water soluble. Conjugated bilirubin is excreted into the intestine in bile. Here, it is metabolized by colonic bacteria to urobilinogen, then to stercobilinogen, and finally stercobilin. The stercobilin gives faeces its brown colour. Some urobilinogen is reabsorbed and excreted in the urine as urobilin.

---

* The AST, ALT, γGT, ALP are not true tests of liver 'function'—the degree of elevation does not correspond with severity of over disease. The albumin and prothrombin tine are better tests of liver 'function' (see Vol.1 Case 1 Chronic Liver Disease).

- Pre-hepatic jaundice is due to increased serum unconjugated bilirubin, and increased urine urobilinogen. The major cause of pre-hepatic jaundice is excess haemolysis.
- Hepatic (or hepatocellular) jaundice is due to liver dysfunction, and thus failure to conjugate bilirubin. The serum unconjugated bilirubin is elevated, but the conjugated bilirubin levels are also usually elevated due to intrahepatic cholestasis from hepatocellular necrosis. Therefore, hepatocellular jaundice usually has a mixed picture.
- Post-hepatic jaundice, due to obstruction of the bile ducts, presents with an elevation in conjugated bilirubin and decreased urine urobilinogen.

How does one diagnose and manage alcoholic hepatitis?

Alcoholic hepatitis is a severe illness, caused by acute liver inflammation due to alcohol. The classical presentation is with fever, jaundice, and elevated leucocyte count. Not all patients have underlying cirrhosis.

Blood tests are very characteristic for alcoholic hepatitis. The AST and ALT are elevated, but rarely greater than 400IU/L. The AST may be elevated greater than the ALT, at a ration of 2:1. The prothrombin time and creatinine may also be elevated. Liver biopsy may be necessary to exclude other causes, but usually will need to done via transjugular liver access because coagulopathy and ascites are contraindications to percutaneous biopsy.

Severity of disease is assessed by scoring systems—the Maddrey discriminant function or Glasgow Alcoholic Hepatitis Score are most widely used.

$$\text{Maddrey's discriminant function} = 4.6 \times (\text{patients PT} - \text{control PT}) + \frac{\text{total bilirubin (μmol/L)}}{17}$$

If Maddrey's discriminant function is greater than 32, this implies severe disease with a 50% mortality at 30 days. These patients may benefit from a trial of steroids or of pentoxifylline (an oral drug with weak anti-TNFα activity), although both these therapies remain controversial because of mixed trial results.

The remainder of the treatment is supportive, including nutrition and treatment of sepsis.

What is the differential diagnosis of liver abnormalities in pregnancy?

Liver diseases unrelated to pregnancy

Pregnant women are predisposed to some diseases which are not specific to pregnancy:

- Thrombotic disease (e.g. Budd-Chiari syndrome)
- Hepatitis E infection—pregnant women are more susceptible to liver failure (15–20%)

Liver diseases specific to pregnancy

- Obstetric cholestasis—occur in the second and third trimesters, and is characterized by intractable pruritus and elevated bile acids. Symptoms tend to recur in subsequent pregnancies. Ultrasound of the bile ducts is typically normal. Ursodeoxycholic acid is safe, and may be of benefit.
- Acute fatty liver of pregnancy (AFLP)—occurs in the latter half of pregnancy, usually the third trimester. The disease is associated with pre-eclampsa in half of patients. The typical presentation is with nausea, vomiting, abdominal pain, and jaundice. Liver failure and complications such as DIC and encephalopathy may occur. Liver enzymes and bilirubin are markedly raised. Liver biopsy is diagnostic, showing fat infiltration, although may not be necessary if the diagnosis is clear clincially. Treatment is delivery of the baby, following supportive intensive care therapy.
- HELLP syndrome (Haemolysis, Elevated Liver enzymes, Low Platelets)—has signiciant overlap with AFLP. Symptoms develop in the third trimester, with abdominal pain, nausea,

and vomiting, and there is a history of pre-eclapmsia in 80% of cases. Haemolysis is microan-giopathic on blood smear along with other laboratory features of haemolysis, although the liver enzymes and bilirubin need not be markedly raised and liver failure is less common than AFLP. Treatment is delivery of the baby. Hypertension and convulsions are managed similarly to patients with pre-eclampsia.

Case 8 ♦ **Abdominal Pain**

INFORMATION FOR THE CANDIDATE

Dear Doctor,

Thank you for seeing this 39-year old lady who has a one-week history of increasingly severe abdominal pain. She tells me the pain is 'like a knife', and comes every day without any association with meals. She is a primary school teacher, and has been unable to work for the past week.

Many thanks for your opinion.

Acquiring the history

Acute abdominal pain may be a medical emergency, and in these cases the history should be taken after initial resuscitation and triage. The scenario in the history-taking section of the MRCP (PACES) is more likely to be a case of chronic abdominal pain, although the technique of goal-oriented history-taking whilst stabilizing a patient may be required in Station 2 of the examination.

The differential diagnosis of chronic abdominal pain is broad, and may be associated with many different physical and psychological symptoms. Therefore, in a PACES station where time is limited, the approach must be to identify the patient's agenda first, before screening for other symptoms.

A. History of presenting complaint:

Begin with open-ended questioning, *'I gather from your doctor you haven't been so well over the past few weeks. Can you tell me what's been happening?'.*

Let the patient describe their story without interruption. During the course of the discussion, ensure that the following characteristics of the abdominal pain are covered, but try to only use focused questions for clarification, or once the patient has finished voicing their concerns.

- Acute or subacute onset: *'Do you remember exactly when the pain started, or did it come on gradually?'*
- Site: *'Where exactly does the pain come on? Can you show me?'.*
- Progression: *'Is the pain constant, or does it come and go in waves?'*
- Nature of pain: *'What sort of pain is it—can you describe it?'; 'Is it more like a sharp stabbing pain, or a dull ache?'.*

- Radiation: *'Does the pain move anywhere from your abdomen?'; 'Does it go through to your back?'*. Abdominal pain radiating to the back is worth asking specifically about, since it is associated with severe conditions such as pancreatitis and aortic aneurysm.
- Severity: *'Can you give me some idea of how bad the pain is? Is it the worst pain you have ever had? Is it worse now, or was it worse when it started?'*
- Relationship to meals, movement, defecation: *'Is it better or worse when you eat/move/open your bowels?'*
- Gastrointestinal symptoms: nausea, vomiting, reflux, bowel habit, weight loss
- Urinary symptoms: frequency, dysuria, haematuria, prostatic symptoms
- Gynaecological symptoms: menstrual and obstetric history, dyspareunia
- Other aggravating and relieving factors: *'Is there anything else that makes it better, or brings it on? How about painkillers—do they help? Which ones have you been taking?'*.

B. Patterns of presentation:

Abdominal pain, perhaps more than any other presentation, may present with a broad range of associated symptoms. The technique of active listening, along with clarification using the above focused questions, will hopefully cover the patient's agenda and yield most of the information required to form a differential diagnosis. However, since the differential is so broad, *pattern recognition* is an essential skill to interpret the patient's symptoms.

Abdominal pain is typically either *visceral* or *somatic:*

- *Visceral pain* is due to stretching of hollow organs, causing a dull, diffuse pain or 'ache'. The localization of visceral pain is imprecise, but in general pain from organs of the foregut (oesophagus, gallbladder, stomach, pancreas, first half of duodenum) is localized to the epigastric area. Pain from midgut organs (second half of duodenum, small intestine, ascending and part of transverse colon) is localized to the periumbilical area. Pain from hindgut organs (transverse colon to anus) is localized to the lower abdomen.
- *Somatic pain* is well-localized and sharp. It is due to inflammation of peritoneum covering abdominal organs.

The character and the site of the pain should lead you to consider the following patterns of presentation:

Right upper quadrant pain

1. Biliary pain is an example of visceral pain—due to postprandial contraction of the gallbladder or bile ducts onto a gallstone. The pain is usually *not* colicky, but is constant and often associated vomiting. Biliary pain may be due to:
   (a) Biliary colic—usually lasts a few hours until the stone falls away back into the gall bladder.
   (b) Cholecystitis—a similar type of pain, although progressive and associated with fever.
   (c) cholangitis—biliary pain, fever, and jaundice (Charcot's triad of cholangitis is fever, jaundice and abdominal pain) (see Case 7 Jaundice).
   (d) sphincter of Oddi dysfunction—a rare condition, which presents with biliary pain without evidence of biliary obstruction. The cause is sphincter of Oddi spasm, and the diagnosis is typically made post-cholecystectomy.

Left upper quadrant pain

2. Splenic pain is also an example of visceral pain. This may be due to splenic infarction or splenic artery aneurysm. Risk factors for splenic infarction are thromboembolism (atrial fibrillation (AF), prosthetic heart valves), haemoglobinopathy or myelproliferative disorders.
3. Atypical pain from myocardial infarction or pneumonia may present with left upper quadrant pain. Ask about associated dyspnoea and radiation of pain to the jaw or arm.

Epigastric pain

4. The most common causes of epigastric pain are acid-related disorders (see Case 2 Dyspepsia). Ask about alarm symptoms, such as dysphagia, weight loss, early satiety, and progressive vomiting.
5. Pancreatic pain is typically 'piercing through to the back'. Patients may use hot water bottles to relieve the pain, or find that sitting forward in the 'pancreatic position' helps. Ask specifically about posture when asking about aggravating and relieving factors. The patient may also have weight loss, steatorrhoea, or diabetes mellitus. Ask about alcohol use and a history of gallstones as risk factors for chronic pancreatitis. Other causes of chronic pancreatitis are hereditary, autoimmune, and drug-induced. Ask about a family history of pancreas problems, a history of autoimmune disease such as systemic lupus erythematosus (SLE) or Sjögren's disease, or drugs such as antiretrovirals, azathioprine or loop and thiazide diuretics.

Lower abdominal pain

6. Irritable bowel syndrome characteristically presents with cramping, colonic pain affecting the left side of the abdomen, and altered bowel habit (see Case 4 Change in Bowel Habit). Colonic pain is visceral in character. The pain is often relieved by defaecation (see below).
7. Colon diverticular disease is usually asymptomatic, unless a complication such as diverticulitis occurs. This causes somatic pain, usually in the left side of the abdomen, with associated fever.

Right iliac fossa pain

8. Appendicitis usually presents with periumbilical, visceral pain (since the appendix is midgut in origin), which localizes to the right iliac fossa when the peritoneum becomes inflamed causing somatic pain.
9. Crohn's disease may cause pain anywhere in the abdomen, but the right iliac fossa is common since Crohn's typically affects the terminal ileum The pain is visceral with associated diarrhoea and weight loss. Stricture formation may cause pain due to obstructive symptoms—ask about intermittent pain and abdominal distension. Crohn's disease may also cause abscesses, resulting in somatic pain and fever.

Pelvic pain

10. Consider gynaecological causes in all female patients. Document menstrual history, contraception and sexual history (see Case 17 Sexually transmitted infection). Ask about the relationship and timing of the pain to menstruation and sexual activity.
11. Renal colic typically presents with flank pain, although ureteric pain radiates to the groin and may resemble iliac fossa pain. (see Case 36 Haematuria). Gout, hyperparathyroidism, sarcoidosis, and Crohn's disease are risk factors for renal calculi.

Central abdominal pain

12. Central abdominal pain is of particular importance, since it may represent life threatening conditions such as mesenteric ischaemia, ruptured aortic aneurysm or pancreatitis. These should be considered in any case of severe central abdominal pain. Acute appendicitis may also present with acute periumbilical pain in the early stages.
13. Mesenteric ischaemia may cause chronic postprandial abdominal pain, leading to weight loss in 30–40% of cases. Midgut ischaemia is due to superior mesenteric artery disease, causing central abdominal pain. Coeliac artery disease typically causes epigastric pain due to foregut ischaemia. Inferior mesenteric artery disease is more likely to cause acute ischaemic colitis, possibly associated with embolic risk factors such as AF.

C. Relevant medical history:

- Ask about a history of gallstones, jaundice, and pancreatic disease.
- Haematological disease (e.g. sickle cell anaemia) may predispose to pigment gallstones and splenic infarction.

- Autoimmune disease is associated with autoimmune pancreatitis.
- Ensure to ask about previous gastroduodenal disease and surgery, and for upper GI and colonic alarm symptoms.

D. Medications and allergies:

Patients may have been using analgesics or antispasmodics for their pain. Take note of:

- Drugs which may cause gastric ulceration—NSAIDs, corticosteroids.
- Drugs which may cause gastro-oesphageal reflux—nitrates, calcium antagonists, theophyllines, bisphosphonates.
- Drugs which may cause pancreatitis—azathioprine, antiretroviral drugs, loop and thiazide diuretics?

E. Social issues:

- Ensure to take a thorough alcohol history (see Case 7 Jaundice for alcohol history).
- Determine the impact of the patient's symptoms on their occupation and daily activities.
- Since irritable bowel syndrome is associated with several psychological symptoms, ask empathetically and openly about the impact of their pain. 'It must be quite a burden to be in severe pain every day. How have you been feeling in yourself?'; 'Did the symptoms come on during a stressful time in your life?'; 'How about now—is there anything else that is worrying you, or that you would like to talk about?'.

Formulating a plan of action

- Explain to the patient that a full clinical examination is required. Investigations will include routine blood and urine tests, as well as a pregnancy test in female patients of child-bearing age.
- Emphasize that further tests may involve an ultrasound, CT scan, or endoscopy, but a follow-up appointment will be arranged first to discuss the results of the blood tests.
- Empirical treatment is unlikely to be helpful without a firm diagnosis, but a trial of proton pump inhibitor (e.g.omeprazole) or antispasmodic (e.g. colpermin) may be tried for an acid-related disorder or irritable bowel syndrome respectively.

Questions commonly asked by examiners

How does one diagnose irritable bowel syndrome?

Irritable bowel syndrome may be diagnosed using the Rome III criteria (Box 1), although if any alarm features are present then further colon investigation is necessary. Furthermore, the pain of irritable bowel syndrome is rarely progressive. Pain that is progressive, or wakes the patient from sleep, requires further investigation, usually with imaging. Many gastroenterologists recommend a baseline abdominal ultrasound in female patients over the age of 40 to exclude ovarian pathology.

Alarm symptoms for colon investigation

- Aged above 65
- Unintentional weight loss
- Change in bowel habit
- Iron-deficiency anaemia
- Rectal bleeding

- Frequent nocturnal symptoms
- Family history of colonic cancer

Box 1 Rome III criteria for the diagnosis of irritable bowel syndrome

The Rome III criteria (2006) for the diagnosis of irritable bowel syndrome require that patients must have recurrent abdominal pain or discomfort at least 3 days per month during the previous 3 months that is associated with two or more of the following:
- relieved by defecation
- onset associated with a change in stool frequency
- onset associated with a change in stool form or appearance

Supporting symptoms include the following:
- altered stool frequency
- altered stool form
- altered stool passage (straining and/or urgency)
- mucous with stool
- abdominal bloating or subjective distension

How would you approach abdominal pain in elderly patients or those with HIV?

Serious causes of abdominal pain must be considered in all elderly patients, with a low threshold for investigation. This is not only because malignancy, hepatobiliary disease, and bowel obstruction are more common in this group, but also because signs such as fever and peritonism are less frequently present.

Abdominal pain in HIV may be drug-related, such as didanosine-induced pancreatitis, or related to the underlying condition. Whilst common causes of abdominal pain may occur, these patients are also at risk of complications of HIV such as enteritis and peritonitis due to bacterial or opportunistic infections, and HIV-associated malignancies such as lymphoma and Kaposi's sarcoma.

Can you think of any other causes of abdominal pain that need to be considered if initial investigations are negative?

1. Vasculitis, particularly polyarteritis nodosa, may cause mesenteric ischaemia and recurrent abdominal pain. A proportion of these patients will present with acute abdominal pain and intestinal perforation. There is no specific test for polyarteritis nodosa, although autoimmune assays such as anti-neutrophil cytoplasmic antibody (ANCA) may rarely be positive. GI lesions may be visible during endoscopy, although they rarely provide histological confirmation of vasculitis, therefore a full thickness intestinal biopsy (not a superficial endoscopic biopsy) may be required.
2. Familial Mediterranean fever presents with acute attacks of abdominal pain, serositis, and fever. Patients may have a family history and the diagnosis can be confirmed by genetic testing.
3. Acute intermittent porphyria may cause acute abdominal pain, and may have associated psychiatric symptoms.

4. Adrenal insufficiency may present with non-specific nausea and abdominal pain, and these symptoms often correlate with the severity of adrenal insufficiency.

Case 9 ◆ Chest Pain

INFORMATION FOR THE CANDIDATE

Dear Doctor,

Thank you for seeing this 53-year old gentleman who has recently started to complain of chest pain. He has had chest pain since returning from holiday in Turkey, and he is concerned that he may have a pulmonary embolus since his mother has suffered from recurrent pulmonary emboli. He has a history of hypertension, although has no other medical history. He is a smoker. A sublingual glyceryl trinitrate (GTN) spray has been helpful on some occasions. A 12-lead ECG taken at our clinic has been unremarkable. I would be grateful for your assessment.

Acquiring the history

Chest pain is a common presenting symptom for acute medical admissions. The differential diagnosis is broad, and it is the history that plays a key role in determining subsequent investigations and management. When taking a history from a patient with chest pain, it is important to be aware of the broad differential diagnosis list and preliminary questioning will appropriately narrow this differential diagnosis. Subsequently, specific targeted questions will lead to the diagnosis.

A. History of presenting complaint:

This is the most important part of the history that will determine the aetiology of chest pain. Initially the questions should be broad, followed by focused questions to help narrow the differential diagnosis.

Characteristic of chest pain

- **Site**
    - **Cardiac ischaemic pain**: central, and may radiate to the jaw, neck, and left arm
    - **Respiratory chest pain**: localizes to the site of pathology, i.e. infection or pneumothorax. However, patient with asthma or obstructive airways disease may complain of central chest pain or tightness, but other features in the subsequent history will help differentiate this from cardiac ischaemia.
    - **Musculoskeletal chest pain**: localizes to site of pathology or injury or may relate to the posterior chest in the region of the spine.
    - **Peptic ulcer disease** and **gastro-oesophageal reflux**: lower chest and epigastrium.
- **Nature**
    - **Cardiac ischaemic chest pain**: dull pressure like sensation that is not pleuritic.
    - **Respiratory** and **musculoskeletal**: sharp and pleuritic

- ◆ **Pericarditis**: sharp and pleuritic.
- ◆ **Nerve root pain**: band like shooting pain around the chest from the back to the anterior chest
- ◆ **Gastro-oesophageal reflux**: sharp and burning-like sensation
- **Radiation**
  - ◆ **Cardiac ischaemic pain**: jaw, neck, and arms (often the left arm)
  - ◆ **Aortic dissection, peptic ulcer disease**, and **pancreatitis**: back
  - ◆ **Nerve root pain**: around the chest wall resulting in a band-like pain sensation
- **Onset, duration and frequency**
  - ◆ *'When did the chest pain start?'* It is important to establish duration of symptoms. In the given scenario, it is important to relate the onset of symptoms in relation to the recent holiday. It is equally important to establish if there were any symptoms prior to or during the holiday. It is often the case that symptoms may have been present for sometime before seeking medical advice and opinion.
  - ◆ *'Does the pain come on suddenly or gradually?'*
  - ◆ *'Is it constant or intermittent?'*
  - ◆ If intermittent, *'How frequently do you experience chest pain?'*

Precipitating factors

- **Exertion**: cardiac ischaemia
- **Deep inspiration**: respiratory, musculoskeletal, and pericarditis
- **Movement**: musculoskeletal
- **Eating**: peptic ulcer disease, gastro-oesophageal reflux
- **Position**: pericarditis, pancreatitis, and gastro-oesophageal reflux (worse lying down); bending forward can exacerbate gastro-oesophageal reflux

Relieving factors

- **Rest**: Cardiac ischaemic pain
- **Sublingual nitrates**: cardiac ischaemic pain and oesophageal spasm
- **Antacid preparation**: peptic ulcer disease and gastro-oesophageal reflux
- **Simple analgesics**: musculoskeletal pain, respiratory pain, and pericarditis
- **Bronchodilators**: asthma and obstructive airways disease

Associated features

- **Cardiac ischaemic chest pain**: nausea, vomiting, sweating, pallor, breathlessness (may be a manifestation of ischaemia or left ventricular dysfunction), palpitations and dizziness (arrhythmias) and symptoms of left ventricular dysfunction (orthopnoea, paroxysmal nocturnal dyspnoea, ankle oedema, and reduced exercise tolerance)-*'Do you ever wake up at night feeling breathless?'* (paroxysmal nocturnal dyspnoea), *'How many pillows do you sleep on at night?'* (orthopnoea)
- **Respiratory tract infection**: cough (productive or non-productive), sputum (colour and consistency), fever, and haemoptysis
- **Pulmonary embolism (PE)**: non-productive cough, haemoptysis, low-grade fever, calf pain, and swelling (indicating underlying deep vein thrombosis)
- **Lung malignancy**: productive cough, haemoptysis, weight loss, and loss of appetite
- **Pericarditis**: cold and flu-like symptoms

- **Peptic ulcer disease**: nausea, vomiting, haematemesis, and melaena
- **Gastro-oesophageal reflux**: acid taste in mouth, dysphagia (oesophageal strictures)
- **Musculoskeletal**: back and joint pains
- **Nerve root pain**: symptoms of underlying occult malignancy (weight loss, loss of appetite, change in bowel habit, noticeable masses or lumps) would indicate underlying metastatic disease; neurological symptoms in lower limbs, urinary and faecal incontinence (spinal cord involvement)

Other factors

- Enquire about any recent history of chest trauma.

B. Relevant past medical and family history:

Past medical history

- **Cardiovascular risk factors** (smoking, hypertension, hypercholesterolaemia, diabetes, family history, previous history of myocardial infarction)
- If risk factors are present, enquire about risk factor control and compliance to therapy. *'Do you remember the last blood pressure measurement?' 'Have you had your cholesterol level checked?'* If so, *'Do you remember what it was?'*
- If previous cardiac history, then enquire about previous myocardial infarction, coronary angiography, coronary angioplasty, or coronary artery bypass graft (CABG) surgery
- **Menopause**—enquire about menstrual cycle in females, as the risk of ischaemic heart disease is increased in the post-menopausal period
- **Thrombotic risk factors** (previous history of thromboembolic disease, thrombophilia, malignancy, immobility, recent surgery or long-haul flight, and oral contraceptive pill use [females])
- **Peptic ulcer disease**—enquire about previous endoscopy
- **Asthma/COPD**
- **Pneumothorax**—recurrence of pneumothorax is common (15–40%) and up to 15% of recurrences can be on the contralateral side

Family history

- **Ischaemic heart disease**—enquire about the age at first presentation (establish risk of premature coronary artery disease)
- **Thrombo-embolic disease**—enquire about thrombophilia

C. Medications:

- Enquire about full drug history and compliance to therapy
- Enquire about any use of medications (including over-the-counter drugs) to alleviate symptoms (sublingual nitrates, simple analgesics, antacids, and bronchodilators)
- Enquire about side-effects of therapy, i.e. cough (ACE inhibitors), headaches (nitrates) and myalgia (statins)
- Oral contraceptive pill use in females increases thromboembolic risk

D. Social issues:

- Smoking habits (cardiovascular risk factor)
- Alcohol consumption (risk factor for peptic ulcer disease and pancreatitis)
- Enquire about job. Heavy lifting and manual labour may contribute to musculoskeletal chest pain and aggravate exertional cardiac ischaemia

- Does the patient drive? A diagnosis of myocardial infarction will have an impact on driving restrictions
- Impact of symptoms on daily life
- Marital status and sexual history. Sexual intercourse may potentiate cardiac ischaemia, and discussion related to this forms an important part of cardiac rehabilitation
- Elicit the patient's concerns about the symptoms

Formulating a plan of action

Explain to the patient that there are possible causes for chest pain and this will warrant further investigation. Given the above scenario the possible causes for chest pain are cardiac ischaemia or PE. In this case it would be appropriate to initially exclude PE. Once this is excluded, only then will it be appropriate to investigate further for myocardial ischaemia.

- Bloods
    - **Anaemia** can be seen in peptic ulcer disease with GI blood loss or in any chronic disease, including malignancy (anaemia can potentiate cardiac ischaemia)
    - **Leucocytosis** and **raised inflammatory markers** would suggest underlying infection
    - **Elevated D-dimer** for suspected PE
    - **Cardiac enzymes** if suspecting myocardial ischaemia.
- ECG
    - **Myocardial ischaemia**: the ECG can be normal at rest in a patient with exertional angina
    - **PE**: sinus tachycardia is the most common finding, often combined with non-specific ST segment and T-wave changes
- Chest radiograph
    - To exclude other causes of chest pain, e.g. pneumothorax, collapse, consolidation. and malignancy.

The following specific tests may be indicated:

- **Doppler USS of the leg** for suspected deep vein thrombosis
- **CT pulmonary angiogram** for suspected PE
- **Exercise ECG** to look for inducible cardiac ischaemia
- **Dobutamine stress echocardiography** to look for inducible ischaemia (if patient unable to perform exercise ECG)
- **Coronary angiography** if there is evidence of inducible ischaemia on exercise ECG or dobutamine stress echocardiography
- **Endoscopy** if suspecting peptic ulcer disease

Questions commonly asked by examiners

What are the causes of pleuritic chest pain?

- PE
- Pneumonia
- Malignancy
- Pleurisy
- Pneumothorax
- Musculoskeletal chest pain
- Pericarditis

What do you understand by the term acute coronary syndrome?

Acute coronary syndromes include unstable angina (USA), non-ST segment elevation myocardial infarction (NSTEMI) and ST segment elevation myocardial infarction (STEMI) (see Figure 9.1[2]). Acute coronary syndromes with persistent ST-elevation (STEMI) generally require urgent reperfusion therapy with thrombolysis or primary percutaneous coronary intervention. Those without persistent ST-elevation represent a continuum from USA to NSTEMI and can be further classified on the basis of troponin release, a biochemical marker of myocardial cell death. This varies between different laboratories and troponin assays used. Troponin levels should be measured after 12 hours from the onset of chest pain.

What is the initial management of acute coronary syndrome?

- Oxygen
- Aspirin 300mg PO
- Clopidogrel 300mg PO
- Sublingual nitrates
- Analgesia (morphine with metoclopramide)

STEMI

- primary percutaneous coronary intervention or thrombolysis*
- beta blocker (contraindications: bradycardia, heart block, hypotension, pulmonary oedema)
- ACE inhibitors
- Statin

---

* Patients receiving thrombolysis with recombinant tissue plasminogen activators (rt-PA) require concurrent unfractionated heparin. Recent evidence suggests that low molecular weight heparin can be used in this setting.[1]

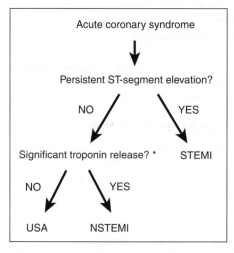

Figure 9.1
MB Iqbal, MA Westwood, and RH Swanton. Recent development in acute coronary syndromes. Clin Med. 2008; 8:42–8.

NSTEMI

- Low molecular weight heparin
- beta blocker (contraindications: bradycardia, heart block, hypotension, pulmonary oedema)
- Glycoprotein IIb/IIIa inhibitors in high risk patients*
- ACE inhibitors
- Statin

What do you know about the TIMI risk score?

This is a risk stratification tool in patients with acute coronary syndrome. A TIMI score ≥ 3 indicates high risk.[2] A score of 1 is assigned for the following 7 factors:

1. **age ≥ 75 years**
2. **≥ 3 risk factors for coronary artery disease**
3. **50% coronary stenosis**
4. **ST segment deviation**
5. ≥ 2 anginal episodes in 24 hours
6. positive troponin
7. aspirin use in the last 7 days

What is the role of an early invasive strategy in patients with USA or NSTEMI?

Recent research has compared clinical outcomes associated with early invasive strategy versus an early conservative therapy in patients with USA or NSTEMI. An early conservative strategy involves aggressive medical therapy, with coronary angiography and revascularization reserved only for patients with recurrent or inducible ischaemia. With this early invasive strategy, all patients undergo early coronary angiography within 12–48 hours of presentation, and revascularization if indicated. Current evidence suggests that a routine early invasive strategy is associated with better long-term outcomes, particularly in high-risk patients. In the TACTICS-TIMI 18 trial,[3] the benefits of an early invasive strategy were only observed in high-risk patients, defined as those with troponin elevation, ST segment deviation or TIMI risk score ≥3. Pooled data from 7 trials has shown that although a routine invasive strategy is associated with higher early mortality during initial hospitalization, it is associated with better *long-term* outcomes with a significant reduction in death, myocardial infarction, recurrent angina, and re-hospitalization.[4]

What do you know about the DVLA guidelines for restrictions on driving following a myocardial infarction?

It is important that patients and doctors are aware of the restrictions on driving following myocardial infarction. Different criteria must be satisfied depending on the type of vehicle driven:

- GROUP 1: cars and motorcycles
- GROUP2: lorries, vans, ambulances, and public transport (including taxi)

The DVLA guidelines for all cardiovascular conditions are summarized in the table.

---

* Patients at high-risk include those with ongoing chest pain, haemodynamic instability, dynamic ST/T wave changes on the ECG and an elevated troponin. Another tool to identify high-risk is a TIMI score ≥ 3.

	GROUP 1	GROUP 2
Angina	Cannot drive if symptoms at rest. Can recommence when symptoms are controlled.	Can drive when free from anginal symptoms for more than 6 weeks and obtains satisfactory exercise ECG (completing stage 3 of the BRUCE protocol) off anti-anginal therapy (≥48 hours).
STEMI	1 month (1 week if percutaneous coronary intervention (PCI))	
NSTEMI	1 month (1 week if PCI)	
CABG	1 month	
Following pacemaker insertion	1 week	6 weeks
Following ICD insertion (primary prevention)	1 month	Cannot drive
Following ICD insertion (secondary prevention)	Can drive after a 6-month shock-free period. Following alteration of anti-arrhythmic medications, cannot drive for 1 month	
Arrhythmia	Cannot drive if arrhythmia causes incapacity. Can recommence when cause identified and controlled for 1 month.	Cannot drive if arrhythmia causes incapacity. Can recommence when cause identified and controlled for 3 months.
Unexplained syncope	Cannot drive if arrhythmia causes incapacity. Can recommence when cause identified and controlled for 1 month. If no cause identified, then can recommence only if free of symptoms for 6 months	Can drive 3 months after if the cause has been identified and treated. If no cause identified, then licence refused/revoked for 1 year.
Simple faint (definite prevocational factors, associaited prodromal symptoms and unlikely to occur at rest)	No restrictions	No restrictions

References

1. Antman EM, Morrow DA, McCabe CH, Murphy SA, Ruda M, Sadowski Z et al; ExTRACT-TIMI 25 Investigators. Enoxaparin versus unfractionated heparin with fibrinolysis for ST-elevation myocardial infarction. N Engl J Med. 2006; 354:1477–88.

2. Iqbal MB, Westwood MA, Swanton RH. Recent developments in acute coronary syndromes. Clin Med. 2008; 8:42–48.

3. Cannon CP, Weintraub WS, Demopoulos LA, Vicari R, Frey MJ, Lakkis N et al; TACTICS (Treat Angina with Aggrastat and Determine Cost of Therapy with an Invasive or Conservative Strategy)-Thrombolysis in Myocardial Infarction 18 Investigators. Comparison of early invasive and conservative strategies in patients with unstable coronary syndromes treated with the glycoprotein IIb/IIIa inhibitor tirofiban. N Engl J Med. 2001; 344:1879–87.

4. Mehta SR, Cannon CP, Fox KA, Wallentin L, Boden WE, Spacek R et al. Routine vs selective invasive strategies in patients with acute coronary syndromes: a collaborative meta-analysis of randomized trials. JAMA. 2005; 293:2908–17.

Case 10 ◆ **Breathlessness**

INFORMATION FOR THE CANDIDATE

Dear Doctor,

Thank you for seeing this 73-year old gentleman who gives a 3-month history of worsening breathlessness on exertion. He previously had unrestricted exercise tolerance, but now becomes extremely breathless on walking 30 yards. He has a history of hypertension, hypercholesterolaemia, diabetes, and previous coronary artery bypass surgery. He has since been free of anginal symptoms.

Many thanks for your opinion.

Acquiring a history

A. History of presenting complaint:

- **Onset, duration and frequency**
  - ◆ It is important to establish the duration of breathlessness
  - ◆ Ask about the breathing prior to this, to establish baseline functional status: *'What was your breathing like 6 months ago?'*
  - ◆ *'Does the breathlessness come on suddenly or gradually?'*
  - ◆ *'Is the breathlessness constant or intermittent?'*
  - ◆ If intermittent, *'How frequently do you experience breathlessness?'*
- **Precipitating factors**
  - ◆ Ask about any factors that precipitate or worsen breathlessness?
  - ◆ *'Is it exertional?' 'Is it present at rest?'*
  - ◆ *'Does lying down make it worse?'* (orthopnoea)
- **Relieving factors**
  - ◆ *'Is it relieved with rest?'*
  - ◆ Enquire about any medications, e.g. sublingual nitrates or inhalers that may have relieved symptoms
- **Associated symptoms**
  - ◆ **Chest pain** suggests underlying cardiac ischaemia, but may rarely be a feature of asthma or COPD. If chest pain is present, it is important to differentiate cardiac ischaemic chest pain from other causes (see Case 9 Chest Pain).
  - ◆ **Palpitations** suggest the presence of underlying arrhythmia (which can be exertional), particular AF/flutter or ventricular arrhythmias. If palpitations are present, then further questioning will be necessary to characterize the arrhythmia (see Case 11 Palpitations) *'Have you measured your pulse during these episodes of palpitations?' 'Are they regular or irregular?'* alternatively, patients may complain of a slow heart rate and bradycardia can manifest as exertional breathlessness
  - ◆ **Pre-syncope or syncope** can be associated with arrhythmia or underlying left ventricular outflow obstruction, i.e. aortic stenosis or hypertrophic obstructive cardiomyopathy
  - ◆ **Orthopnoea** indicates left ventricular dysfunction. It is important to note that a history of orthopnoea can often be elicited in patients with COPD with good left

ventricular function. This is primarily because of a hyper-inflated chest, and patients rely predominantly on vertical chest expansions and diaphragmatic excursion for breathing

- **Paroxysmal nocturnal dyspnoea** indicates left ventricular failure. *'Do you ever wake up at night feeling breathless?'*
- **Oedema** indicates congestive cardiac failure. Cor pulmonale can be seen in patients with good left ventricular function, but with pulmonary hypertension due to advanced lung disease, i.e. COPD or interstitial lung disease. Enquire about sites of fluid retention, i.e. abdominal distension (ascites) and scrotal oedema in males. If there is a history of leg swelling, enquire about asymmetry—asymmetrical leg swelling may suggest deep vein thrombosis thereby implicating PE (thromboembolic disease) as a cause of breathlessness
- **Respiratory symptoms**, i.e. cough, sputum, wheeze, and haemoptysis suggest underlying respiratory disease. A dry non-productive cough may indicate interstitial lung disease. A productive cough may indicate infection, suppurative lung disease or malignancy. Haemoptysis can occur in PE, infection, and malignancy. Haemoptysis can also be seen in patients with pulmonary congestion, especially with mitral stenosis. Wheeze signifies asthma or COPD
- **Thyroid disease**. Hyperthyroidism can cause breathlessness. Enquire about weight loss, heat intolerance, tremor, sweating
- **Neurological symptoms**. Neuromuscular weakness can result in breathlessness: Guillain-Barre Syndrome (recent respiratory or diarrhoeal illness, progressive ascending weakness and ptosis) and myasthenia gravis (fatiguability, diplopia, ptosis). Fatiguability is characterized by symptoms being worse at the end of the day
- **Vasculitic symptoms** (fever, joint aches, muscle aches, and rashes) would suggest pulmonary vasculitis
- **Renal disease**. Renal failure can lead to breathlessness as a result of fluid retention and/or metabolic acidosis. Enquire about uraemic symptoms, particularly restlessness and pruritus. Ask about urinary symptoms, particularly any noticeable reduction in urine output

- **Exercise tolerance**
  - It is important to quantify reduction in exercise tolerance.
  - Establish pre-morbid, and then current functional status and exercise tolerance.
  - This can be used to establish New York Heart Association (NYHA) functional class: I (unrestricted), II (breathless on heavy exertion), III (breathless on mild exertion), and IV (breathless at rest).
- Other factors
  - Enquire about any recent history of chest trauma (pneumothorax).

B. Relevant previous medical and family history:

Medical history

- **Cardiac disease**
  - Enquire about cardiovascular risk factors (smoking, hypertension, hypercholesterolaemia, diabetes, family history, previous history of myocardial infarction)
  - If risk factors are present, enquire about risk factor control and compliance to therapy. *'Do you remember the last blood pressure measurement?' 'Have you had your cholesterol level checked?'* If so, *'Do you remember what it was?'*
  - If previous cardiac history, then enquire about previous myocardial infarction, coronary angiography, coronary angioplasty, or CABG surgery.

- Enquire about pre-existing left ventricular dysfunction or previous echocardiography. *'Have you ever had an ultrasound scan of the heart'* If so, *'What did it show?'*
- Enquire about any history of valvular heart disease. *'Have you ever been told that you have heart murmur?' 'Is there a history of rheumatic fever?'*
- **Respiratory disease**
  - History of chronic lung diseases, i.e. asthma, COPD, bronchiectasis, interstitial lung disease, sarcoidosis (ask about fever, joint aches, and painful nodules on the legs)
  - Thrombotic risk factors (previous history of thromboembolic disease, thrombophilia, malignancy, immobility, recent surgery or long-haul flight, and oral contraceptive pill use).
- **Thyroid disease**
- **Renal disease**

Family history

- **Ischaemic heart disease**—enquire about the age at first presentation (establish risk of premature coronary artery disease)
- **Cardiomyopathy**—familial dilated or hypertrophic cardiomyopathy
- **Thrombo-embolic disease**—enquire about thrombophilia
- **Primary pulmonary hypertension**

C. Medications:

- Enquire full drug history and compliance to therapy
- Oral contraceptive pill use in females increases thromboembolic risk
- Enquire about any use of medications (including over-the-counter drugs) to alleviate symptoms (sublingual nitrates and bronchodilators)
- Appetite suppressors (e.g. fenfluramine) are associated with pulmonary hypertension

D. Social issues:

- Smoking habits (cardiovascular risk factor)
- Alcohol consumption (risk factor for dilated cardiomyopathy)
- Enquire about job. Heavy lifting and manual labour may aggravate breathlessness.
- Impact of symptoms on daily life
- Elicit the patient's concerns about the symptoms

Formulating a plan of action

Explain to the patient that there are possible causes for exertional breathlessness which are primarily cardiac or respiratory and this will warrant further investigation.

- Pulse oximetry
- Bloods
  - **Anaemia** can be potentiate cardiac ischaemia and cardiac failure
  - **Leucocytosis** and **raised inflammatory markers** would suggest underlying infection
  - **D-dimer** for suspected PE
  - **Cardiac enzymes** if suspecting myocardial ischaemia
  - **BNP** for heart failure
- ECG
  - **Myocardial ischaemia**: the ECG can be normal at rest in a patient with exertional angina
  - **Arrhythmia**: AF/flutter or ventricular arrhythmias can be easily detected

- ◆ **PE**: sinus tachycardia is the most common finding, often together with non-specific ST and T-wave changes
- Chest radiograph
  - ◆ Cardiomegaly and pulmonary congestion (left ventricular dysfunction)
  - ◆ To exclude other causes of chest pain, e.g. pneumothorax, collapse, consolidation, and malignancy.

The following specific tests may be indicated:

- **Echocardiogram**: to assess ventricular function, valvular heart disease, pulmonary artery systolic pressure and to detect shunts or a pericardial effusion
- **Ambulatory ECG monitoring:** to detect paroxysmal arrhythmia
- **Exercise ECG** to look for inducible cardiac ischaemia
- **Dobutamine stress echocardiography** to look for inducible ischaemia (if patient unable to perform exercise ECG)
- **Coronary angiography** if there is evidence of inducible ischaemia on exercise ECG or dobutamine stress echocardiography.
- **CT pulmonary angiogram** for suspected PE
- **Lung function tests**: obstructive or restrictive lung defect if suspecting respiratory disease
- **CT chest** if suspecting interstitial lung disease or lung malignancy
- **Arterial blood gas** to confirm hypoxia and/or metabolic acidosis

Questions commonly asked by examiners

What is the role of a d-dimer measurement in patients with suspected thromboembolic disease?

The d-dimer may be elevated in infection or with underlying malignancy. However, a negative d-dimer reliably excludes PE if there is a low pretest probability. However, a low d-dimer doesn't exclude PE if the pretest probability is moderate or high.

When should you consider a ventilation-perfusion (V-Q) scan as a first-line investigation for PE?

V-Q scan should only be considered as a first-line investigation for PE, if the chest radiograph is normal and there is no significant cardiopulmonary disease. In this setting, a normal V-Q scan reliably excludes PE, but an intermediate scan should be followed up by CT pulmonary angiography (which remains the gold standard).

What do you know about BNP?

This is one of the four known natriuretic peptides (ANP, BNP, CNP, and DNP) that is released from ventricles (left ventricle > right ventricle) during volume or pressure overload. Its physiological effects include dilatation of the arteries and veins, diuresis, and natriuresis. Normal levels are less than 100pg/mL. It has a negative predictive value of at least 96%, so heart failure can be confidently ruled out for patients in the normal range. The positive predictive value of BNP for diagnosing heart failure is 90%, as an elevated BNP value can be seen with renal failure, pulmonary hypertension, and PE.

What is the management of left ventricular systolic dysfunction?

Diuretics are useful in relieving congestive symptoms, especially in acute decompensated stages of heart failure. All patients with left ventricular systolic dysfunction should be started on ACE inhibitors provided there are no contraindications, irrespective of functional status. If they are not tolerated, then angiotensin II receptor blockers can be used. A rise in creatinine up to 20% can be expected after starting an ACE inhibitor or angiotensin receptor blocker. If the creatinine level rises by > 20%, the ACE inhibitor should be discontinued and underlying renovascular disease should be considered. The presence of hypotension is not an absolute contraindication to starting ACE inhibitors. Patients often have low blood pressure readings in the context of a low cardiac output. Therapy may be initiated in patients with systolic blood pressures as low as 90mmHg, provided they do not become symptomatic as a result of hypotension. This also applies to other pharmacotherapeutic agents in heart failure.

Beta blockers should not be commenced in the acute stages of heart failure. Once considered a contraindication, there is now overwhelming data to support the use of β-blockers in stable heart failure. They should be initiated with NYHA class I–II status. However, they may be used cautiously in patients with NYHA class III–IV status. Beta blockers that are licensed for use in heart failure include bisoprolol, carvedilol, metoprolol, and nebivolol. Current guidelines suggest that all patients with stable heart failure should initially be started on an ACE inhibitor, followed by initiation of β-blockers therapy.

Spironolactone should be used for patients in NYHA class III–IV status. It is important to monitor the renal function and for hyperkalaemia (given that such patients may also be on ACE inhibitors or angiotensin II receptor blockers).

Digoxin should be used as a first-line treatment with ACE inhibitors in all patients with heart failure and AF. For patients in NYHA class III–IV status in sinus rhythm, digoxin has been shown to improve symptoms and reduce hospitalization, but without a reduction in mortality.

For patients with NYHA III–IV status, who are on maximal medical therapy (ACE inhibitor, β-blockers, spironolactone, and digoxin) with evidence of interventricular conduction delay (LBBB; QRS > 120mm), these patients may be considered for cardiac resynchronization therapy (biventricular pacemaker).

Further Reading

1. National Institute for Health and Clinical Excellence. Management of chronic heart failure. London: NICE; 2003.

2. National Institute for Health and Clinical Excellence. Cardiac resynchronization therapy for the treatment of heart failure. London: NICE; 2007.

Case 11 ◆ **Palpitations**

INFORMATION FOR THE CANDIDATE

Dear Doctor,

Thank you for seeing this 43-yearold female who complains of intermittent palpitations associated with light-headedness. She has no significant medical history and takes no regular medications. She works as a financial analyst and has an extremely stressful job. She has a large caffeine intake, which can range from 8 to 10 mugs of coffee per day. There is no family history of ischaemic heart disease, but her mother has a long-standing diagnosis of atrial fibrillation, and suffered a stroke as a complication. She is extremely anxious and concerned that she may have developed AF. A resting 12-lead ECG at the surgery showed normal sinus rhythm.

Thank you for your help.

Acquiring the history

Although the cause of palpitations is usually benign, they may occasionally herald an underlying life-threatening cardiac disorder. Since the differential diagnosis is broad, the focus of the history is to distinguish the minority of patients who require extensive diagnostic testing and management.

A. History of presenting complaint:

Age of onset

Consider supraventricular tachycardias (SVTs) in young patients presenting with a history of palpitations in childhood or adolescence. AF is the commonest arrhythmia occurring in patients over 65 years. ventricular tachycardia (VT) also occurs more commonly with age because of the higher incidence of structural heart disease, although congenital long QT syndromes may present in childhood and adolescence.

Character of the palpitations

- **Nature of palpitations.** Various terminologies are used to describe palpitations, although these descriptors are generally non-specific. Ask the patient an *open* question about the sensation they experience: '*What do the palpitations feel like?*'
  - *'Racing or tapping heart'* suggesting a fast arrhythmia.
  - *'Missed or extra beats'* followed by a *'Pounding or more forceful beat'* are indicative of ventricular ectopic beats.
  - *'Pounding in the neck'* or *'Everything stopped for a moment'* may suggest atrioventricular dissociation or bradycardia. The pounding feeling in the neck is due to cannon A waves which suggest atrial contraction against closed atrioventricular valves. Rapid and regular pounding in the neck is most typical of re-entrant supraventricular arrhythmias, particularly atrioventricular nodal re-entry tachycardia (AVNRT).
- **Rate and rhythm**
  - *'Are the palpitations fast or slow?' Do you take your pulse at the time, if so what was it?'*
  - *'Are the palpitations regular?'* Some patients may be able to tap out the rhythm they experience during episodes, although *do not insist on this* since it is not always a useful exercise. Rapid, regular palpitations favour sinus tachycardia, SVT, and VT. Irregular palpitations suggest AF and extrasystoles.
- **Time course, onset and frequency of palpitations**
  - *How long have you had the palpitations?'* Palpitations occurring since childhood strongly favour SVT.
  - *'How often do you experience the palpitations?'*
  - *'Do the palpitations occur gradually or suddenly?'* Sinus tachycardia is more likely to have a gradual onset and termination
  - *'How long do the episodes last?'*
- **Precipitants**
  - *'Is there anything that triggers the episodes—such as exercise, stress, alcohol or coffee?'* These can aggravate any type of arrhythmia. Exercise can precipitate VT and polymorphic VT in long QT syndrome. The latter can also be triggered by emotion and sudden arousal.
  - *Ask specifically about cocaine and amphetamine use.*
  - Recent illness can precipitate AF; ask about these during systems review.
- **Termination.** *'How do the palpitations stop—have you tried stopping them by straining or holding your breath?'* SVTs can be terminated by Valsalva manoeuvres. Ectopic beats terminate with exercise.

Associated symptoms

- Dyspnoea occurs with most arrhythmias.
- Syncope and presyncope are signs of haemodynamic compromise necessitating intervention.
- Chest pain, nausea, and sweating are signs of myocardial ischaemia associated with a tachyarrhythmia, which also requires urgent treatment.
- Exertional dyspnoea, orthopnoea, paroxysmal nocturnal dyspnoea, ankle swelling, and reduced exercise tolerance indicate cardiac failure. Determine whether these symptoms have worsened following the onset of palpitations, since tachyarrhythmias and bradyarrhythmia may aggravate cardiac failure.

Relevant medical and family history:

Past medical history

- **Thyrotoxicosis**—weight loss, heat intolerance, tremor, sweating.
- **Hypothyroidism**—weight gain, cold intolerance, fatigue, constipation.
- **Hypoglycaemia**—hunger, headache, irritability, confusion, and sweating.
- **Phaeochromocytoma**—headaches, flushing, tremor, and excessive sweating.
- **Cardiac disease**—myocardial infarction, angina, known arrhythmias, valvular disease, and other structural cardiac disease.
- **Cerebrovascular disease** is a complication of inadequately treated AF.
- **Vascular risk factors**—hypertension, hyperlipidaemia, and diabetes mellitus.
- **Psychiatric illness** such as anxiety disorders.
- **Asthma**—treatment with β agonists can precipitate sinus tachycardia.

Family history

A family history of cardiac disease and sudden death is particularly relevant in younger patients presenting with palpitations. Hypertrophic cardiomyopathy and long QT syndrome are inherited conditions that can present with palpitations, syncope, and sudden death due to VT.

C. Medications:

Take a thorough drug history enquiring about medications that can precipitate palpitations. These are:

- β agonists
- Theophylline
- Levothyroxine
- Sympathomimetics such as monoamine oxidase inhibitors
- Drugs that prolong the QT segment may precipitate polymorphic VT
    - Antiarrhythmic drugs—quinidine, disopyramide, amiodarone, sotalol
    - Macrolide antibiotics—erythromycin, clarithromycin, azithromycin
    - Antihistamines—terfenadine
    - Psychotropic drugs—phenothiazines, butyrephenones, SSRIs, and tricyclic antidepressants.
    - GI motility agents—cisapride, domperidone
- Recreational drugs such as amphetamines and cocaine increase sympathetic drive causing palpitations.

D. Social issues:

- Ask specifically about alcohol and caffeine consumption.
- Ask about smoking habits.

- Determine the impact of the symptoms on daily activities.
- Does the patient drive?
- Elicit the patient's concerns about their symptoms.

Formulating a plan of action

- Explain to the patient that a clinical examination and ECG will be required in order to help determine the cause of the palpitations.
- Reassure the patient that the cause is likely to be benign, and further tests may not be required if the examination and ECG are normal. However, further investigation may be warranted to rule out structural heart disease, identify a possibly treatable arrhythmia, or to reassure the patient.
- Consider the following investigations:
  - **Blood count** may indicate an anaemia causing a sinus tachycardia. An infection precipitating or aggravating atrial arrhythmias is suggested by a leucocytosis or elevated CRP.
  - **Urea, creatinine, electrolytes** (including potassium, calcium, magnesium, and phosphate)—any electrolyte disturbances can precipitate arrhythmias either directly or by prolongation of the QT interval.
  - **Thyroid function tests** will indicate hypo/hyperthyroidism.
  - **Cardiac enzymes and 12-hour troponin level** if the history or ECG suggests myocardial ischaemia.
  - **Plain chest radiograph** may reveal signs of heart failure, chest infection, or mitral valve disease causing left atrial enlargement.
  - **Ambulatory ECG monitoring**—A 12-lead ECG is diagnostic in identifying the underlying arrhythmia *during* symptoms, however ambulatory ECG monitoring is required for recurrent, unexplained palpitations. The patient must record their symptoms for appropriate analysis of the ECG recording, since not all asymptomatic arrhythmias require treatment.
  - **Echocardiography** will demonstrate underlying structural heart disease, valvular disease, and left ventricular dysfunction.
  - **Exercise ECG** is indicated in patients who experience palpitations on exercise.
  - **Electrophysiological studies (EPS)** are indicated in patients in whom a tachycardia is suspected but has not been confirmed by non-invasive investigations. Ablation of causative pathways can also be performed during the procedure.
  - **Cardiac MRI** (magnetic resonance imaging) may be used in selected patients to investigate for cardiomyopathies.
- Other investigations to consider in the evaluation of palpitations as guided by the history
  - **D-Dimer and/or CT pulmonary angiogram** maybe considered if the history is suggestive of a pulmonary embolus triggering sinus tachycardia or AF.
  - **Urinary catecholamine metabolites** will be raised in the presence of a phaeochromocytoma.
  - **Implantable loop recorders** are small devices that can be implanted subcutaneously that can record continuously for up to 3 years. These are useful for detecting infrequent arrhythmias.

Questions commonly asked by examiners

What are the causes of AF?

The common causes of AF are:

- Cardiac
  - ◆ Ischaemic heart disease
  - ◆ Hypertension
  - ◆ Mitral valve disease
  - ◆ Congestive cardiac failure
- Non-cardiac
  - ◆ Thyrotoxicosis
  - ◆ Acute illness, e.g. pneumonia, PE
  - ◆ Alcohol
  - ◆ Idiopathic AF

How is AF distinguished from ventricular ectopic beats clinically?

Ventricular ectopic beats disappear with exercise, whereas in AF the rhythm remains unchanged.

How is AF classified?

AF is classified into three categories according to the mode of termination of the arrhythmia:

1. Paroxysmal AF terminates spontaneously without intervention.
2. Persistent episodes of AF terminate with either electrical or pharmacological cardioversion.
3. Permanent AF does not revert to sinus rhythm despite electrical or pharmacological cardioversion.

What are the management strategies for haemodynamically stable persistent and permanent AF?

Management of AF consists of rhythm and/or rate control and anticoagulation to prevent thromboembolic events. Anticoagulation is discussed below.

Rhythm control

There is no significant difference in overall mortality in patients receiving rhythm or rate control therapy. However, the rhythm control strategy is often associated with adverse effects of anti-arrhythmic agents which can be proarrhythmic. Recent NICE guidelines[1] recommend rhythm control as the first-line treatment for persistent AF in:

- young patients (<65 years)
- symptomatic patients
- lone AF
- AF secondary to a treated precipitant, i.e. infection
- patients with congestive cardiac failure (restoration of atrial contraction can contribute 20% to cardiac output)

Sinus rhythm can be restored with electrical or pharmacological cardioversion after at least 4 weeks of therapeutic anticoagulation with warfarin (Target INR: 2–3). The recurrence rate of AF is approximately 50% and therefore post-cardioversion medical treatment is often required for maintenance of sinus rhythm. First-line treatment is with standard β-blockers. Sotalol and flecainide are second-line options; the latter is contraindicated in structural heart disease.

Amiodarone is considered when there is treatment failure with other agents. In some situations, a further attempt at cardioversion may be an option, often with concurrent anti-arrhythmic therapy. Rhythm control is unlikely if left atrial diameter is greater than 5cm, as these patients have a low chance of successful cardioversion and a high chance of recurrence of AF. In such cases, a rate control strategy is more appropriate.

Rate control

The rate control strategy is appropriate in patients with failed attempts at cardioversion, permanent AF and in persistent AF in whom warfarin anticoagulation is contraindicated (thus unable to receive cardioversion). First-line drugs for ventricular control are standard β-blockers and non-dihydropyridine calcium channel blockers (verapamil and diltiazem). Digoxin is added if further rate control is required, and amiodarone may be considered if there is failure of treatment.

Other options

Device therapy can be considered as an option for rhythm control under specialist care. Atrial pacing aims to suppress atrial ectopics that initiate the arrhythmia. Atrial defibrillators attempt to cardiovert episodes of AF. Radiofrequency ablations to the left atrium or pulmonary veins are used in selected cases. In patients with permanent AF and difficult rate control despite optimum rate control therapy, ablation of the AV node with implantation of permanent pacemaker is an option.

What is the role of anticoagulation in the management of AF?

The incidence of stroke in the presence of AF is 5% per year and the risk is increased with the presence of other vascular risk factors, warranting the need for thromboprophylaxis.[2] The risk of stroke is stratified into high, moderate, and low risk groups, taking into consideration contraindications to antithrombotic treatment and the presence of other risk factors for stroke (age >75 years, history of thromboembolic disease, hypertension, diabetes mellitus, valvular heart disease, left ventricular dysfunction, and thyrotoxicosis). Pooled data from trials comparing anti-thrombotic therapy with placebo has shown that warfarin reduces the risk of stroke by 62% and aspirin, alone, reduces the risk by 22%. Overall, in high risk patients, warfarin is better than aspirin in preventing strokes, with a relative risk reduction of 36%. Warfarin has been shown to be more effective at stroke prevention than combination antiplatelet therapy (clopidogrel and aspirin).[3] However, aspirin may be appropriate in younger patients with no risk factors, or if there is a contraindication to warfarin. Please refer to the algorithm below for anticoagulation in AF.[4]

What is the role of implantable cardioverter defibrillators (ICDs) in the management of ventricular arrhythmias?

ICDs are implantable devices which monitor heart rhythm, and can either pace, cardiovert or defibrillate depending on the indication. Their role in the prevention of sudden cardiac death due to ventricular arrhythmias has been reviewed by NICE:[5]

- *Secondary prevention of sudden cardiac death—patients with one of:*
  - ⬥ ·a previous cardiac arrest due to VT or ventricular fibrillation (VF)
  - ⬥ sustained VT causing syncope or significant haemodynamic compromise
  - ⬥ sustained VT without haemodynamic compromise, with a LVEF <35%
- *Primary prevention of sudden cardiac death—patients with a history of previous (>4 weeks) MI (myocardial infarction) and **either***
  - ⬥ LVEF <35% with non-sustained VT on ECG monitoring and electrophysiological testing, **or**
  - ⬥ LVEF <30% and prolonged QRS interval.

Differential diagnosis of palpitations

Cardiac causes
Supraventricular arrhythmias
- Atrial tachycardia
- Atrial fibrillation and atrial flutter
- Supraventricular tachycardias (SVTs)
  - Atrioventricular re-entry tachycardia (AVRT) and Wolff-Parkinson-White (WPW) syndrome
  - Atrioventricular nodal re-entry tachycardia (AVNRT)

Ventricular tachyarrhythmias
- Sustained ventricular tachycardia
- Non-sustained ventricular tachycardia
- Normal heart ventricular tachycardia
- Polymorphic VT (Torsades de Pointes)

Atrial and ventricular ectopic beats
Bradycardia
- Intermittent atrioventricular block
- Sinoatrial node disease

Non-cardiac causes
Anaemia
Thyrotoxicosis (causes AF and sinus tachycardia)
Hypothyroidism (causes bradycardia)
Metabolic
- Hypoglycaemia
- Phaeochromocytoma

Drugs
- Caffeine
- Alcohol
- β-agonists
- Thyroxine

Anxiety/panic attacks
Physiological
- Exercise
- Pregnancy

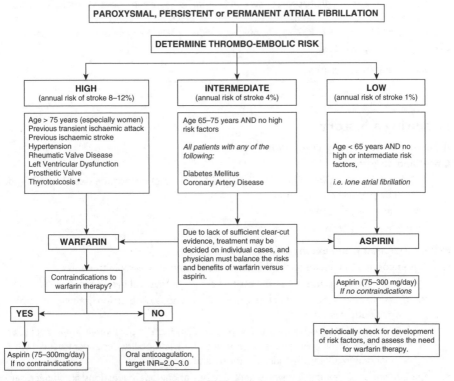

Figure 11.1 Algorithm for anticoagulation in atrial fibrillation.
Adapted from Iqbal et al. Recent developments in atrial fibrillation. BMJ 2005; 330:238–243.

References

1. National Institute for Clinical Excellence. The management of atrial fibrillation. London: NICE; 2006.

2. Lip GYH *et al.*, Antithrombotic treatment in atrial fibrillation. Heart. 2006; 92: 155–61.

3. Connolly S *et al.*, Clopidogrel plus aspirin versus oral anticoagulation for atrial fibrillation in the Atrial Fibrillation Clopidogrel trial with Irbesartan for prevention of vascular events (ACTIVE): a randomised controlled trial. Lancet. 2006; 367:1903–12.

4. Iqbal MB *et al.* Recent developments in atrial fibrillation. BMJ 2005; 330:238–243.

5. National Institute for Health and Clinical Excellence. Implantable cardioverter defibrillators for arrhthymias. London: NICE; 2006.

Case 12 ◆ Ankle Swelling

INFORMATION FOR THE CANDIDATE

Dear Doctor,

Thank you for seeing this 69-year old woman who gives a 6-month history of worsening ankle swelling. She has noticed a gradual reduction in exercise tolerance, which she attributes to her ankle swelling. There is no history of chest pain, orthopnoea, or paroxysmal nocturnal dyspnoea. She has a history of asthma, rheumatoid arthritis, diabetes, and hypertension. Her medications include aspirin 75mg OD, salbutamol inhaler 2 puffs PRN, ibuprofen 400mg TDS, metformin 500mg TDS, gliclazide 80mg BD, amlodipine 5mg OD, and furosemide 40mg OD.

I am very grateful for you opinion.

Acquiring a history

A. History of presenting complaint:

Onset and duration

- 'When did the ankle swelling first start?' If acute (<72 hours) onset, then deep vein thrombosis should be strongly considered.

- 'Was it gradual and sudden?'

- 'Has it been progressive or intermittent?'

Pattern, symmetry, and extent of involvement

- It is important to enquire about the pattern and symmetry early in the history.

- Remember the key causes of asymmetrical versus symmetrical involvement:

   ◆ *Asymmetrical*: venous thrombosis, lower limb venous obstruction, trauma, infection, lymphoedema, and arthritis

   ◆ *Symmetrical*: congestive cardiac failure, cor pulmonale, hypoalbuminaemia (nephrotic syndrome, chronic liver disease, poor nutrition), immobility, dependent oedema, lymphoedema, hypothyroidism, arthritis, and drugs

- Enquire about the extent of involvement. Start by asking open questions, and if necessary use closed questions: 'Is it confined to the joints?' (arthritis); 'How far up the legs/thighs does the swelling extend?'; 'Is there swelling of your groin?' (scrotal and/or penile swelling in males); 'Is there abdominal swelling?'

- Ask if the oedema is pitting in nature. 'Does pressing on the swelling with your fingers leave finger marks?' Lymphoedema and oedema secondary to hypothyroidism is often non-pitting in nature. Early lymphoedema can be associated with pitting oedema.

Aggravating factors

- Dependant oedema or oedema due to venous insufficiency is often worse at the end of the day.
- Although a full drug history will be taken later, it is important to clarify if the onset of the ankle oedema coincides with any drugs that may have been prescribed for other medical conditions, i.e. calcium antagonists for hypertension.
- Enquire about trauma, animal bites, and stings.

Relieving factors

- Dependant oedema or oedema due to venous insufficiency is relieved by leg elevation and/ or compression stockings.
- Ask if diuretics have been prescribed, and if so, 'Have the diuretics reduced the ankle swelling?'

Other features

- 'Is there any associated leg weeping or oozing?'
- 'Is there any skin discoloration?' A brown haemosiderin discoloration over the medial aspect of the ankle suggests venous insufficiency. Erythema and tenderness suggests active inflammation, i.e. arthritis or cellulitis.
- Enquire about any trophic changes to the skin, suggesting previous ulceration.

Associated features

- **Deep venous thrombosis**: calf pain and tenderness. It is important to enquire if the oedema is painful. Pain is associated with deep vein thrombosis. Oedema secondary to chronic venous insufficiency, congestive cardiac failure, and renal disease can cause low-grade aching. Lymphoedema is usually painless.
- **Cellulitis**: erythema, tenderness, fever
- **Arthritis**: joint aches, tenderness, and swelling
- **Cardiac failure**: exertional breathlessness, orthopnoea, and paroxysmal nocturnal dyspnoea. Enquire about symptoms of cardiac ischaemia, i.e. exertional chest pain
- **Cor pulmonale**: enquire about symptoms of respiratory disease, i.e. chronic cough, sputum, haemoptysis; obstructive sleep apnoea (snoring, daytime somnolence, large collar size)
- **Chronic liver disease**: jaundice, pruritus, abdominal swelling, haematemesis, and melaena
- **Malabsorption**: enquires about symptoms of inflammatory bowel disease (weight loss, bloody diarrhoea, joint aches, and rash on legs [erythema nodosum]), and Coeliac disease (intolerance to gluten).
- **Nephrotic syndrome**: periorbital and generalized oedema, breathlessness (pleural effusions), nausea, vomiting.
- **Hypothyroidism**: goitre, weight gain, cold intolerance, fatigue, and constipation
- **Extrinsic venous compression**: is there any history to suggest underlying occult malignancy? Ask about weight loss, loss of appetite, change in bowel habit, and unusual bumps/ lumps (lymphadenopathy).
- **Renal disease**: Renal failure can result in fluid retention and breathlessness. Enquire about uraemic symptoms, particularly restlessness and pruritus. Ask about urinary symptoms, particularly any noticeable reduction in urine output.

Exercise tolerance
- It is important to quantify reduction in exercise tolerance.
- Establish pre-morbid, and then current functional status and exercise tolerance.
- This can be used to establish New York Heart Association (NYHA) functional class: I (unrestricted), II (breathless on heavy exertion), III (breathless on mild exertion), and IV (breathless at rest).

B. Relevant previous medical and family history:

Medical history
- **Cardiac disease**
  - Enquire about cardiovascular risk factors (smoking, hypertension, hypercholesterolaemia, diabetes, family history, previous history of myocardial infarction)
  - If risk factors are present, enquire about risk factor control and compliance to therapy. *'Do you remember the last blood pressure measurement?' 'Have you had your cholesterol level checked?'* If so, *'Do you remember what it was?'*
  - If previous cardiac history, then enquire about previous myocardial infarction, coronary angiography, coronary angioplasty, or CABG surgery.
  - Enquire about pre-existing left ventricular dysfunction or previous echocardiography. *'Have you ever had an ultrasound scan of the heart'* If so, *'What did it show?'*
  - Enquire about any history of valvular heart disease. *'Have you ever been told that you have heart murmur?'; 'Is there a history of rheumatic fever?'*
- **Respiratory disease**
  - History of chronic lung diseases, i.e. asthma, COPD, bronchiectasis, interstitial lung disease, sarcoidosis (ask about fever, joint aches, and painful nodules on the legs). Vasculitis symptoms may implicate pulmonary vasculitis as a cause of pulmonary hypertension and cor pulmonale.
  - Thrombotic risk factors (previous history of thromboembolic disease, thrombophilia, immobility, recent surgery or long-haul flight, and oral contraceptive pill use). Chronic thromboembolic disease is an important cause of pulmonary hypertension, leading to cor pulmonale.
  - Obstructive sleep apnoea can cause cor pulmonale.
- **Rheumatological disease**
  - History of arthritis—enquire about distribution of arthritis. Does it correlate with sites of swelling?
  - Enquire about systemic lupus erythematous (arthralgia, myalgia, and facial rash) and systemic sclerosis (arthralgia, myalgia, rash, skin changes). Limited cutaneous systemic sclerosis is associated with pulmonary hypertension.
  - Enquire about previous hip and knee replacements. This can result in pitting localized oedema.
- **Thyroid disease**
  - Hypothyroidism is assocaited with generalized subcutaneous oedema.
  - Graves' disease can cause hypothyroidism and hyperthyroidism, as well as pretibial myxoedema. Pretibial myxoedema in its extreme form can resemble lymphoedema.
- **Renal disease**
- **Nephrotic syndrome**
- **Chronic liver disease**
- **Malabsorption**
  - Enquire about Crohn's disease, ulcerative colitis, and Coeliac disease

- **Lymphoedema**
  - Previous surgery and irradiation (damage to lymphatic drainage)
- **Venous insufficiency**
  - Previous history of deep vein thrombosis or varicose veins.

Family history

- **Ischaemic heart disease**—enquire about the age at first presentation (establish risk of premature coronary artery disease)
- **Cardiomyopathy**—familial dilated or hypertrophic cardiomyopathy
- **Thrombo-embolic disease**—enquire about thrombophilia

C. Medications;

- Complete a full drug history and compliance to therapy.
- Enquire about complications of medications.
- Calcium antagonists, long-term steroids, hydralazine minoxidil, methyldopa, thiazolinediones (pioglitazone and rosiglitazone), monoamine oxidase inhibitors, and NSAIDs can cause fluid retention.
- Oral contraceptive pill and HRT use in females increases thromboembolic risk.
- Appetite suppressors, i.e. fenfluramine are associated with pulmonary hypertension.
- Nephrotoxic medications can potentiate and aggravate renal failure. (eg. Nsaids, penicillins, gentamicin, sulphonamides, ACE inhibitors, ciclosporin).

D. Social issues:

- Smoking habits (cardiovascular risk factor)
- Alcohol consumption (risk factor for dilated cardiomyopathy and chronic liver disease)
- Impact of symptoms on daily life
- Elicit the patient's concerns about the symptoms

Formulating a plan of action

Explain to the patient that there are possible causes for ankle oedema. It is important to exclude drug causes of ankle oedema and dependent oedema. This should be clear from the history. Subsequent investigations will reflect possible underlying causes. Preliminary screening investigations include:

- Bloods
  - **Anaemia** can potentiate cardiac ischaemia and cardiac failure
  - **Leucocytosis** and **raised inflammatory markers** would suggest underlying infection, i.e. cellulitis
  - **Urea and electrolytes (U&Es)**: renal failure
  - **D-dimer** for suspected thrombo-embolic disease
  - **Cardiac enzymes** if suspecting myocardial ischaemia
  - Brain natriuretic peptide (**BNP**) if suspecting cardiac failure
  - **LFT and clotting if suspecting chronic liver disease**
  - **Autoimmune profile** and **rheumatoid factor** if suspecting rheumatological disease
  - **Albumin**: hypoalbuminaemia is seen in nephrotic syndrome, chronic liver disease, advanced chronic illnesses, and poor nutritional status.
  - **Lipid profiles**: hypercholesterolaemia may be seen in nephrotic syndrome
  - **Thyroid function tests**

- **Urinalysis** to demonstrate proteinuria (nephrotic syndrome)
- **ECG**
  - **Myocardial ischaemia**: the ECG can be normal at rest in a patient with exertional angina
  - **Right heart strain**: cor pulmonale
- **Chest radiograph**
  - Cardiomegaly and pulmonary congestion (left ventricular dysfunction)
  - Pleural effusions in conditions of fluid retention (congestive heart failure, nephrotic syndrome, chronic liver disease)
  - Chronic respiratory disease: interstitial lung disease, obstructive airways disease

The following specific tests may be indicated:

- **Echocardiogram**: to assess ventricular function, valvular heart disease, pulmonary artery systolic pressure, and to detect shunts and pericardial effusions.
- **CT pulmonary angiogram** for suspected PE (chronic thrombo-embolic disease)
- **Lung function tests**: obstructive or restrictive lung defect if suspecting respiratory disease
- **HRCT chest** if suspecting interstitial lung disease as a cause of cor pulmonale
- **Doppler US scan of leg**: if suspecting deep vein thrombosis
- **24 hour urine collection, or urinary protein: creatinie ratio for proteinuria**: nephrotic range proteinuria is defined as ≥ 3g in 24 hours
- **Venography:** if suspecting IVC obstruction of extrinsic venous compression as a cause of ankle oedema
- **Renal ultrasound scan**: small kidneys with thin cortices indicates chronic renal disease
- **Right heart catheterization** can be considered in patients with pulmonary hypertension
- **Abdominal and pelvic ultrasound** to exclude pelvic masses causing venous compression
- **CT chest, abdomen, and pelvis** if considering extrinsic venous compression due to underlying malignancy
- **Lymphoscintigraphy** can be helpful to distinguish lymphoedema from venous insufficiency. This is performed by injecting a radioactive tracer into the first web space and monitoring lymphatic flow with a gamma camera.

Questions commonly asked by examiners

When should diuretics be used in patients with ankle oedema?

- Loop diuretics can be used to reduce lower limb oedema in patients with congestive cardiac failure, cor pulmonale, nephrotic syndrome, and renal failure (see Case 10-Breathless, for management of cardiac failure).
- Patients with ascites and lower limb oedema due to chronic liver disease require high doses of spironolactone often in conjunction with loop diuretics.
- Patients with chronic venous insufficiency should only have diuretics after leg elevation and compression stocking have failed. Diuretics can be used in severely affected patients but only sparingly and briefly.
- Diuretics should not be used in patients with lymphoedema.

What is the management of lymphoedema?

Generally, the treatment for lymphoedema is disappointing. Diuretics are generally not helpful.

- General measures:
  - Exercise
  - Leg elevation
  - Compressive garments

* Treatment of cellulitis (prophylactic antibiotics may be indicated with recurrent cellulitis)
* Specific measures:
    * Manual lymphatic drainage
    * Intermittent pneumatic compression devices
    * Surgery to relieve lymphatic obstruction

What is the treatment of chronic venous insufficiency?

* Leg elevation
* Knee-high compression stockings to provide 30–40mmHg pressure at the ankle. This is contra-indicated in significant peripheral vascular disease
* Intermittent pneumatic compression pumps
* Diuretics can be used for short periods only in severely affected patients for short periods of time. As venous insufficiency is not truly a condition with fluid overload, prolonged diuretic use can predispose to renal impairment.

How common is lower limb oedema in patients taking calcium antagonists?

Up to 50% of patents taking calcium antagonists develop oedema. Dihydropyridines (amlodipine and nifedipine) are more likely to precipitate oedema than non-dihydropyridines (verapamil and diltiazem).

Case 13 ◆ **Cough**

INFORMATION FOR THE CANDIDATE

Dear Doctor,

This 52-year old gentleman presents with a 4-month history of a daily cough. He also reports frequent episodes of a runny nose and sneezing throughout the year. He was diagnosed with essential hypertension several months ago, and his only medications are Lisinopril and Ranitidine. Clinical examination is unremarkable. He is a non-smoker and is finding the cough troublesome at night.

Many thanks for your opinion.

Acquiring the history

A. History of presenting complaint:

Onset of symptoms

The cause of cough can be classified by the onset and duration. Acute cough has a duration of less than three weeks, most likely caused by acute respiratory tract infection. Other causes of acute cough are exacerbation of COPD, pneumonia, asthma, PE, and, rarely, inhaled foreign body. The presence of stridor and choking suggests upper airway obstruction which requires immediate attention.

Subacute cough is present for between three and eight weeks, and chronic cough for greater than eight weeks.

Age of onset
The most common cause of chronic cough in childhood is asthma, although in adults gastro-oesophageal reflux and upper airway syndromes (e.g. postnasal drip) are also common.

Characteristics
- **Frequency of cough**: daily, intermittent, and seasonal
- **Temporal pattern**: *'Is there a particular time in the day when the cough is the worst?'*
  - Cough that is worse in the morning suggests chronic bronchitis
  - A nocturnal cough may indicate asthma, gastro-oesophageal reflux, or left ventricular failure
  - Cough during or after meals favours aspiration or gastro-oesophageal reflux
- **Progression**: Ask about any *change* in the character or frequency of the cough over time. This could signify a new problem. Consider lung cancer in a smoker with a change in the nature of a chronic cough.

Precipitating factors. *'Does anything in particular trigger or aggravate the cough?'*
Ask specifically about the association of the cough with
- Food or drink suggesting gastro-oesophageal reflux or aspiration.
- Change in posture. For example a cough that is worse on bending forwards or lying flat also suggests gastro-oesophageal reflux.
- Irritants such as dust, pollen, animals, fumes, vapours, and cigarette smoke may precipitate rhinitis or extrinsic asthma.
- Cold weather and exercise can exacerbate the symptoms of asthma.

Associated symptoms
- **Sputum production**: determine the quantity, character, and colour of sputum.
  - Clear or grey sputum is seen with chronic bronchitis
  - Purulent yellow/green sputum suggests acute infection of any cause
  - Rusty or brown coloured, foul smelling and tasting sputum is characteristic of bronchiectasis
  - Frothy, pink sputum occurs with left ventricular failure
- Conversely, a dry cough may be a feature of viral upper respiratory tract infection, gastro-oesophageal reflux or interstitial lung disease.
- **Haemoptysis**: determine the quantity expectorated in a 24-hour period. Blood tinged sputum occurs with acute infection of any cause and left ventricular failure. A variable amount of haemoptysis occurs with lung cancer and tuberculosis.
- **Chest pain**
  - pleuritic pain is a feature of acute infection or PE
  - chest 'tightness' occurs with asthma and COPD
  - central chest pain of cardiac origin will point towards left ventricular failure secondary to a myocardial infarction
  - musculoskeletal chest pain, similar in nature to pleuritic pain, may be the result of rib fractures secondary to severe paroxysms of coughing.
- **Dyspnoea**
  - Sudden onset of breathlessness suggests asthma, PE, acute pulmonary oedema, or foreign body inhalation
  - Subacute onset of breathlessness is suggestive of pneumonia, aspiration, COPD, asthma
  - Gradually progressive dyspnoea is characteristic of COPD and left ventricular failure
  - Orthopnoea and paroxysmal nocturnal dyspnoea favour left ventricular failure

- ◆ Enquire about dyspnoea on exertion and quantify exercise tolerance 'How far can you walk before your breathing stops you?' or 'How many flights of stairs can you manage without stopping?'.
- **Wheeze**: 'Do you have a wheeze; that is, a whistling sound when you breathe?'. Wheeze occurs with asthma, COPD, and cardiac failure and Churg-Strauss Syndrome.
- **Nasal symptoms**: upper airway syndromes are a common cause of chronic cough. This is due to postnasal drip stimulating cough receptors in the pharynx and larynx. Causes of postnasal drip include allergic rhinitis, perennial non-allergic rhinitis, sinusitis, and acute nasopharyngitis. Ask about:
  - ◆ Rhinorrhoea or nasal discharge
  - ◆ Nasal congestion
  - ◆ Throat clearing, irritation and sensation of 'dripping' at the back of the throat
  - ◆ Sneezing
  - ◆ Facial pain suggesting sinusitis
- **Hoarseness**. Ask the patient 'Have you, or others, noticed any change in the quality your voice?' Hoarseness of voice results from vocal cord paralysis due to laryngitis, laryngeal malignancy, or bronchogenic carcinoma invading the recurrent laryngeal nerve.
- **Gastrointestinal symptoms**. Determine the presence of symptoms suggestive of gastro-oesophageal reflux. These are
  - ◆ Retrosternal burning
  - ◆ Dyspepsia or retrosternal pain that is worse on lying down
  - ◆ Acid brash

Vomiting or regurgitation shortly after swallowing food suggests aspiration.

- **Other symptoms**
  - ◆ Recent upper respiratory tract infection suggest a postinfectious cause or postnasal drip syndrome
  - ◆ Weight loss and anorexia occurs in malignancy, advanced COPD, bronchiectasis, and cystic fibrosis
  - ◆ Fever and night sweats suggest an infective cause. Consider tuberculosis in patients with these symptoms and a chronic cough
  - ◆ Skin rash (erythema nodosum) and eye symptoms such as redness and pain are manifestations of sarcoidosis
  - ◆ Purpuric rash or mononeuritis multiplex on the background of asthma or rhinitis, suggest Churg-Strauss syndrome
  - ◆ Associated urinary stress incontinence
  - ◆ Episodes of syncope associated with cough

B. Relevant medical and family history:

Past medical history:
- Ask about respiratory illnesses such as childhood asthma, recurrent chest infections, COPD, previous tuberculosis, and sinusitis.
- Enquire about a personal and family history of atopy: hayfever, eczema, and asthma.
- Ask about acid-related GI disorders, such as dyspepsia or peptic ulcer disease.
- Ask about cardiac disease and vascular risk factors which may suggest congestive cardiac failure.

Family history
- atopy
- lung cancer
- tuberculosis

C. Medications and allergies:
- Take a thorough drug history and note the use of:
  - ACE inhibitors frequently cause cough. The onset is usually within one week of commencing therapy, but can occur up to six months later.
  - NSAIDs and aspirin which trigger asthma.
  - β-blockers may cause bronchoconstriction and exacerbate the symptoms of asthma.
- Note any medications that may exacerbate gastro-oesophageal reflux and these are:
  - nitrates
  - calcium channel blockers
  - theophylline
  - bisphosphonates
- Is the patient allergic to house dust, pollen, animals, and other possible triggers for rhinitis and extrinsic asthma?
- How often does the patient use inhalers for known asthma/COPD?

D. Social issues:
- Ask about the impact of the cough on the patient's quality of life. Determine if the cough interferes with daily activities, work, exercise, and sleep.
- Take a thorough occupational history to determine any triggers for the cough. Ask about exposure to solvents, fumes, vapours, animals, and dusts which can trigger occupational asthma, and also cause the dry cough associated with interstitial lung diseases such as extrinsic allergic alveolitis and pulmonary fibrosis.
- Has the patient been exposed to asbestos?
- Smoking history is essential as smoking is the single most important risk factor in the development of COPD, lung, and laryngeal cancer.
- Enquire about travel abroad, in particular travel to areas where tuberculosis is endemic.
- Ask about exposure to animals which can cause extrinsic allergic alveolitis
- Ask about contact with others with similar symptoms, and patients with tuberculosis.
- Ask openly about the patient's own concerns regarding their symptoms: '*Is there anything in particular that you are worried this may be?*'

Formulating a plan of action
- Explain to the patient that a full clinical examination is required.
- Reassure the patient that the cause is very likely to be upper-airway related, asthma or acid reflux. In patients who are non-smokers, are not taking ACE inhibitors, have a normal radiograph, and no progression in their symptoms, these three causes account for virtually all causes of chronic cough.
- Explain that cough medicines may relieve the symptom, particularly of cough following viral respiratory infections, but that codeine-containing formulations may cause drowsiness affecting driving, and should also be avoided in supparative lung conditions, such as bronchiectasis or cystic fibrosis, where expectoration is essential.
- Explain that a trial of therapy may be preferable to extensive investigation in the first instance. Nasal decongestants and nasal inhalers may relieve postnasal symptoms, however antihistamines may cause drowsiness and a dry mouth. Acid suppressants or bronchodilator inhalers may also be indicated, however remember to check adequacy of inhaler technique.

- Consider the following investigations as directed by the history, or when there is failure of trial therapies such as nasal decongestants, bronchodilators, or antacids.

  ♦ **Peak flow monitoring** will demonstrate reversible bronchoconstriction and diurnal variation in asthma.

  ♦ **Sputum culture** for microscopy, culture, and sensitivity, including Ziehl-Nielsen stain for mycobacteria.

  ♦ **Blood tests:**

    – White cell count and CRP for infection. Eosinophilia will be seen in allergic causes and Churg-Strauss syndrome

    – ESR may be elevated in malignancy, infection, and inflammatorydisease

    – Serum calcium may be raised in sarcoidosis

    – Serum ACE for sarcoidosis

    – Autoantibody screen : cytoplasmic anti-neutrophil cytoplasmic antibody (c-ANCA) may be positive in Churg-Strauss syndrome

    – Arterial blood gas if pulse oximetry demonstrates hypoxia, or if there is respiratory distress.

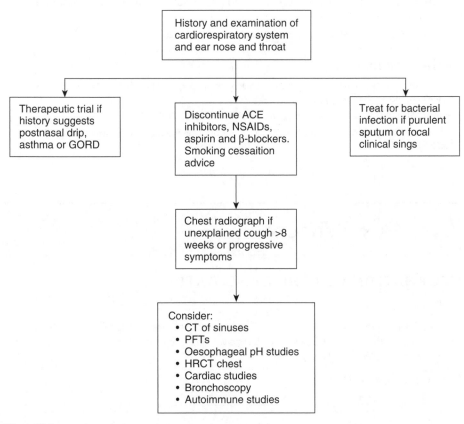

Figure 13.1

- **Imaging:** A plain chest radiograph should be performed in all cases of chronic cough. Also consider:
    - High-resolution CT of the thorax for interstitial lung disease
    - CT of the sinuses
- **Lung function tests:** Spirometry will reveal obstructive or restrictive lung diseases
- **Fibreoptic laryngoscopy and bronchoscopy** is indicated in patients with:
    - suspected malignancy, for biopsies of lesions and/or transbronchial fine needle aspiration of mediastinal lymph nodes
    - interstitial lung disease, for bronchoalveolar lavage and/or transbronchial lung biopsy
    - recurrent chest infections, to obtain bronchial washings for microbiological identification of organisms.
- **Gastrointestinal investigations**: upper gastrointestinal endoscopy or 24-hour oesophageal pH monitoring.

Questions commonly asked by examiners

What is the definition of chronic bronchitis?

Chronic bronchitis is typically a symptom of COPD, and is not necessarily caused by infection. It is defined clinically as a persistent cough that produces sputum and mucus, for at least three months in two consecutive years.

See Case 15 Carcinoma of the Lung and Case 12 COPD in Volume 1

Further reading

1. Morice AH *et al*. Recommendations for the management of cough in adults, British Thoracic Society Guidelines, Thorax. 2006; 61(Suppl I):i1–i24.
2. Morice AH *et al*. Cough 1: Chronic cough in adults Thorax. 2003, 58:901–7.
3. McGarvey LPA Cough 6: Which investigations are most useful in the diagnosis of chronic cough? Thorax. 2004; 59:342–6.

Case 14 ◆ **Wheeze**

INFORMATION FOR THE CANDIDATE

Dear Doctor,

Thank you for seeing this 30-year old gentleman with a recent onset wheeze. He tells me that he had asthma as a child. There is no other past medical history of note and he is not on any regular medications. He is a smoker and works in a paint factory.

Many thanks for your opinion.

Acquiring the history

Wheeze in adults has a wide differential diagnosis and should not always be attributed to asthma.

A. History of presenting complaint:
Age of onset
Details of symptoms

Begin with an open question to determine the patient's symptoms, avoiding jargon such as 'inspiratory' or 'expiratory'. Ask them what they mean by a 'wheeze'. The correct definition is a high-pitched sound with a musical quality heard in inspiration and expiration and caused by airway obstruction, although patients may use the term to describe other respiratory symptoms such as cough or breathlessness.

Onset of symptoms

Enquire about the onset of symptoms that can help narrow the differential diagnosis:

- Acute onset wheeze, often with a clear precipitant, should raise the possibility of anaphylaxis, acute exacerbation of asthma or COPD, aspiration syndromes, PE and foreign body. The latter is far more common in children.
- Subacute wheeze may be caused by respiratory tract infections, PE, or left ventricular failure.
- Chronic wheeze is suggestive of causes with a longstanding underlying pathology such as asthma, COPD, and lung carcinoma.

Associated symptoms

- **Respiratory symptoms:**
  - *Cough.* Ask about the duration and progression of the cough. A chronic non-productive cough that is troublesome at night, occurring together with wheeze and dyspnoea, is the classical presentation of asthma. However, even with these typical features, other respiratory and non-respiratory conditions are common in adults.
  - *Dyspnoea.* Enquire about the onset of associated shortness of breath and quantify exercise tolerance. *'When you have the wheeze, how many flights of stairs can you walk before stopping because of shortness of breath?'*
  - *Chest tightness* occurs with asthma and COPD. Pleuritic chest pain is indicative of pneumonia or PE.
  - *Haemoptysis* is suggestive of PE or lung carcinoma. If PE is suspected, ask about leg swelling and pain as well as the presence of risk factors for venous thromboembolism (previous history, family history of thrombophilia, recent surgery, recent long haul journey, immobility and use of oral contraceptive pill in women).
  - *Change in voice.* Ask the patient if they or others have noticed a change in the character of their voice, suggesting bronchogenic carcinoma causing recurrent laryngeal nerve compression, laryngeal disease, or GORD causing laryngeal inflammation.
  - *Constitutional symptoms* of fever, weight loss, and night sweats raise the possibility of infection or malignancy.
- **Cardiac symptoms**
  - Cardiac chest pain, dyspnoea, orthopnoea, paroxysmal nocturnal dyspnoea, and ankle swelling suggest heart failure as a cause.
- **Other**
  - Urticaria, tongue swelling, angioedema, abdominal pain, and sudden-onset nausea and vomiting suggest anaphylaxis.

- History of rhinitis (nasal congestion, rhinorrhoea, and sneezing) with typical symptoms of asthma (wheeze, dyspnoea, and chest tightness) suggest Churg-Strauss syndrome. These features may precede other signs such as palpable purpuric rash and mononeuritis multiplex.
- Although rare, carcinoid syndrome should be considered in patients with intermittent wheeze and dyspnoea with accompanying head and facial flushing. Other features are abdominal pain and chronic diarrhoea.
- Ask about symptoms suggestive of GORD: retrosternal burning, acid brash and regurgitation, which are worse on lying flat or bending forwards.

Progression of symptoms

Ask about the chronology of symptoms and progression. Symptoms of asthma are usually intermittent, with exacerbations caused by obvious precipitants (see below). Asthma is likely if the symptoms are reversible with bronchodilators and conventional asthma therapy. Symptoms that are unremitting with optimal bronchodilator and oral therapy should raise the possibility of an alternative diagnosis.

Precipitants

Ask openly about potential triggers for the patient's symptoms: *'Have you noticed anything that triggers your symptoms?'* The following are environmental triggers for asthma:

- viral illness
- cigarette smoke
- pollen
- house dust mite
- animal dander
- cold air and pollutants
- exercise
- emotional stress

Anaphylaxis will be suggested by preceding ingestion of nuts or other foodstuffs, wasp/bee sting, or administration of medication.

Is the patient a known asthmatic?

If the patient is a known asthmatic presenting with deteriorating symptoms, take a detailed account to determine the disease severity.

- *'In what way are the symptoms worse than usual?'*
- The control of symptoms can be determined by asking the following three questions validated by the Royal College of Physicians:
    - *'Have you had difficulty sleeping because of your asthma symptoms (including cough)?'*
    - *'Have you had your usual asthma symptoms during the day (cough, wheeze, chest tightness, or breathlessness)?'*
    - *Has your asthma interfered with your usual activities (housework, work, and school)?'*
- Other questions to ask to assess disease severity are:
    - *'Do you get symptoms on exercise?'*
    - *'What is your best peak expiratory flow rate reading? Has this changed recently?'*
    - *'What treatment are you on? Inhalers? Oral treatment? Home nebulizers? Have you needed the salbutamol inhaler more than usual?'*
    - *'How many times in the last year have you had an asthma attack? Have you previously been admitted to ITU because of asthma?'*

B. Relevant medical and family history:

Past medical history

- Atopy—eczema and allergic rhinitis, which are associated with intrinsic asthma
- A history of cardiac disease and the presence of vascular risk factors may suggest left ventricular failure in the presence of other cardiac symptoms.
- GORD
- Previous anaesthetic—endotracheal intubation or tracheostomy may result in laryngeal or tracheal injury and consequent stridor or wheeze.

Family history

- Atopy—the triad of eczema, allergic rhinitis, and intrinsic asthma are heritable traits.

C. Medications and interactions:

- Ask about drugs that induce bronchoconstriction
  - ◆ Aspirin and NSAIDs
  - ◆ β-blockers
- Allergies to medications and other substances as precipitants.
- Ask women about the use of the oral contraceptive pill as a risk factor for venous thromboembolism
- Inhaled and smoked cocaine can precipitate an exacerbation of asthma.

D. Social issues:

- Obtain a detailed occupational history, including the nature of the current job and its impact on the patient's symptoms.
  - ◆ Determine the exact nature of the work and document exposure to potential precipitants of occupational asthma: industrial dusts, chemicals (especially ammonia and platinum), fumes, flour, animals, mould and hay.
  - ◆ Ask specifically if the symptoms *improve* when away from work.
  - ◆ Enquire about possible exposure to asbestos for underlying mesothelioma or bronchogenic carcinoma.
- Determine the impact of the patient's symptoms on daily activities. General questions may be *'Are the symptoms restricting you from doing the housework?'; 'Have you had to take time off work because of your symptoms?'* Determine the financial implications for the patient.
- Obtain a smoking history and ask about exposure to passive smoke. Cigarette smoke is a precipitant of asthma and is the single most important aetiological risk factor for COPD, bronchogenic, and laryngeal carcinoma.
- Ask about exposure to animals and pets as triggers.
- Ask openly about the patient's concerns regarding their symptoms *'Is there anything in particular you are worried may be causing these symptoms?'*. Lung cancer is a common concern for patients with new-onset respiratory symptoms.

Formulating a plan of action

- Explain to the patient that a full clinical examination will be required.
- If there are no constitutional symptoms, reassure the patient that lung cancer is unlikely. Explain the most likely cause (see below).
- All patients presenting with wheeze must have objective measurement of airflow obstruction by spirometry. Note that spirometry can be normal between episodes of asthma, therefore serial peak flow measurements may be required to illustrate diurnal variability of

airway obstruction in asthma. A diurnal variation of greater than 20% from baseline measurements is highly suggestive of asthma.

- The diagnosis of asthma is based upon the presence of two or more of the characteristic symptoms of asthma (wheeze, dyspnoea, cough, and chest tightness) *with* objective demonstration of airflow obstruction, reversibility and/or hyperresponsiveness.[1]

Patients are categorised into three groups based on the likelihood of a diagnosis of asthma:

- **High probability of asthma** suggested by clinical features and demonstration of airflow obstruction on spirometry (FEV_1:FVC <0.70). Patients are initially treated with a therapeutic trial of bronchodilator or steroids (inhaled or oral). Asthma is likely if there is a positive response to therapy. Bronchodilator response testing is less sensitive than a trial of steroid therapy, therefore an initial negative response to bronchodilators should lead to a trial of steroids.

- **Intermediate probability of asthma *with* demonstration of airflow obstruction** also warrants a trial of bronchodilator or steroid therapy. An improvement in FEV_1 >15% or >200ml after bronchodilator administration confirms a diagnosis of asthma. A response >400ml is more specific. A negative response requires further testing with assessment of airway responsiveness with methacholine/histamine or exercise challenge. If this is negative then COPD is likely, although approximately 15% of patients with COPD have a positive response to bronchodilator reversibility testing.

- **Intermediate probability of asthma *without* demonstration of airflow obstruction**. Patients with normal spirometry should have further investigation before a trial of treatment, such as airway responsiveness testing. Since these are sensitive tests, normal results provide strong evidence against a diagnosis of asthma.

- **Low probability of asthma *or* negative responses to reversibility and airway challenge**. Consider the following investigations in such patients to look for other possible causes:

  - **Blood tests**
    - Blood count—an elevated eosinophil count may be seen in asthma. An elevated sputum eosinophil count (>2%) is highly sensitive for asthma, and also present in Churg-Strauss syndrome.
    - CRP and/or ESR will be raised in infection, Churg-Strauss syndrome, and malignancy.
    - Autoantibody screen—P-ANCA titre may be present in Churg-Strauss syndrome.

  - **Imaging**
    - CXR is indicated in patients with atypical features, or with additional signs and symptoms.
    - Contrast enhanced CT scan of the thorax (or HRCT scan) is indicated when alternative respiratory conditions are suspected.

  - **Fibreoptic bronchoscopy**
    - Bronchoalveolar lavage has a role in the diagnosis of interstitial lung disease. Bronchoscopy also has a role in the management of lung carcinoma and foreign body.

  - **Echocardiography** is indicated for assessment of left ventricular function and structural heart disease as a cardiac cause is possible.

  - **Gastrointestinal investigations:** upper gastrointestinal endoscopy and oesophageal pH monitoring if GORD is suspected.

  - **Tests for carcinoid syndrome:** 24 hour urinary excretion of 5-Hydroxyindole Acetic Acid and/or serotonin levels.

◆ **Laryngoscopy** if upper airways disease is suspected.
◆ **Exhaled nitric oxide (NO) analysis:** Patients with asthma have higher concentrations of NO in their expirate than non-asthmatics, reflecting eosinophilic airway inflammation. These patients are more likely to have asthma and to respond to steroids.

Table 14.1 Differential diagnosis of wheeze—modified from BTS guidelines[1]

With airflow obstruction on spirometry	*Without* airway obstruction on spirometry
• Asthma	• Chronic cough syndromes
• COPD	• Hyperventilation syndromes
• Bronchiectasis/cystic fibrosis	• Vocal cord dysfunction
• Allergic bronchopulmonary aspergillosis (ABPA).	• Rhinitis
• Lung cancer	• Gastroesophageal reflux disease (GORD)
• Sarcoidosis	• Left ventricular failure ('cardiac wheeze')
• Anaphylaxis	• Pulmonary fibrosis
• Foreign body	
• Laryngo-tracheal stenosis	
• Churg-Strauss syndrome	
• Carcinoid syndrome	
• Drug induced bronchoconstriction e.g. NSAIDs, β-blockers.	

Questions commonly asked by examiners

How do you define asthma?

Asthma is a chronic inflammatory airways disease associated with airway hyperresponsiveness that leads to widespread *reversible* airflow obstruction resulting in episodes of wheeze, chest tightness, dyspnoea, and cough.

How is chronic asthma managed?

The management of asthma is stepwise to achieve optimum control of symptoms and is based on the British Thoracic Society guidelines (2008):

General measures

• Patient education about disease process, compliance, inhaler technique, peak flow monitoring, self-management, and management of exacerbations.
• Avoidance of known precipitants
• Smoking cessation
• Immunizations against influenza and pneumococcal pneumonia +H1N1
• Prompt treatment of exacerbations by stepping up treatment, appropriate antibiotics, and steroids.

Drug treatment

• **Step 1 Mild intermittent asthma**
   Inhaled short acting β_2 agonist as required

- **Step 2 Regular preventer therapy**
  Add on inhaled steroid 200–800mcg/day
- **Step 3 Initial add on therapy**
  Add on long acting β_2 agonist (LABA). Continue if a good response is seen with the addition of LABA, if not discontinue and increase the dose of inhaled steroid.
- **Step 4 Persistent poor control**
  Options include:
  1. Increase dose of inhaled steroid up to 2000mcg/day
  2. Add on a fourth drug: leukotriene receptor antagonist, theophylline, or oral β_2 agonist.
- **Step 5 Continuous or frequent use of oral steroids**
  1. High dose inhaled steroid up to 2000mcg/day
  2. Daily oral prednisolone (lowest possible dose)
  3. Referral for specialist input and monoclonal antibody therapy

Which patients are referred for specialist input?

- Patients on step 4 or 5 therapy
- Patients suspected to have occupational asthma
- Patients with a high risk of asthma related deaths. These are patients who are admitted to hospital for treatment of exacerbations and those previously requiring ITU an/or mechanical ventilation.

How would you manage acute asthma?

- Assess the severity of asthma.
  - **Acute severe asthma** is characterized by:
    - PEFR 33–50% of best or predicted measurement
    - Respiratory rate >25
    - Heart rate >110bpm
    - Unable to complete sentences
  - Features of **life-threatening asthma** are:
    - PEFR <33% of best or predicted measurement
    - SaO_2 <92%
    - Poor respiratory effort, cyanosis, silent chest
    - Arrhythmia, hypotension
    - Confusion, exhaustion, coma
    - ABG: acidosis, PaO_2 <8Kpa, normal or raised $PaCO_2$
    - Hypercapnia suggests **near-fatal asthma**
- High flow oxygen to maintain SaO_2 94–98%
- Oxygen driven nebulized salbutamol 5mg (every 15 minutes if failure to respond initially or features of life-threatening asthma present) and ipratropium bromide 500mcg (4–6 hourly)
- Continuous salbutamol nebulization if failure to respond.
- Steroids IV hydrocortisone 200mg or prednisolone 40mg daily for 5 days.
- Intravenous magnesium sulphate 1.2–2g once only indicated in patients who do not respond to bronchodilator treatment.
- Consider intravenous salbutamol and aminophylline infusion.
- Mechanical ventilation is necessary in patients who fail to respond to the above treatment with poor respiratory effort, progressive hypoxia, hypercapnia, confusion, drowsiness, or exhaustion.

What are the common causes of occupational asthma?

Several hundred agents have been reported to cause occupational asthma.[1] The most common are: isocyanates, flour, latex, animals, aldehydes, and wood dust.

The most frequently affected professions are: paint sprayers, bakers, nurses, animal handlers, welders, and timber workers.

Occupational asthma presents with symptoms of airflow limitation, similar to allergic asthma. However, this must be distinguished from extrinsic allergic alveolitis (EAA), which is also caused by exposure to occupational agents. EAA is a result of an immunological reaction to an inhaled agent affecting the pulmonary parenchyma rather than the airway. The most frequent agents are agricultural dusts or microorganisms, affecting farming and poultry workers in particular. Acute EAA causes fever, cough, and dyspnoea. Chronic EAA is similar to pulmonary fibrosis, with cough dyspnoea and digital clubbing. Wheeze is typically absent.

References

1. British Thoracic Society guidelines. British guideline on the management of asthma. May 2008.

2. British Thoracic Society guidelines. Emergency oxygen use in adult patients, October 2008.

Case 15 ◆ **Haemoptysis**

INFORMATION FOR THE CANDIDATE

Dear Doctor,

This 68-year old gentleman presents with frequent episodes of 'coughing up blood'. He has had a nephrectomy in the past for a renal cell carcinoma. He is a lifelong smoker and has recently returned from a holiday in India. He is worried that he may have lung cancer.

Many thanks for your opinion.

Acquiring the history

A. History of presenting complaint:

The history should aim to distinguish true haemoptysis (blood originating from the lower respiratory tract), from bleeding from the nasopharynx or upper gastrointestinal tract. Causes of haemoptysis include:

- **Respiratory**
  - Infection: Pneumonia, tuberculosis, lung abscess, acute bronchitis, bronchiectasis, aspergillosis
  - Neoplastic: Bronchogenic carcinoma, metastases, Kaposi's sarcoma
  - Vascular: PE, Wegner's granulomatosis, Goodpasture's syndrome, Hereditary Haemorrhagic Telangiectasia (HHT)
- **Cardiac**
  - Pulmonary oedema
  - Mitral stenosis

- **Other**
  - Bleeding disorders
  - Anticoagulants
  - Thoracic endometriosis (catamenial haemoptysis)

Age of onset

Consider lung cancer in patients over 50 years of age presenting with haemoptysis especially with a strong smoking history. Pulmonary-renal syndromes and HHT should be considered in younger patients.

Characteristics of haemoptysis

- **Onset and duration**. Sudden onset haemoptysis suggests acute pathology such as a PE or pulmonary haemorrhage.
- **Frequency of and number of previous episodes**
- **Colour**
  - fresh blood
  - pink suggests a small amount of blood. Seen in pulmonary oedema and mitral stenosis
  - brown/rusty indicates mucopurulent sputum rather than haemoptysis, suggestive of pneumonia or bronchiectasis
  - black indicates melanoptysis seen in pneumoconiosis
- **Quantity**. Determine the volume of blood loss per 24 hours in measures of teaspoons/cups. Haemoptysis of greater than 200ml per 24 hours indicates a poorer prognosis.

Associated symptoms

- **Cough and sputum production**. Establish the onset of these symptoms. Acute or subacute onset of cough with productive sputum suggests infection of any cause. Blood streaked sputum in small quantities is a feature of chronic bronchitis. Chronic purulent sputum production with streaks of blood is seen in bronchiectasis.
- **Dyspnoea** may be respiratory or cardiac in origin. Sudden onset of shortness of breath with haemoptysis occurs following massive pulmonary embolus and occasionally infection. Sudden onset or progressive dyspnoea with pink, frothy sputum suggests pulmonary oedema or mitral stenosis. Note that profuse haemoptysis may occur with mitral stenosis due to pulmonary hypertension and rupture of bronchial vessels, or due to anticoagulation for AF. In such patients also ask about exercise tolerance, orthopnoea, and paroxysmal nocturnal dyspnoea.
- **Chest pain**. Pleuritic pain is caused by an infection or a PE.
- **Fever, rigors, and night sweats** occur with any infective process. Swinging fevers are characteristic of a lung abscess and profuse night sweats occur with tuberculosis.
- **Hoarseness of voice and dysphagia** may occur with compression of adjacent thoracic structures by a bronchogenic carcinoma and in mitral stenosis due to an enlarged left atrium.
- **Weight loss and anorexia** are non-specific features of malignancy and tuberculosis.
- **Rash, arthralgia, and myalgia** are also features of Wegner's granulomatosis and SLE.
- **Bleeding** from elsewhere may suggest bleeding disorders of any cause. Epistaxis occurs with Wegner's granulomatosis and HHT, whilst haematuria and massive haemoptysis suggest pulmonary-renal syndromes.
- **Leg pain, swelling, and erythema** are symptoms suggestive of a DVT and may indicate a PE. Determine the presence of any risk factors for venous thromboembolism such as prolonged immobility, long haul journeys, recent surgery, underlying malignancy, use of the oral contraceptive pill, and a personal or family history of venous thromboembolism.

- In women, ask if the haemoptysis is cyclical occurring during menstruation suggesting catamenial endometriosis (ectopic endometrial tissue—a rare cause of moderate to severe haemoptysis).
- **Gastrointestinal symptoms.** The presence of nausea, vomiting, epigastric pain, and malaena differentiates haemoptysis from haematemesis.

B. Relevant medical and family history:

Past medical history:

- Ask about recurrent chest infections that suggest bronchiectasis or cystic fibrosis.
- Previous history of childhood rheumatic fever suggests mitral stenosis.
- Bleeding disorders
- Malignancy may suggest metastases or a predisposition to venous thromboembolism
- Intracranial haemorrhage which may suggest the presence of cerebral arteriovenous malformations (AVM) which occur in association with HHT. Gastrointestinal bleeding is also a feature of HHT.
- Enquire about chronic liver disease as a cause of coagulopathy or haematemesis which could be mistaken for haemoptysis. In addition, a history of peptic ulcer disease may point towards an upper gastrointestinal bleed rather than haemoptysis together with other symptoms in the history.
- Immunosuppression from any cause will predispose to opportunistic lung infections and reactivation of tuberculosis.

Family history:

- Lung malignancy
- Tuberculosis
- HHT has an autosomal dominant mode of inheritance
- Bleeding disorders and thrombophilia

C. Medications and interactions:

- Ask about the use of anticoagulant and antiplatelet therapy
- Ask specifically about the use of the oral contraceptive pill—a risk factor for venous thromboembolism
- Determine the use of recreational drugs. Cocaine in particular is associated with pulmonary haemorrhage and infarction.

D. Social issues:

- Smoking is the single most important risk factor for the development of lung carcinoma.
  - Obtain a thorough occupational history to determine possible exposure to asbestos. As well as mesothelioma, asbestos exposure also increases the risk of bronchogenic carcinoma.
  - Enquire about travel abroad, particularly to areas where tuberculosis is endemic. Similarly ask about any contact with tuberculosis.
  - Patients are likely to be concerned about lung cancer—sensitively address their concerns, and reassure them about alternative, treatable diagnoses and the need for further investigations.

Formulating a plan of action

- Explain to the patient that the cause of the haemoptysis will be determined by investigations.
- Explain the possible causes suggested by the history.

Imaging:

Chest radiography is the key initial investigation, since it may suggest specific causes such as malignancy, focal infection, or possible mitral valve disease. The chest X-ray is normal in 5–10% of patients with malignancy.

Abnormal findings on the CXR are typically followed by **fibreoptic bronchoscopy** for visualization and sampling of abnormal tissue.

If the chest radiograph is normal, **contrast enhanced CT scan** of thorax and abdomen is the investigation of choice to exclude lesions not seen on plain radiography. The presence, site, size, and number of lesions can be determined as well assessment of nodal involvement, which determines the stage of disease and further investigation and management.

Other investigations to consider:

* **Sputum** for microbiology (gram and Ziehl-Nielsen stain), culture, and cytology. Three samples should be sent to the laboratory for suspected tuberculosis.
* **Blood tests**
    * Blood count to determine the degree of blood loss. A raised white cell count and CRP may suggest infection.
    * ESR will be raised in infection, malignancy, and vasculitis
    * Clotting screen for coagulopathies. Cross-match blood if there is massive blood loss
    * LFTs may be deranged in metastatic lung cancer or liver failure
    * Urea, creatinine, and electrolytes for assessment of renal function in suspected pulmonary-renal syndromes.
    * Corrected calcium may be raised in lung malignancy
    * Consider a D-dimer in suspected cases of PE
    * Autoantibody screen:
        – ANCA is positive in Wegner's granulomatosis (c-ANCA) and microscopic polyangitis (perinuclear anti-neutrophil cytoplasmic antibody (p-ANCA)) and usually negative in Polyarteritis Nodosa
        – Anti-glomerular basement membrane antibody (anti-GBM) is positive in Goodpasture's Syndrome
* **Urinalysis**. The presence of red cell casts will indicate glomerulonephritis of pulmonary-renal syndromes.

Questions commonly asked by examiners

Which population groups are at high risk of developing tuberculosis

* New migrants to the UK or travellers from endemic regions (sub-Saharan Africa, Asia, Eastern Europe)
* Low socioeconomic status—associated with crowded living conditions, homelessness, and poor healthcare.
* Immunocompromised individuals: HIV positive, patients on immunosuppressants and chemotherapy.
* Healthcare workers

How is suspected active pulmonary tuberculosis diagnosed?

When active pulmonary TB is suspected, the following investigations should be initiated:

* Plain chest radiograph may reveal features consistent with TB and should prompt further investigations for a definitive diagnosis.
* Sputum smear microscopy. Diagnosis is made on at least one out of three positive early morning sputum samples with either Ziehl-Nielsen staining or auramine flurorescence microscopy

for acid fast bacilli whilst waiting for culture results. Specificity is greater for spontaneously expectorated sputum than induced sputum or bronchial alveolar lavage specimens.

- Sputum culture for acid fast bacilli using solid culture medium (Lowenstein-Jensen) for growth and liquid media (BACTEC or MGIT) for rapid sensitivities. Molecular nucleic acid amplification tests are then undertaken to confirm the mycobacterium species.
- PCR techniques are employed to detect multiple drug resistant strains of M. *tuberculosis*. Detection of *rpo* gene suggests rifampicin resistance.

Treatment must be initiated *before* confirmation of TB by culture if there is a high clinical suspicion of TB, although treatment may be altered if drug resistance is found following culture.

How is active pulmonary TB treated and what monitoring is required for patients on anti-tuberculous treatment?

The standard six month regimen for the treatment of active TB consists of

- Isoniazid and rifampicin for six months
- Pyrizinamide and ethambutol for the first two months of therapy only

Treatment can be monitored on an outpatient basis and patients are admitted when the diagnosis is uncertain, there is suspicion of multi-drug resistant TB, or poor social circumstances may lead to poor compliance.* Patient isolation is necessary for smear-positive patients without risk of multi-drug resistant TB until two weeks of anti-tuberculous treatment is complete. Patients with high risk or confirmed multi-drug resistant TB should be nursed in a negative pressure room with barrier nursing techniques. Patients who do not have a productive cough, or are smear-negative on sputum microscopy, do not require isolation unless immunocompromised/HIV patients are on their ward or at home.

Monitoring of clinical and blood parameters are necessary before and during anti-tuberculous treatment to detect side-effects of treatment. All patients should have baseline and ongoing:

- Blood tests including FBC, renal, and LFTs (hepatotoxicity occurs with all the drugs, and nephrotoxicity and blood dyscrasias are seen with rifampicin).
- Visual acuity, colour vision, and fundoscopy (optic neuritis may occur with ethambutol treatment)
- Assessment of peripheral nervous system for neuropathy (peripheral neuropathy is a side effect of isoniazid which is reduced with concurrent use of pyridoxine).

Remember to advise the patient that if they develop jaundice, altered vision or parasthesiae, to stop their medication and seek medical attention immediately. Also advise them that rifampicin will make their urine and eye secretions turn red, hence they should avoid contact lenses. They should also use barrier contraception. Finally, explain that rifampicin has the potential to interact with other drugs (enzyme-inducer), and they should check the suitability of any new drugs with their docor or pharmacist.

What is the management of known TB contacts?

- Contacts who have had a BCG vaccination are investigated with:
  - ♦ Mantoux test if under 35 years of age. Chemoprophylaxis is commenced in those with a positive Mantoux *and* IFN-γ test** (if available) *and* normal clinical examination/chest X-ray.
  - ♦ Chest X-ray if over 35 years.

---

* Directly observed therapy can be initiated to improve treatment adherence in patient groups in whom compliance is an issue (alcoholics, homeless, drug abusers).

** IFN-γ tests measure the release of IFN-γ by T lymphocytes following exposure to mycobacterial antigens, since high levels suggest recent exposure or active infection by TB. These tests may be more sensitive than tuberculin skin testing for screening or predicting active TB infection in immunosuppressed patients (e.g. patients with renal failure).

- Contacts who have not have had BCG vaccination are investigated with a Mantoux test.
  - A positive Mantoux test *and* IFN-γ test (if available) *and* normal clinical examination/ chest X-ray requires chemoprophylaxis.
  - BCG vaccination is given in Mantoux negative contacts if under 35 years of age.

Abnormal chest X-ray appearances warrant further investigation to exclude active TB in all cases.

Who is offered BCG vaccination?

BCG vaccination is no longer recommended as part of the childhood vaccination programme at age 10–14 years. Criteria for vaccination are:

- Healthcare workers who are Mantoux negative
- Contacts of TB aged under 35 years who are Mantoux negative
- New UK entrants from high endemic areas
- Neonates born in high incidence areas of the UK with a family history of TB
- Children aged 1 month–16 years at high risk *and* Mantoux negative

Further reading

1. National Institute for Health and Clinical Excellence. Tuberculosis. Clinical diagnosis and management of tuberculosis, and measures for its prevention and control (NICE guidance). London: NICE; March 2006.

Case 16 ◆ Fever in the Returning Traveller

INFORMATION FOR THE CANDIDATE

Dear Doctor,

Thank you for seeing this 21-year old gentleman who has recently returned from a six week expedition in Kenya and Tanzania. He has had fever and rigors for the last two weeks, and I am concerned he has malaria. There is no significant past medical history of note. Please could you see and advise.

Many thanks for your opinion.

Acquiring the history

A. History of presenting complaint:

- Symptoms should initially be evaluated as if the patient had not travelled. Patients can acquire routine infections during travel, or may have been unwell prior to departure. Ask about:
  - **Cardiovascular**: palpitations, chest pain, dyspnoea
  - **Respiratory**: dyspnoea, cough, purulent sputum, pleuritic pain
  - **Ear nose and throat:** earache, headache, facial pain, sore throat
  - **Abdominal:** abdominal pain, nausea, vomiting, diarrhoea, constipation, haematochezia, urinary symptoms, jaundice
  - **Neurological:** headache, neck stiffness, photophobia, rash, weakness, altered conscious level

- ◆ **Dermatological:** rash, oral ulceration, alopecia, nail fold infarcts
- ◆ **Genitourinary:** genital ulceration, genital discharge, rash, urinary symptoms
- ◆ **Musculoskeletal:** joint pain, joint swelling, joint stiffness
- The timing and onset of symptoms is vital in the returning traveller, to establish the possible incubation period of an infectious illness (see the first question below). Carefully document the following points:
- Symptoms **preceding** travel
- Time, onset, and geographical location of symptoms occurring **during** travel
- Time and onset of symptoms occurring **after** return from travel

B. Travel history:

Illnesses such as malaria, dengue fever, or rickettsial infections, occur in focal geographical distributions. Therefore a clear geographical history, as well as modes of transportation and journey routes, is essential to establish the risk of infectious illness. The risk of viral haemorrhagic fevers is influenced by staying in rural areas, the presence of rodents, or sleeping in rural dwellings without concrete floors. Ask about:

- Dates of travel
- Duration of stay in each geographical location
- Nature of area—urban or rural
- Nature of accommodation—camping, rural dwelling, guesthouse, hotel
- Means of transportation

C. Activities and exposures during travel

Sexual contact with new partners is common during travel, and may cause blood-borne virus infection, or other sexually transmitted diseases. Exposure to animals, freshwater, or soil may be a route of acquisition of parasitic or helminthic infection. Ask carefully about:

- Sexual contacts—type of encounter (heterosexual, homosexual), number of partners, barrier protection
- Animal contact—exposure to birds, rodents; shared living quarters with animals; activities such as hunting, skinning
- Insect exposure—bites from mosquitoes, flies, ticks
- Needle and blood exposure—shared needles, tattoos, piercings, dental or medical care abroad
- Food and drink—raw food, unpasteurized milk, tap water
- Soil or water contact—freshwater lakes, watersports, areas of flooding, digging or excavation

D. Relevant medical and family history:

- Ask about conditions which predispose to immunosuppression, such as HIV *"Have you ever had a HIV test? what was the result?"*.
- Specifically ask about relevant surgery, such as previous splenectomy.

E. Medications, vaccines, and chemoprophylaxis:

- Ask about medications which are immunosuppressive, such as corticosteroids.
- Ask about over-the-counter medications and antipyretic use.
- Vaccination history must be documented, since it influences the risk of certain infectious diseases. Ask specifically about:
  - ◆ Typhoid
  - ◆ Hepatitis A
  - ◆ Hepatitis B
  - ◆ Tetanus and diphtheria

- ◆ Meningococcus—subtypes A, C, Y, W-135
- ◆ Influenza
- ◆ Yellow fever
- ◆ Polio (for travellers to Africa and Asia)
- • Ask specifically about malaria prophylaxis:
  - ◆ Drug regimen of malaria prophylaxis
  - ◆ Compliance with malaria prophylaxis
  - ◆ Duration before and after travel that malaria prophylaxis was continued for (ideally two weeks before travel, and four weeks after, depending on regimen).

Formulating a plan of action

- • Explain that a diagnosis will require blood tests, and possibly further investigations such as a HIV test or imaging. Although treatable infectious conditions are possible, the majority of travellers with a fever have a non-specific, self-limiting febrile illness.
- • Explain that if the patient has spent any time in a malarious region, then three separate thick and thin blood films will be required to exclude malaria, even if they have taken chemoprophylaxis.
- • Suggest an initial workup of FBC, liver enzymes, blood cultures, three thick and thin blood films for malaria, and a chest radiograph. Also suggest a stool culture and microscopy if the patient has diarrhoea.
- • Specific investigations for malaria include: FBC ($\downarrow$ Hb, platelets), clotting (DIC), glucose (hypoglycaemia), Ure (renal failure), urinalysis (haemoglobinria causing blackwates fever"). ABG (acidosis) and lactate.
- • Ensure the patient understands travel precautions for his next trip, including visiting a travel clinic prior to travel, food and water precautions, insect avoidance, safe sexual practice, and malaria chemoprophylaxis.
- • Consider early notification to the Health Protection Agency if a serious transmissible disease is possible (see the first question below).

Questions commonly asked by examiners

Which diseases manifest soon after exposure, and which may occur months after travel?

The differential diagnosis of fever in the returning traveller can be stratified by the interval between exposure, and onset of symptoms.

Short incubation (less than 10 days)

- • Dengue fever
- • Influenza
- • Typhoid*
- • Legionnaire's disease*
- • Acute HIV seroconversion
- • Meningococcal infections*
- • Rickettsial infections*

Medium incubation (less than 1 month)

- • Amoebic liver abscess
- • CMV
- • Hepatitis A

- Schistosomiasis
- Toxoplasmosis

Long incubation (greater than 3 months)
- Brucellosis
- Bartonellosis
- Histoplasmosis
- Lyme disease
- Malaria*
- Tuberculosis*
- Syphilis

Which clinical signs require urgent attention?

Haemorrhagic manifestations, respiratory distress, haemodynamic instability, or features of neurological infection such as neck stiffness, photophobia, altered conscious level or focal neurological deficit, require urgent medical intervention.

What is the presentation of typhoid fever, and how has the management changed over recent years?

Salmonella typhi, and *Salmonella paratyphi*, are the causes of typhoid and paratyphoid fever respectively. They occur when sanitation is poor, or drinking water is contaminated.

The incubation period is short. The onset is characterized by fever and dry cough, rather than constipation or other gastrointestinal symptoms. Later symptoms, after 7–10 days, include diarrhoea, rash, or complications such as intestinal bleeding and perforation.

The diagnosis is usually made from blood cultures, with a yield of greater than 60% within 24 hours. Stool cultures may represent asymptomatic carriage rather than infection. Emerging quinolone resistance has been the major change in therapy over recent years. The first line treatment is now a 3rd generation cephalosporin.

What is the management of severe falciparum malaria?

Plasmodium falciparum is increasingly resistant to chloroquine in endemic areas. Therefore, artemisinin derivatives or quinine are the preferred first line treatments. The WHO recommend artemisinin derivatives (artesunate, artemether, artemotil) for uncomplicated as severe falciparum malaria.)

Cerebral malaria, pulmonary oedema, acute renal failure, severe intravascular haemolysis, or haemoglobinuria are features of severe malaria. Any of these features, or a parasite count greater than 3% of all red cells, or the presence of schizonts on a blood film, must be treated with intravenous quinine. Other aspects of management include maintenance of blood glucose levels, correction of anaemia by transfusion, and avoidance of convulsions with prophylactic anticonvulsants. Pulmonary oedema may require positive-pressure ventilation. Acute renal failure normally responds to conservative treatment.

What are the Rickettsial illnesses, and how do they present?

Rickettsial illnesses are tick- or lice-borne infections causing systemic diseases in humans. The most common is Rocky Mountain spotted fever, which is endemic in the Rocky Mountains, and the east coast of the USA.

All these illnesses have a short incubation period. The onset is characterized by fever and frontal headache. The pathology is of an endovascultitis, which causes a rash and bleeding diathesis.

---

* Statutory notifiable diseases (The Public Health (Infectious Diseases) Regulations 1988)

Whilst the rash is non-specific, with maculopapular and petechial features, patients may have an eschar from a preceding tick bite.

The diagnosis is by serological tests, most commonly an IgM immunoassay. The treatment of choice is doxycycline, for up to 14 days.

Why are the viral haemorrhagic fevers important?

Viral haemorrhagic fevers (VHFs) are a group of viral infections, in which severe haemorrhage is a clinical feature. These include dengue fever, yellow fever, Lassa fever, Marburg disease, and Ebola virus.

These infections cause a severe systemic disease, with fever, sore throat, headache, arthralgia, and progressive multi-organ dysfunction. Specific features such as rash, diarrhoea, or renal failure may occur. Haemorrhage is usually due to platelet deficiency or dysfunction, and disseminated intravascular coagulation.

Lassa fever, Marburg disease, and Ebola virus have a significant mortality, and are highly transmissible through body fluids. Therefore, any clinical suspicion should prompt contact with the local Health Protection Agency, and transfer to an infectious diseases unit with isolation facilities.

Further Reading

1. Guidelines for the treatment of malaria. Geneva: World Health Organization, 2006.

Case 17 ◆ Sexually Transmitted Infection

INFORMATION FOR THE CANDIDATE

Dear Doctor,

Thank you for seeing this 32-year old gentleman who presents with a few days history of penile discharge and dysuria. He has a regular partner of many years. He has recently returned from a business trip to Europe, and is concerned that he may have contracted a sexually transmitted infection.

Many thanks for your opinion.

Acquiring the history

The fundamental components of the diagnosis of sexually transmitted infection (STI) are history taking (sexual and general medical history), examination, and investigations. Taking a sexual history requires excellent communication skills to establish rapport and create a safe environment for the patient to be honest and open with the interviewer. The generic skills of empathy and appropriate non-verbal communication are paramount, as are emphasizing confidentiality, signposting, and gaining consent to proceed with the interview, and using gender-neutral language (e.g. 'partner') to avoid appearing judgemental. Asymptomatic patients may also present with a request for STI screening, and in this case a thorough history is important for risk assessment and appropriate investigations.

A. History of presenting complaint:

Sexually transmitted infections present differently in men and women. Following the history of the presenting complaint, the remainder of the history is common to both genders.

Male symptoms

- **Penile discharge**. *'Have you noticed a discharge from the penis? Is it worse in the morning?'* Penile discharge is always pathological and an STI is the likely cause. Ask about duration, amount, frequency, and colour. Often the discharge is more noticeable after holding urine and a thick, green discharge is indicative of gonorrhoea.
- **Dysuria.** *'Do you have pain when you pass urine?'* Dysuria is a common symptom accompanying urethral discharge and is indicative of an STI.
- **Scrotal swelling and pain.** Ask about sudden onset of testicular pain, swelling, tenderness, and associated fever and vomiting to exclude testicular torsion. Epididymo-orchitis is a complication of chlamydial and gonococcal infection.
- **Abdominal and/or pelvic pain** can be caused by prostatitis. Ask about associated symptoms such as urinary frequency, hesitancy, dribbling, and occasionally acute urinary retention.
- **Anal symptoms.** Ask about rectal bleeding, anal discharge, painful defecation, and tenesmus. These may be caused by STIs acquired during receptive anal intercourse, such as gonorrhoea or lymphogranuloma venereum (caused by *Chlamydia trachomatis*). Other anorectal conditions such as anal fissures, haemorrhoids, and pruritis ani are also associated with anal intercourse.
- **Ulcers.** *'Have you noticed any ulcers, blisters or sores on the penis, anal region or elsewhere for example the mouth, or fingers?'; 'Are they painful?'*
- **Rashes and warts.** *'Have you noticed a rash in the genital area or elsewhere on the body?'; 'Is it red, raised or itchy?'*

Female symptoms

- **Vaginal discharge.** This is a common symptom in women, and therefore not pathognomonic of sexually transmitted infection. Ask about the following:
  - ◆ *Duration.* *'How long have you had the discharge?'*
  - ◆ *Amount and frequency.* *'How much discharge do you pass?'; 'Does the amount increase mid-cycle, after menstruation, or after sexual intercourse?'; 'Do you have the discharge all month?'; 'Do you have to wear sanitary protection?'* Clear discharge of variable amount during the menstrual cycle is physiological and not associated with other symptoms. Prolonged discharge suggests an alternative cause. Profuse discharge is associated with trichomoniasis and bacterial vaginosis. The latter is also associated with increased amount and frequency of discharge after menstruation and sexual intercourse.
  - ◆ *Colour and consistency.* A thick white discharge is typical of candidiasis, grey discharge suggests bacterial vaginosis, yellow or frothy discharge is distinctive of trichomoniasis, mucopurulent discharge occurs with chlamydia and gonococcal infections, and physiological discharge is clear.
  - ◆ *Odour.* *'Does the discharge have a foul smell?'* Bacterial vaginosis has a typically strong odour often described as 'fishy'.
  - ◆ *Blood.* *'Is the discharge blood stained?'* Bleeding can occur with infective and gynaecological causes.
- **Soreness.** *'Is the vaginal or vulval area sore?'* Genital soreness is highly suggestive of infection.
- **Dysuria.** *'Does it hurt when you pass urine?'* Dysuria is associated with infection with Chlamydia and gonorrhoea, and also urinary tract infections. Enquire about other urinary symptoms such as frequency and nocturia. Determine the site of dysuria (urethral versus vulval) by asking *'When you pass urine, does it hurt in the area where it comes out, or around the outside of your vagina?'* Chlamydia and gonorrhoea cause urethral dysuria whereas vulval dysuria (vulval soreness), suggests candidiasis or trichomoniasis.
- **Pruritis.** *'Does the vaginal or vulval area itch?'* Pruritis is usually associated with candidiasis.
- **Ulcers.** *'Have you noticed any sores or blisters in the genital region or elsewhere on your body such as mouth, fingers, buttocks?'* Establish if the ulcers are painful or painless to narrow

your differential diagnosis. Consider neoplasia in ulcers that are progressive over several months.

- **Rashes and warts.** *'Have you noticed a rash in the genital, anal, or other areas of the body?'*; *'Is it red, raised or painful?'*; *'Does it itch?'*

- **Gynaecological symptoms.** These symptoms can occur with both STIs and gynaecological conditions. Ask about:
  - *Abdominal and pelvic pain*—onset, duration, site, radiation, aggravating and relieving factors, associated symptoms, and severity.
  - *Dyspareunia*—*'Do you experience any pain during sexual intercourse?'*; *'Is it deep in your abdominal area or lower around the vaginal or vulval area?'*; Deep dyspareunia is associated with pelvic infection, pelvic inflammatory disease, or gynaecological causes such as endometriosis. Superficial dyspareunia is suggestive of infective causes or vaginal disease.
  - *Intermenstrual and/or postcoital bleeding*— *'Do you bleed in between periods or after sexual intercourse?'* Although gynaecological conditions must be excluded, these symptoms are frequenctly the result of *Chlamydia* and gonorrhoea.
  - Ask about last cervical smear test, any abnormal results and treatment.

- **Menstrual history.** Ask about last menstrual period, regularity of cycle, and menorrhagia.

- **Contraceptive history.** Ask specifically about contraceptive methods used, missed pills, and episodes of unprotected sexual intercourse.

Systemic symptoms

- Fever, malaise, night sweats (bacterial infection, Behcet's disease, lymphoma, HIV)
- Sore throat (can be caused by infections acquired through the practice of oral sex)
- Myalgia
- Arthralgia and arthritis (Behcet's disease, reactive arthritis)
- Conjunctivitis (Behcet's disease, reactive arthritis)
- Mouth ulcers (Behcet's disease)
- Jaundice (viral hepatitis)

Sexual history

Establish risk of STIs, in particular HIV by taking a detailed sexual history. Ask specifically about:

- **Last sexual contact.** *'When did you last have sex and/or sexual intercourse?'*
- **Gender.** *'Was this with a male or female partner?'*
- **Type of partner**. *'Was this with a regular, casual, or unknown partner?'*
- **Country of origin of partner.** *'Where is your partner from?'*
- **Type of sexual activity.** *'What type of sex did you have—vaginal, anal, oral, or other?'*
- **Use of condoms.** *'Did you use condoms throughout?'*; *'Were there any breaks or splits in the condom?'*
- **Number of partners in the last 3 months.** *'Have you had sex with anyone else apart from this partner in the last three months?'* Three months is the window period for most STIs. If the answer is yes, note the above details for each partner.
- **Sex industry.** *'Have you had sex with a sex worker?'*
- **Past history of STIs.** *'Have you had a sexually transmitted infection before?'*
- **Previous HIV tests.** *'Have you had a HIV test before?'*; *'When was your last test?'*
- **Previous hepatitis A/B vaccination.** *'Have you had vaccinations for hepatitis infection before?'*

B. Relevant medical and family history:

Obtain a thorough past medical and family history. In particular enquire about gynaecological conditions in women.

C. Medications and interactions:

- Ask the patient about any regular medications and allergies.
- Determine the use of any recreational drugs, in particular intravenous drug use.

D. Social issues:

- Ask about smoking habits and alcohol intake.
- Enquire about travel and sexual activity abroad.
- Ask about tattoos and where these were done.
- Does the patient donate blood? When did the patient last donate blood?
- Determine the patient's social setup. Does the patient have support from family and friends?
- Elicit the patient's concerns and expectations of their symptoms.

Formulating a plan of action

- Explain to the patient that sexually transmitted infections are a likely cause for the patient's symptoms and that a clinical examination followed by investigations are required to confirm the diagnosis and type of infection present.
- Discuss the investigations and inform the patient which results will be available today and when the remainder will be available.
- Explain the 'window period' for HIV tests. Explain that because seroconversion takes up to three months, a positive test today means that the infection was acquired more than 3 months ago. If the patient may have been exposed to infection in the last 3 months the test will need to be repeated at the correct time from exposure. Offer the patient pre-test counselling with a health advisor.
- Partner notification should be discussed with the patient once an STI is confirmed. Discuss possible approaches with the patient and provide contact slips that the patient can give to sexual contacts to attend the genitourinary clinic. This is a patient referral. In the event of the patient being unable to do this, offer a provider referral which involves the clinic contacting the sexual partners without disclosing that the patient has provided their details.
- Arrange a follow up appointment for results and if appropriate response to treatment.

Consider the following investigations

Specific investigations in men

- **Urine sample**
1. First catch sample for Chlamydia nucleic acid amplification test (NAAT)
2. Mid-stream urine sample for suspected urinary tract infections. Urinalysis will be positive for nitrites, leucocytes and blood.
- **Urethral swabs.** Microscopy for pus cells and polymorphs. Culture for gonorrhoea and NAAT for Chlamydia.
- **Rectal swabs** for microscopy and culture for gonorrhoea.
- **Throat swabs** for culture for gonorrhoea.

Specific investigations for women

- **Mid stream urine sample** for microscopy, culture, and sensitivities. Culture for gonorrhoea, Chlamydia NAAT. Consider a pregnancy test. Urinalysis may be positive for nitrites and leucocytes suggesting a urinary tract infection.
- **Vaginal swabs.** Vaginal wall swabs. Microscopy may reveal candida and clue cells (indicative of bacterial vaginosis). A wet film is obtained for Trichomonas Vaginalis. Swabs are also taken for pH and culture. A high pH >4.5, presence of clue cells, and a positive Whiff test are diagnostic of bacterial vaginosis.

- **Cervical swabs.** A high vaginal swab is taken for microscopy and culture for gonorrhoea. An endocervical swab is taken for Chlamydia NAAT. Consider a smear test for cytology in patients over 25 years.
- **Urethral swabs.** Taken for microscopy and culture for gonorrhoea and Chlamydia NAAT.
- **Throat swabs** for gonorrhoea.

Other tests

- **Skin samples.** Sample the base of ulcers and other skin lesions for herpes simplex viral culture or antigens, dark ground microscopy for primary or secondary syphilis.
- **Hepatitis screen:** hepatitis surface antigen, hepatitis core antibody, and anti hepatitis C virus (HCV) antibodies in high risk groups.
- **HIV test.** Rapid testing for HIV-1 and 2 antibodies, p24 antigen and PCR.
- **Syphilis serology.** Screening tests are EIA, FTA, and TPHA (see below).

Questions commonly asked by examiners

What are the causes of male urethral and female vaginal discharge?

Male	Female
Infective	**Physiological**
• Gonorrhoea	**Pathological**
• Chlamydia	**1. infective**
• Non-specific urethritis	• STI: Chlamydia, gonorrhoea
• Trachomoniasis	• Non STI: candidiasis, Bacterial vaginosis, Trachomoniasis
• Ureaplasma urealycitum infection	**2. Non-infective**
• Herpes simplex virus	• Ectropion
Non-infective	• Polyp
• Cystitis	• Atrophic vaginalis
• Prostatitis	• Carcinoma
• Reactive arthritis/Reiter's sydrome	

What are the causes of genital ulcers?

Painless	Painful
Solitary	**Multiple**
• Primary syphilis (chancre)	• Chancroid (*Hameophilus ducreyi*)
• Lymphogranuloma venereum (*Chalmydia trachomatis L1-3*)	• Herpes simplex infection
• Donovanosis (Granuloma inguinale, *Klebsiella*)	• Behcet's syndrome
• Carcinoma	• Balanitis (*Trichomonas, Candida*)
• Lichen sclerosis	• Lichen planus
Multiple	
• Secondary syphilis	

What is the natural history of syphilis and how is it diagnosed?

Syphilis is a sexually transmitted infection caused by the spirochete *Treponema pallidum*.

Syphilis infection can be classified into:

- Early infection: primary or secondary

- Latent infection: early latent (<2 years of infection) and late latent (>2 years post-infection)
- Tertiary

Primary syphilis is characterized by the appearance of a painless, genital ulcer called a chancre. The chancre appears 9–90 days after infection and heals spontaneously within 10 weeks.

Secondary syphilis is suggested by non specific systemic symptoms such as fever, malaise, and myalgia, followed by widespread maculopapular rash, other skin lesions such as condylomata lata in the anogential regions, hepatitis, arthritis, and generalized lymphadenopathy. Other features include iritis, meningitis, and nephritic syndrome, although these are rare. These symptoms may resolve spontaneously but recur without treatment.

Latent syphilis is not characterized by any symptoms and these patients progress to tertiary syphilis. Serology is positive.

Tertiary syphilis occurs 5–15 years post-infection and presents as gummatous disease (granulomatous skin, mucous membrane, and visceral lesions), neurosyphilis (meningitis, tabes dorsalis, taboparesis-), and cardiovascular syphilis (aortitis, aortic aneurysm, and aortic imcompetence).

Diagnosis is made by

1. Dark ground microscopy of samples from chancre, and other skin lesions
2. Serology. Serological tests for syphilis include:
   - *Specific tests*: *T pallidum* enzyme immunoassay (EIA), *T pallidum* haemagglutination (TPHA), and absorbed fluorescent treponemal antibody (FTA) tests. These are useful for screening for syphilis and confirming the diagnosis as they remain positive through-out life. EIA and FTA are the first to rise in primary syphilis infection. Titres rise three to four weeks after infection. TPHA begins to rise from four to eight weeks post-infection.
   - *Non-specific tests*: Venereal Disease Reference Laboratory (VDRL) and Rapid Plasmin Reagin (RPR) tests. These are raised in infection and are therefore only used to monitor response to treatment and diagnose reinfection. Note that false positive tests arise with a number of conditions such as measles, mumps, herpes viruses, rheumatoid arthritis, and autoimmune conditions.

Case 18 ◆ HIV Treatment

INFORMATION FOR THE CANDIDATE

Dear Doctor,

Thank you for seeing this HIV-positive 36-year old gay man who has recently started antiretroviral therapy. He has had a fever, rash, and abdominal pain for the last 3 days, and I am concerned he may have an HIV-related illness.

Many thanks for your help.

Acquiring the history

HIV infection and the use of highly active antiretroviral therapy (HAART) are increasingly prevalent, and HIV-related illness is a common reason for medical admission. Therefore, the ability to take an HIV-related history and a basic knowledge of HIV complications and HAART therapy are expected of the MRCP (PACES) candidate. The approach is similar to that employed in other sensitive cases, such as when acquiring the sexual history. The generic skills of empathy, signposting, non-verbal communication, and emphasizing confidentiality are essential. Gender-neutral language (e.g. 'partner') should also be used to avoid appearing judgemental. Whilst there are specific aspects of HIV disease that must be documented during this history, the importance of *open questioning* must not be overlooked. This is easily done in patients with chronic illnesses, such as HIV, where the 'disease-history' may lead the candidate to overlook the reason for presentation.

A. Presenting complaint:

Begin with open questioning to explore the patient's agenda for the visit, despite the referral letter stating the history of HIV. *'Your doctor has asked me to discuss your fevers and rash with you. Is there anything else you would like to talk about today?'.*

History of presenting complaint:

Fever and rash in HIV: Begin by evaluating symptoms as in a patient without HIV infection:

- **Cardiovascular**: palpitations, chest pain, dyspnoea
- **Respiratory**: dyspnoea, cough, purulent sputum, pleuritic pain
- **Ear nose and throat**: earache, headache, facial pain, sore throat
- **Abdominal**: abdominal pain, nausea, vomiting, diarrhoea, constipation, haematochezia, urinary symptoms
- **Neurological:** headache, neck stiffness, photophobia, weakness, altered conscious level
- **Dermatological:** characteristics of rash (see below) oral ulceration, alopecia, nail fold infarcts
- **Genitourinary:** genital ulceration, genital discharge, urinary symptoms
- **Musculoskeletal:** joint pain, joint swelling, joint stiffness

Also assess the timing and onset of the fever, along with diurnal variation—are they mainly night sweats?

Rashes are common in HIV, and may be due to bacterial, fungal, or viral infections, as well as drug reactions or malignancy. Ask about the following characteristics of the rash:

- site and distribution
- onset and duration
- itch or tenderness
- bleeding or discharge
- mucosal involvement—oral ulceration or diarrhoea. (Stevens-Johnson syndrome and Toxic Epidermal Necrolysis are more common in HIV infection)
- associated tongue swelling, lip swelling, or wheeze. (Urticaria is also more common in HIV.)

Background of HIV infection

Ask openly about the patients HIV infection; *'Tell me about your HIV—how have things being going?'.*

Follow this up with closed questioning to cover the background of their infection. Most patients are well educated about their disease, and will know their CD4 count, viral load, and drug regimens.

- HIV exposure history: date and place of diagnosis, route of exposure (if known). *'When were you diagnosed with HIV?'*; *'Do you know how you contracted it?'.*
- Most recent CD4 count and viral load. *'What was your most recent CD4 count and viral load?'*
- Nadir CD4 count and peak viral load. *'What is the lowest the CD4 count has been?'*; *'And the highest viral load?'.*
- Any drug resistance known about.
- Current and previous HAART therapy.

- Any previous opportunistic infections (OIs). *'Have you had any infections since contracting HIV?'*; *'Do you know if they were related to your HIV?'*.
- Any adverse reactions to HAART or drugs used for OI prophylaxis. *'Have you had any rashes or other reactions to the drugs you are taking?'*.
- Current HIV physician or unit.

Ask specifically about certain OIs:

- Any possibility of exposure to TB? Any TB contacts? Previous BCG? History of positive tuberculin skin test?
- Any history of hepatitis? Previous hepatitis B vaccination (requires at least 3 injections—confirm how many the patient has received)?

Sexual history

This does not need to be extensive if the patient does not have genitourinary symptoms, and taking an extensive sexual history in a gay HIV patient may risk him feeling 'stereotyped'. However, disseminated gonococcal infection acquired through sexual contact remains a differential diagnosis of fever and rash in HIV, therefore attempt to obtain the following as a minimum:

- Current sexual activity—gender of partner, number of partners in last 3 months, type of partner (regular, casual, sex-worker).
- Current sexual practices—vaginal, anal, oral, use of barrier contraception.
- Past history of STIs.

B. Relevant medical history and review of symptoms:

- Document all past hospitalizations and illnesses. Ask about OIs as stated above.
- Ask about blood transfusions and blood products, especially before 1985 (HIV testing introduced) or 1990 (hepatitis C testing introduced).
- Ask openly about mood and psychiatric symptoms. *'How has your mood been lately?'*; *'Do you feel low within yourself on most days?'* (see Case 40 Deliberate Self Harm). Attempt to cover the following areas:
    - depression
    - anxiety
    - past or current psychiatric treatment
    - past psychiatric admission
- Consider the following symptoms during systems review:
    - **Constitutional:** weight loss, loss of appetite, lymph node enlargement
    - **Eyes:** change in vision (including blurring, diplopia, or loss of vision)
    - **Head, ears, nose, throat:** headache, dysphagia, odynophagia, hearing loss, dental pain, oral ulcers
    - **Respiratory:** breathlessness, cough, haemoptysis
    - **Cardiovascular:** chest pain
    - **Abdominal:** nausea, vomiting, diarrhoea, perianal symptoms (pain, itch, rash)
    - **Gynaecological:** menstrual history, cervical smear history, intermenstrual bleeding.
    - **Musculoskeletal:** muscle wasting, muscle weakness, joint swelling
    - **Neurological:** difficulty in concentration, parasthesiae, or numbness

C. Medications and interactions:

- Document all current prescription and non-prescription medicines. Many complementary and alternative medicines have cytochrome p450 enzyme inducing or inhibiting effects (e.g. Echinacea is theoretically an enzyme inhibitor and may increase HAART drug levels).

- Ask about vaccination history. Aside from routine childhood immunizations, hepatitis A, hepatitis B, and pneumococcal vaccines are recommended for HIV-infected persons. These should be given early in the disease course to maximize efficacy. Live vaccines should be avoided if the CD4 count is less than 200/mm^3

D. Substance use history

- Ask about current and previous use of drugs. *'What about drugs—have you ever injected?'*; *'What about other drugs, like cocaine, marijuana, ecstasy, or amphetamines?'*; *'Do you use prescription drugs like benzodiazepines?'*.
- *'How often are you using these drugs?'*; *'How much are you spending a day/week?'*
- *'Are you sharing needles with anyone?'*
- *'How are you managing to pay for the drugs?'*; *'Are you exchanging sex for drugs?'*
- *'Have you ever had treatment for a drug or alcohol habit?'*; *'How did that go—have you used since?'*

E. Social issues:

- Enquire about cigarette smoking and lifestyle. Ischaemic heart disease is a major complication of HIV infection (see below).
- Also ask about current alcohol intake—liver disease is also more common in patients with HIV, especially those with hepatitis C co-infection.
- Ask about occupation, and how the patient is supporting himself financially. Ensure the patient has adequate housing.
- Travel history and place of birth (see Case 16 Fever in the Returning Traveller>
- Enquire about family and partners. Does the patient's partner know about their infection? (see Station 4, Confidentiality and Information Sharing section). Enquire about the stability of personal relationships (domestic violence screening), *'I can see things have been stressful for you lately—how are things between you and your partner?'*.
- Does the patient have children or dependents? If so, how are they being supported? If the patient is a female of child-bearing age, ask about family planning and plans for future pregnancies.
- End of life issues may be considered if the patient has advanced disease. Ask sensitively whether the patient has considered a living will, or arrangements for dependent children.

Formulating a plan of action

- Ensure that you have addressed the patient's own concerns about their symptoms and their HIV, *'What do you think is causing these symptoms?'*; *'Is there anything that we haven't discussed that you are worried about?'*.
- Explain that a full examination and blood tests will be necessary to determine the diagnosis.
- If appropriate, congratulate the patient on their compliance with HAART therapy and OI prophylaxis, and use the opportunity to re-emphasize the importance of compliance in HIV.
- Also emphasize the importance of attending a healthcare practitioner with even trivial symptoms, because of the potential for drug interactions between HAART and over-the-counter remedies.

Questions commonly asked by examiners

Which OIs and HIV-related tumours should be considered at different stages of HIV infection?

- **CD4 count 200–350 cells/mm^3**
  - Pulmonary tuberculosis
  - Pneumococcal pneumonia
  - Oral/vaginal candidiasis

- ◆ Oral hairy leukoplakia
- ◆ Cervical intraepithelial neoplasia II–III
- ◆ Kaposi's sarcoma
- **CD4 count <200 cells/mm³**
  - ◆ Oesophageal candidiasis
  - ◆ Mucocutaneous herpes simplex
  - ◆ Cryptosporidium diarrhoea
  - ◆ Disseminated/miliary tuberculosis
  - ◆ *Pneumocystis jirovecii* pneumonia (formerly *Pneumocystis carinii*)
- **CD4 count <100 cells/mm³**
  - ◆ Atypical *Mycobacterium* infection (e.g. *Mycobacterim avium intracellulare*)
  - ◆ Progressive multifocal leucoencephalopathy
  - ◆ Cerebral toxoplasmosis
  - ◆ Non-Hodgkin's lymphoma
  - ◆ Primary CNS lymphoma
  - ◆ Cryptococcal meningitis
  - ◆ CMV retinitis or colitis
  - ◆ HIV-associated dementia

What do you know of prophylaxis for OIs?

Chemoprophylaxis is prescribed for the following conditions:

- *Pneumocystis jirovecii* pneumonia—trimethoprim-sulphamethoxazole (1 double-strength tablet daily), if CD4 count <200 cells/mm³ or past history of *Pneumocystis jirovecii* pneumonia. Side effects include fever, rash, and bone narrow suppression. Alternatives for patients with side effects are dapsone or nebulized pentamidine. Nebulized pentamidine is also recommended for pregnant women during the first trimester.
- *Toxoplasmosis*—trimethoprim-sulphamethoxazole (1 double-strength tablet daily), if CD4 count <100 cells/mm³ and toxoplasma seropositive, or eye involvement regardless of CD4 count. An alternative for patients with side effects is dapsore-pyrimethamine with folic acid.
- *Mycobacterium avium complex*—azithromycin (120mg weekly), if CD4 count <50 cells/mm³.
- *Cytomegalovirus* consider ganciclovir for patients with a CD4 count below 50 cells/mm³ and seropositivity. Seronegative patients should be advised to recevie CMV-negative blood products.

Which drug reactions can cause fever and rash in HIV?

Abacavir may cause a hypersensitivity syndrome, predicted by HLA genotype 570*1 in Caucasians. This reaction usually occurs within 6 weeks of starting the drug, but may occur anytime and may be fatal. The symptoms are skin rash with two of the following: fever, diarrhoea, nausea, vomiting, abdominal pain, breathlessness, or malaise. If a reaction to abacavir is suspected, the drug should be stopped immediately, and alternative antiretroviral therapy commenced by a HIV physician.

Efavirenz may also cause fever, rash, and liver toxicity.

Can you think of any other differential diagnoses for fever and rash in HIV?

- Bacterial infection
  - ◆ *Staphylococcus aureus* may affect intravenous drug users, patients with recent venous catheters or may cause secondary infection of ulcerated or oedematous skin (e.g. due to Kaposi's sarcoma). The associated rashes are impetigo, folliculitis, cellulitis, or abscesses. Disseminated staphylococcal infection may also cause endocarditis, osteomyelitis, or hepatosplenic abscesses.

- ◆ *Neisseria gonorrhoea* infection in HIV is related more to sexual behaviour than immunosuppression. Disseminated gonococcal infection may cause fever, rash, tenosynovitis, and migratory polyarthralgia. The rash is typically painless and pustular over the back and trunk, but may also involve the palms and soles. Rarely, the infection can disseminate to other organs causing pericarditis, endocarditis, and meningitis.
- ◆ Secondary syphilis in HIV usually presents in a similar manner as in immunocompetent individuals—typically with rash, lymphadenopathy and fever (see Case 17 Sexually Transmitted Infection).

- Viral infection
  - ◆ Acute HIV infection may cause an infectious mononucleosis-type syndrome with a maculopapular rash, sore throat, arthralgia, diarrhoea, and aseptic meningitis.
  - ◆ Varicella zoster virus infection may reactivate in HIV, causing a shingles.
  - ◆ Parvovirus can cause fever, arthritis, and a reticular rash on the trunk. Parvovirus may also affect immunocompetent individuals, but infection is more likely to be chronic in HIV.
  - ◆ Hepatitis B infection may be acquired at the same time as HIV due to shared modes of transmission, and acute infection may cause fever, rash, arthralgia, and arthritis as well as hepatitis.

- Fungal infection. Systemic fungal infection is an important differential for fever and rash in any immunocompromised patient. The list of candidate organisms is long, therefore histopathological and microbiological specimens are essential for diagnosis. For example, *Cryptococcus neoformans* may cause meningitis and pneumonia in HIV, although 10% of patients also have cutaneous lesions.

Aside from OIs, which medical conditions are exacerbated by HIV infection?

Cardiovascular disease

With the advent of effective anti-retroviral therapy for HIV, the incidence of cardiovascular disease is increasing as patients are living longer.[1] This is thought to be due to a pro-atherogenic effect of the virus, as well as dyslipidaemia induced by HAART. The dyslipidaemia may be an isolated finding, or part of the HIV-associated lipodystrophy syndrome of fat redistribution, insulin resistance, and hyperlipidaemia. Protease inhibitors (PIs) in particular are associated with dyslipidaemia and lipodystrophy.

The treatment of these metabolic abnormalities is difficult in patients taking PIs, although the endpoints for therapy are the same as in non-HIV patients. After initial dietary modification, and possibly altering HAART therapy to minimize dyslipidaemia, statin therapy may be indicated. However, statins are metabolized by cytochrome p450 3A4 (CYP3A4), and PIs decrease the activity of CYP3A4, thus potentially causin statin toxicity if they are co-administered. Low dose Atorvastatin may be used in this case, since it is only partially metabolized by CYP3A4.

Renal disease

HIV-associated renal disease is also rising due to the success of HAART. Afro-Caribbeans are are at greatest risk. The major causes are HIV-associated nephropathy, interstitial nephritis due to the drugs used for OI prophylaxis, and direct toxicity of anti-retrovirals (e.g. Tenofovir—acute renal injury, Fanconi syndrome, nephrogenic DI; Indinavir—crystalluria, renal calculi).

Liver disease

Liver disease is also a major cause of death in HIV. This is mainly due to HIV and hepatitis C co-infection. Co-infection is associated with increased HCV RNA levels, increased hepatic inflammation and fibrosis, and more rapid progression to end-stage liver disease. This is compounded by reduced HCV treatment response rates among HCV/HIV co-infected persons.

Moreover, antiretroviral therapy is often associated with a paradoxical increase in HCV RNA levels, as well as hepatotoxicity.

References

1. Use of nucleoside reverse transcriptase inhibitors and risk of myocardial infarction in HIV-infected patients enrolled in the D:A:D study: a multi-cohort collaboration. D:A:D Study Group. Lancet 2008; 26(9622):1417–26.

Case 19 ◆ **Diabetes Mellitus**

INFORMATION FOR THE CANDIDATE

Dear Doctor,

Thank you for seeing this 55-year old lady who has been diabetic for many years. She has been on insulin for the last 16 years, but has a persistently elevated HbA1c and also suffers with recurrent hypoglycaemic attacks. She has had an ulcer on her right leg for 18 months, and is also registered blind. She takes bendroflumethiazide 2.5mg daily and simvastatin 20mg daily for blood pressure and lipid control.

Many thanks for your opinion.

Acquiring the history

Diabetes mellitus is a condition that lends itself to a structured history, focused on a variety of risk factors and complications that must be assessed prior to agreeing a management plan. However, the importance of *open questioning* must not be overlooked, especially in circumstances where the past medical history of the patient is known and may influence the interviewing technique of the physician.

A. Presenting complaint:

Begin with open questioning to explore the patient's agenda for the visit, despite the referral letter requesting a review of diabetes management. *'Your doctor has asked me to discuss your diabetes treatment with you, but is there anything else you would like to talk about today?'* This strategy is useful for all *follow-up* clinical encounters in a specialist clinic.

History of presenting complaint: Background of diabetes

- *Type and estimated duration of diabetes?* The distinction between type 1 and type 2 diabetes is important for management and monitoring of complications. Typically, patients with type 2 diabetes may be older, have an elevated BMI and may have been treated with diet-control or oral agents prior to insulin. Distinguishing the type of diabetes may be difficult in young patients with an elevated BMI treated with insulin (these patients may have genetic defects causing diabetes—see below), and in older patients with late-onset diabetes who require insulin (these patients may have latent autoimmune disease of the adult, LADA—see below).
- *Control of diabetes mellitus?*
  - ◆ Current symptoms of hypergylcaemia: polyuria, polydipsia, nocturia, weight loss, blurred vision, recurrent cutaneous sepsis, utis balanitis, pruritus vulvae.

- Recent diabetic control: ask about home glucose monitoring. Patients may provide a record of capillary glucose measurements, or ask directly about the range of readings. For correct interpretation of these values, the time and relation to meals of each reading must be known. Enquire about last HbA1c reading, and if the patient knows their target (ideally <6.5%) for adequate control (assessing the level of the patient's understanding of their condition).

- Record admissions with DKA or HONK. Previous DKA was thought to be pathognomic for type 1 diabetes, however it is becoming increasingly recognized that DKA can occur in type 2 diabetes (ketosis-prone type 2 diabetes mellitus), typically in obese Afro-Caribbean patients. Treatment is as for type 1 patients with ketoacidosis.

- Current treatment of diabetes mellitus:
    - Insulin? Clarify type of insulin, regimen and dosing in relation to meals (see below). Ask which injection sites are used, and about any associated skin problems. Document duration of insulin treatment. Clarify method of dose adjustment and compliance. Some patients with type 1 diabetes in the UK may be enrolled in the Dose Adjustment for Normal Eating programme (DAFNE), which educates individuals to adjust their insulin dose by carbohydrate intake and lifestyle.[1] This programme has been associated with better glycaemic control and quality of life.
    - Oral hypoglycaemic agents? Clarify dose and frequency, and ask about duration of therapy with each agent and previous agents. Enquire about specific side effects with each drug (see below).
    - Ask about previous dietetic consults and compliance with dietetic advice.
    - Ask about participation and compliance with a structured exercise regime.

- Hypoglycaemia: Does the patient have episodes of hypogylcaemia? How often do these occur? What is the reason for these episodes? Does the patient have hypoglycaemia unawareness (i.e. does the patient lack the adrenergic warning signs of hypoglycaemia)? Does the patient require assistance for the treatment of these episodes?

History of presenting complaint: Complications of diabetes mellitus

- Macrovascular Disease
    - **Coronary artery disease**: chest pain, breathlessness, orthopnoea, paroxysmal nocturnal dyspnoea, ankle oedema, previous percutaneous coronary intervention (PCI) or CABG?
    - **Peripheral vascular disease**: cold extremities, claudication, previous vascular bypass surgery?
    - **Cerebrovascular disease**: visual disturbances, neurological deficit, previous transient ischaemic attack (TIA), or stroke?
- Microvascular Disease
    - **Retinal disease**: any recent visual symptoms or deterioration in vision? Results of last eye and retinal examinations? Any previous retinal treatment?
    - **Renal disease:** any history of renal disease? Results of last urine protein and serum creatinine?
    - **Neuropathy:** ask about known neuropathy and symptoms of neuropathy, 'Do you have problems with the feeling in your arms or legs?'; 'Does it ever feel as if you are walking on cotton wool?'.
    - **Autonomic neuropathy:** ask sensitively about marital problems and erectile dysfunction, 'Is your health affecting your marriage in any way?'; 'Have you had any problems with your erection during sex?'

- ◆ **Foot disease:** any known foot ulcers or lesions? Ask about foot care, *'Do you walk barefoot or wear slippers around the house?'*; *'Do you see a chiropodist regularly?'*; *'Do your shoes fit properly?'*.
- **Hypertension**: defined as >130/80mmHg in patients with diabetes. Ask about therapy and compliance.
- **Hyperlipidaemia**: ask about most recent lipid levels, therapy, and compliance. Target is total cholesterol <4.0mmol/L.

(See Volume 1, Case 8 Nephrotic Syndrome and Case 146 Diabetic Retinopathy and Volume 2, Case 1 Hypertension.)

B. Relevant medical and family history:

- Ask about conditions which predispose to diabetes:
  - ◆ Previous gestational diabetes or recurrent stillbirth (see below).
  - ◆ Family history of early-onset diabetes: genetic defects of beta cell function (e.g. hepatic nuclear factor genes, glucokinase gene) account for 2–5% of patients under 25 with type 2 diabetes. Inheritance is autosomal dominant.
  - ◆ Pancreatic disease: chronic pancreatitis, cystic fibrosis, and hereditary haemochromatosis.
  - ◆ Endocrine disease: Cushing's syndrome, acromegaly, phaechromocytoma (cat-echolamine excess causing hyperglycaemia), rare glucagons-secreting tumours.
  - ◆ History of organ transplantation: tacrolimus may cause post-transplant diabetes

C. Medications and interactions:

- Look for drugs which can cause hyperglycaemia:
  - ◆ glucocorticoids
  - ◆ oral contraceptives
  - ◆ thiazide diuretics
  - ◆ atypical antipsychotics
  - ◆ tacrolimus
  - ◆ HIV protease inhibitors
- Beta blockers have traditionally been avoided in diabetes mellitus, due to the theoretical risk of impairing adrenergic hypoglycaemia awareness. The GEMINI trial[2] showed that the use of carvedilol as a second-line anti-hypertensive was safe and decreased progression to microal-buminuria. However, metoprolol has been associated with a worsening of glycaemic control[2,3].

D. Social issues:

- Enquire about cigarette smoking and lifestyle as major contributors to CHD and other vascular complications. Ensure a thorough dietetic history has already been documented.
- Ask about occupation, and how the patient is supporting himself financially.
- Ask about disability and activities of daily living. In particular, ask about visual impairment, mobility, and ability to administer subcutaneous insulin.
- If the patient drives, ensure they have informed the DVLA of their diagnosis.
- Assess occupational risk, in particular commercial driving, use of heavy machinery, and hypoglycaemia awareness.
- If female of child-bearing age, ask about family planning and plans for future pregnancies.
- Enquire openly about mood—depression is more common in diabetic patients, particularly the elderly.

Formulating a plan of action

- Explain the importance of control of diabetes mellitus to prevent complications. Emphasize the benefits of patient education and self-monitoring in addition to regular reviews and annual screening programmes to prevent complications.

- Emphasize the role of diet and lifestyle modification, and negotiate goals for dietary modification and weight loss.
- Offer counselling to support smoking cessation.
- If the patient already monitors their capillary glucose at home, reinforce the purpose of this, and ensure the patient correctly inteprets and acts upon readings. If the patient does not monitor their diabetes, it is unlikely you will be expected to outline the process. This should be done as part of a structured education process.
- If the patient is on insulin, ensure the patient understands dose titration, management of hypoglycaemia, and has access to telephone support from their local diabetic service.
- Outline the plan of regular monitoring of blood pressure, lipids, and renal function, and annual retinal photography.
- Emphasize the need for proper footcare, including avoidance of injuries and walking barefoot, care when cutting nails, daily washing, and self-examination and correctly fitted footwear.
- Tell the patient that a follow-up appointment will be given to discuss the changes to management and the results of tests.

Questions commonly asked by examiners

How would you approach the management of a patient with type 2 diabetes mellitus?

What are the benefits of tight glycaemic control in diabetes mellitus?

In type 1 diabetes, the *Diabetes Control and Complications trial (DCCT)*[5] randomized 1441 patients to standard treatment or 'intensive control' (HbA1c 8.9% versus 7.4%). After treatment for a mean 6.5 years, patients were found to have a significantly decreased incidence of eye disease, renal disease, and neuropathy, and a non-significant reduction in macrovascular disease. The subsequent *Epidemiology of Diabetes Interventions and Complications trial (EDIC)*[6] found a significant reduction in cardiovascular disease in patients from the DCCT trial who had been offered intensive treatment.

In type 2 diabetes, the *UK Prospective Diabetes Study (UKPDS)*[7] confirmed a similar benefit of intensive glucose control (HbA1c 7.9% versus 7.0%) on microvascular disease, reducing the incidence by 25% over 10 years. However, there was no improvement in macrovascular disease. Indeed, unlike type 1 diabetes, subsequent studies (ACCORD, ADVANCE) have not found an improvement in macrovascular disease with tight glycaemic control, and the ACCORD study found excess mortality from cardiovascular disease and other causes in patients receiving intensive treatment (HbA1c <6%).

In summary, a HbA1c of 6.5–7.5% is appropriate for most patients due to the benefits in preventing microvascular complications of diabetes mellitus, although less stringent control may be appropriate for patients with recurrent hypoglycaemia or significant co-morbidity.

What are the major contraindications and adverse effects of metformin?

Metformin is contraindicated in patients with a serum creatinine >150μmol/L due to a theoretical risk of lactic acidosis; and should be used with caution in any patient with impaired renal function. Gastrointestinal side-effects, such as bloating and diarrhoea, affect one-third of patients on metformin. Strategies to minimize these are gradual escalation of dose and trial of extended-absorption preparations.

What are the major contraindications and adverse effects of thiazolidinediones?

Significant oedema affects 5% of patients, and up to 15% of patients also on insulin and sulphonylureas. For this reason, moderate/severe heart failure (NYHA grade 3/4) is the major

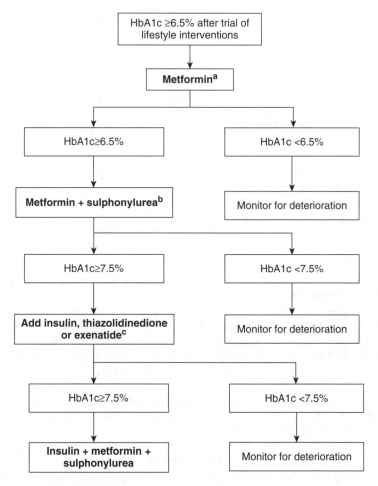

HbA1c ≥6.5% after trial of lifestyle interventions

↓

Metformin[a]

HbA1c≥6.5% | HbA1c <6.5%

Metformin + sulphonylurea[b] | Monitor for deterioration

HbA1c≥7.5% | HbA1c <7.5%

Add insulin, thiazolidinedione or exenatide[c] | Monitor for deterioration

HbA1c≥7.5% | HbA1c <7.5%

Insulin + metformin + sulphonylurea | Monitor for deterioration

[a]Consider sulphonylurea if:
• not overweight, or
• metformin is not tolerated/contraindicated, or
• rapid therapeutic effect is required due to symptoms of hyperglycaemia

[b]Consider substituting thiazolidinedione:
• for sulphonylurea if hypoglycaemia is a problem
• for metformin if not tolerated/contraindicated

[c]Consider thiazolidinedione if insulin not tolerated or high BMI. Consider exentatide if very high BMI (>35kg/m² —see below)

Figure 19.1
Modified from NICE guidelines:[4]

contraindication. Both rosiglitazone and pioglitazone have also been associated with an increased risk of fracture, particularly of the upper limbs.

Do you know of any novel therapies for type 2 diabetes?
Glucagon-like peptide 1 (GLP-1) is a gastrointestinal peptide that affects glucose metabolism by delaying gastric emptying, regulating postprandial glucagons release, reducing food intake, and

enhancing glucose-dependent insulin action. GLP-1 is metabolized by the enzyme dipeptidyl peptidase IV (DPP-IV).

GLP-1 based therapies for the treatment of type 2 diabetes have been developed, acting either as GLP-1 analogues or DPP-IV inhibitors.

- *GLP-1 analogues:* Exenatide is a subcutaneously-administered GLP-1 analogue, which augments the effect of insulin (the incretin effect). Several studies have demonstrated improvements in HbA1c and associated weight loss. Potential side effects are nausea, worsening of diabetic gastroparesis and increased risk of hypoglycaemia when used with sulphonylureas.

  NICE guidelines currently recommend consideration of Exenatide for patients with an elevated BMI (>35kg/m^2) and inadequate glycaemic control after a trial of metformin and a sulphonylurea.

- *DPP-IV inhibitors:* these agents (Sitagliptin and Vildagliptin) can be administered orally, and have been shown to improve HbA1c when combined with other oral hypoglycaemic agents, although their place in the management of type 2 diabetes is yet to be established.

References

1. National Institute for Health and Clinical Excellence. Diabetes (types 1 and 2)—patient education models. London: NICE; February 2006.

2. Bakris GL, Fonseca V, Katholi RE et al. Metabolic effects of carvedilol vs metoprolol in patients with type 2 diabetes mellitus and hypertension: a randomized controlled trial. JAMA. 2004; 292:2227–36.

3. Gress TW, Nieto FJ, Shahar E et al. Hypertension and antihypertensive therapy as risk factors for type 2 diabetes mellitus. Atherosclerosis Risk in Communities Study. N Engl J Med. 2000; 342:905–12.

4. National Institute for Health and Clinical Excellence The management of type 2 diabetes. London: NICE; May 2008.

5. The effect of intensive treatment of diabetes on the development and progression of long-term complications in insulin-dependent diabetes mellitus. The Diabetes Control and Complications Trial Research Group. N Engl J Med. 1993; 329:977–86.

6. Nathan DM, Cleary PA, Backlund JY et al. Intensive diabetes treatment and cardiovascular disease in patients with type 1 diabetes. N Engl J Med. 2005; 353:2643–53.

7. Intensive blood-glucose control with sulphonylureas or insulin compared with conventional treatment and risk of complications in patients with type 2 diabetes (UKPDS 33). UK Prospective Diabetes Study (UKPDS) Group. Lancet. 1998; 352:837–53.

Case 20 ◆ **Neck Lump**

INFORMATION FOR THE CANDIDATE

Dear Doctor,

Thank you for seeing this 18-year old student who presents with a 6-month history of a firm, painless neck lump. She also reports fever, night sweats, and weight loss. She has been otherwise well, with no past medical history of note.

Many thanks for your opinion.

Acquiring the history

The broad differential diagnosis of a neck lump in adults includes medical and surgical causes. Causes of neck lumps include (see Volume 1, Case 97 Goitre>):

- **Cervical lymphadenopathy (85% of all cases)**
- **Thyroid disease (8%)**
  - ◆ Goitre: Grave's disease, Multinodular goitre, Hashimoto's thyroiditis, subacute thyroiditis
  - ◆ Solitary nodule
  - ◆ Adenoma
  - ◆ Thyroid cancer: medullary thyroid carcinoma, multiple endocrine neoplasia type 2
- **Other (7%)**
  - ◆ Congential: branchial, thyroglossal, and dermoid cysts
  - ◆ Neoplastic: head and neck cancer
  - ◆ Vascular: carotid artery aneurysm, chemodectoma
  - ◆ Cervical rib
  - ◆ Salivary gland disease: parotitis, submandibular calculi, neoplasms

A. History of presenting complaint:

Age of onset

The aetiology of a neck lump varies with age.

- Congenital and inflammatory conditions are common in patients under 16.
- Infective, inflammatory, and malignant conditions occur with decreasing frequency in patients between 16 and 40 years.
- The prevalence of malignancy increases with age and should be excluded in patients over 40 presenting with a neck lump.

Mode of onset

Begin by asking *'When did you first notice the lump?'* to determine onset and duration.

- A sudden appearance of a lump suggests an infective process
- Lumps presenting for months to years may suggest a benign cause. In this case, it is important to determine what brought the lesion to medical attention: any *changes* in the characteristics of the lump or development of associated symptoms?

Characteristics of the lump

- **Site**
  - ◆ *'Where is the lump?* Midline lumps are usually congenital or a thyroid goitre in aetiology.
- **Size.** Ask the patient
  - ◆ *'How big was the lump when you first noticed it?'*
  - ◆ *'Has the lump changed in size over time?'*. Determine the rate of change if the lump has increased in size over time. A rapidly expanding lump over a few days indicates an infective process. A lump that increases progressively over a few months suggests malignancy.
- **Number**
  - ◆ *'How many lumps can you feel?'* Multiple lumps suggest lymphadenopathy.
  - ◆ *'Have you noticed <u>similar</u> lumps elsewhere—face, armpit, elbows, groin?'* Presence elsewhere suggests generalized lymphadenopathy.
  - ◆ *'Have you noticed any <u>other</u> lumps elsewhere, such as the breasts or testicles?'* suggesting a primary malignant site.
  - ◆ *'Have you noticed any facial swelling?'* indicative of lymphadenopathy, salivary gland disease or head and neck malignancy.

- **Shape**
- **Consistency**
  - *'How does the lump feel—firm, soft, rubbery, or smooth?'*
- **Mobility**
  - *'Can you move the lump under the skin?'*
    - A mobile lump in all planes suggests a lipoma, cyst, or reactive lymph node.
    - An immobile, firm lump is highly suggestive of a malignant lymph node.
    - A neck lump mobile in the horizontal plane only suggests a carotid-body tumour, or chemodectoma, with involvement of the carotid sheath.
  - *'Does the lump move when you swallow?'* A midline lump which moves upwards with swallowing is characteristic of a thyroglossal cyst or goitre.
  - *'Can you feel the lump beating?'* A pulsatile neck mass suggests a carotid artery aneurysm or chemodectoma.
- **Aggravating factors**
  - Alcohol can exacerbate lymph node related pain in Hodgkin's lymphoma. This occurs within a few minutes of alcohol ingestion and occurs at sites of bony involvement and lymphadenopathy.
  - Pain worse before or during eating is related to salivary gland pathology: parotitis, submandibular calculi, and salivary gland neoplasms. Carcinoma of the parotid gland can involve the facial nerve as it innervates the facial muscles, therefore enquire about facial weakness and loss of taste.

Associated symptoms

Ask specifically about the following symptoms:

- **Symptoms related to the lump itself**
  - Pain and tenderness are features of reactive lymph nodes, subacute thyroiditis, and haemorrhage into a thyroid nodule or adenoma.
  - Skin changes, such as surrounding erythema and warmth, suggest an infective cause.
- **Thyroid symptoms**
  - weight change
  - cold or heat intolerance
  - tremor
  - palpitations and excessive sweating
  - skin changes
  - diplopia, painful eye movements
  - change in bowel habit
  - menorrhagia/oligomenorrhoea in women
- **Ear, nose, and throat symptoms**
  - ask about recent sore throats or tonsillitis suggesting reactive lymphadenopathy
  - earache and discharge favour an ear infection
  - mouth ulcers or lumps may suggest infection or malignancy
  - dental problems may give rise to a palpable dental abscess
- **Constitutional symptoms** suggest malignancy or infection
  - weight loss and anorexia
  - fevers and night sweats occur with haematological malignancy and tuberculosis
  - pruritis occurs in Hodgkin's lymphoma
  - malaise

- **Respiratory symptoms**
  - Shortness of breath, stridor and cough, which are *worse* on lying down, indicate compression of the trachea by a large neck mass such as a goitre.
  - Haemoptysis and chronic cough may suggest underlying bronchogenic carcinoma with metastatic lymph node deposits.
- **Gastrointestinal symptoms**
  - *'Have you noticed a change in the quality or pitch of your voice?'* Dyphonia and hoarseness of the voice favour laryngeal or bronchogenic carcinoma with invasion of the recurrent laryngeal nerve.
  - Dysphagia may be the result of compression of the oesophagus from a large neck mass or due to underlying oesophageal malignancy. Ask if the dysphagia is to solids, liquids, or saliva to establish the extent of involvement.
  - Abdominal pain, nausea, vomiting, early satiety, change in bowel habit, or haematochezia suggests an underlying gastrointestinal malignancy with lymph node involvement (typically left supraclavicular node, or *Virchow's* node).
- **Cardiovascular symptoms**
  - Dizziness and syncope are symptoms that may suggest a chemodectoma
- **Neurological symptoms**
  - Ask about limb weakness, sensory disturbance, dysphasia, and amaurosis fugax. TIAs occur with carotid artery aneurysms and compression of the carotid artery by a chemodectoma.
  - Upper limb paraesthesiae from a cervical rib.
- **Other**
  - Rash, dry cough, and eye symptoms are features of sarcoidosis.

B. Relevant medical and family history:

Past medical history
- Causes of polyglandular lymphadenopathy:
  - tuberculosis
  - cancer of any type
  - infectious mononucleosis—EBV, CMV, human herpesvirus-6 (HHV-6), toxoplasma, bartonella
  - SLE
- Thyroid disease
  - Hypertension may be secondary to phaeochromocytoma, as part of multiple endocrine neoplasia 2 with associated medullary thyroid cancer.

Family history
- Tuberculosis
- Cancer of any type. Consider familial medullary carcinoma and multiple endocrine neoplasia 2 in patients with a family history of thyroid cancer.

C. Medications:
- Ask about drugs that can cause lymphadenopathy:
  - Allopurinol
  - Phenytoin
  - Atenolol
  - Cephalosporins
- Lithium and anti-thyroid drugs can lead to the development of a goitre.

D. Social issues:

- Cigarette smoking is the most important risk factor for laryngeal, bronchogenic, and gastrointestinal malignancies, and is also a risk factor for Graves' disease.
- Ask about travel abroad, especially to areas where tuberculosis is endemic.
- Enquire about HIV risk factors:
  - Sexual activity
  - intravenous drug use
  - transfusion of blood and blood products
- Contact with animals such as cats which is a risk factor for toxoplasmosis and bartonella
- Elicit the patient's ideas and concerns about their symptoms and diagnosis.

Formulating a plan of action

- Explain to the patient that a full clinical examination is required.
- Discuss the possible causes of the neck lump suggested by the history and explain the need for investigations.
- Consider the following investigations as directed by the history:
  - **Throat swab** for culture and sensitivity.
  - **Sputum culture** for acid fast bacilli.
- **Blood tests**
  - Blood count. A microcytic anaemia may occur with a gastrointestinal malignancy and normocytic normochromic anaemia with haematological malignancy. A raised white cell count with a neutrophilia indicates an infection; lymphocytosis occurs with leukaemia and non-Hodgkin's lymphoma. Eosinophilia, neutrophilia, and lymphopenia may occur in Hodgkin's lymphoma.
  - ESR is non-specific and is raised in infection, inflammation, and malignancy.
  - Blood film for cell morphology.
  - Thyroid function tests.
  - Thyroid autoantibodies—anti-thyroid peroxidase and anti-thyroglobulin antibodies are raised in autoimmune thyroid disease.
  - Calcitonin levels are elevated in medullary thyroid cancer.
  - LFTs may be deranged in metastatic disease or liver involvement in haematological malignancies.
  - Serum ACE will be raised in sarcoidosis
  - Viral serology for CMV and Epstein-Barr virus (EBV)
  - Paul-Bunnell/Monospot test for infectious mononucleosis
  - HIV test
- **Imaging**
  - Plain chest radiograph may reveal a cervical rib, hilar lymphadenopathy, pulmonary tuberculosis, lung cancer, or retrosternal extension of a goitre.
  - Ultrasound scan of the neck to allow distinction between types of neck lump.
  - Ultrasound guided fine-needle aspiration cytology or core needle biopsy of lymph nodes and thyroid nodules.
  - Radioisotope scan of thyroid gland may be indicated if the cause of thyrotoxicosis is indeterminate. Of the 'cold' nodules, 5% are malignant and 25% are indeterminant.
  - Contrast enhanced CT scan of neck to establish the dimensions and extent of neck swelling and involvement of adjacent structures; CT of chest or abdomen if broncho-genic carcinoma or gastrointestinal malignancy is suspected.

- **Other investigations to consider**
  - ◆ Excision lymph node biopsy is diagnostic for haematological malignancy.
  - ◆ Bone marrow aspirate or biopsy for staging of non-Hodgkin's lymphoma.
  - ◆ Carotid dopplers if carotid arterial disease is suspected.
  - ◆ Gastrointestinal endoscopy for suspected gastrointestinal malignancy.

Questions commonly asked by examiners

What are the causes of cervical lymphadenopathy?

Cervical lymphadenopathy can be classified as localized or generalized.

Localized	Generalized
Infection	**Haematological malignancy**
• Upper respiratory tract infection, ear infection	**Infection**
• Tonsilllitis	• Tuberculosis
• Dental abscess	• HIV
• EBV	• EBV
• CMV	• Toxoplasmosis
• Hepatitis	• Cat-scratch disease (bartonella)
Malignancy	**Inflammatory**
• Haematological: lymphoma and leukaemia	• Sarcoidosis
• Metastatic spread from gastrointestinal tract, breast, lung, melanoma and head and neck cancer.	• SLE
	Drugs
	• Phenytoin
	• Allopurinol
	• Atenolol
	• Cephalosporins

What is the differential diagnosis of an infectious mononucleosis syndrome?

1. EBV
2. CMV
3. HIV seroconversion
4. Toxoplasmosis
5. HHV-6

Aside from fever and lymphadenopathy, what are the other clinical manifestations of infectious mononucleosis?

1. Splenomegaly—splenic rupture has been reported, and patients should be advised to avoid contact sports and vigorous exercise for six weeks
2. Rash—a generalized maculopapular rash is occasionally seen, and is more common following amoxicillin administration.
3. Neurological symptoms—Guillain-Barré syndrome, cranial nerve palsies, meningoencephalitis, aseptic meningitis, and transverse myelitis have been reported.

What is DRESS syndrome?

Drug Reaction with Eosinophilia and Systemic Symptoms (DRESS), or Drug Hypersensitivity Syndrome (DHS), is a further differential for infectious mononucleosis. The syndrome is a severe reaction to a drug(s), causing fever, rash, and systemic features. The pathogenesis is thought to involve co-infection with human herpesvirus 6 (HHV-6). A high fever is the initial symptom, followed by a maculopapular rash and organ involvement manifested as eosinophilia and abnormal LFTs. Lymphadenopathy is present in 75% of cases. The most common drugs to cause this reaction are allopurinol and anti-epileptics such as phenytoin, carbamezapine, and phenobarbital.

How is Hodgkin's Lymphoma diagnosed and classified?

The presence of multinucleated Reed-Sternberg cells with reactive infiltrate of inflammatory cells (lymphocytes, eosinophils, neutrophils, and plasma cells) on histological examination of a lymph node is pathognomonic of Hodgkin's lymphoma. The Reed-Sternberg cells stain positive for CD30 and CD15.

The histological appearance allows classification of Hodgkin's lymphoma into 5 types:

1. Nodular sclerosis*
2. Mixed cellularity*
3. Lymphocyte depleted
4. Lymphocyte rich
5. Nodular lymphocyte predominant (Reed-Sternberg cells are absent)

How is Hodgkin's lymphoma staged?

The Cotswolds system (modified Ann Arbor) is used for staging of Hodgkin's lymphoma

Stage I	Involvement of one lymph node area
Stage II	Involvement of two lymph node areas on the same side of the diaphragm
Stage III	Involvement of lymph nodes on both sides of the diaphragm
Stage IV	Extranodal disease (bone marrow, liver)

The presence of systemic symptoms such as fevers, night sweats, and weight loss is indicated by the suffix B, otherwise the suffix A indicates the absence of these symptoms.

What is the management of Hodgkin's lymphoma?

The management of Hodgkin's lymphoma is determined by the stage of the disease and the presence or absence of B symptoms. Treatment involves radiotherapy and/or chemotherapy. ABVD (see below) is the gold standard chemotherapy regime used to treat advanced disease or disease with B symptoms. Other regimes include alternating COPP–ABVD, escalated BEACOPP which has been shown to have a better overall 5 year survival rate than COPP–ABVD, and Stanford V with radiotherapy.

*   Stage IA & IIA is treated with involved field radiotherapy alone and short course of chemotherapy.
*   Stage IB, IIB, III, IV disease is treated with combination chemotherapy
*   Relapsed disease is responsive to high dose combination chemotherapy with stem cell transplantation, with survival rates reaching 80%.

ABVD	Adriamycin, bleomycin, vinblastine, dacrabazine
COPP	cyclophosphamide, Oncovin (vincristine), prednisolone, procarbazine
BEACOPP	bleomycin, etoposide, doxorubicin, cyclophosphamide, Oncovin(vincristine), prednisolone, procarabazine
Stanford V	doxorubicin, vinblastine, mechlorethamine, vincristine, bleomycin, etoposide, prednisolone, and radiotherapy.

Further reading

1. Thomas R et al. Part I: Hodgkin's Lymphoma—molecular biology of Hodgkin and Reed-Sternberg cells. Lancet Oncol. 2004; 5:11–18.

2. Diehl V et al. Part II: Hodgkin's Lymphoma—diagnosis and treatment. Lancet Oncol. 2004; 5:19–26.

---

* Most common histological types comprising 70–85% of all cases.

Case 21 ◆ Weight Gain

INFORMATION FOR THE CANDIDATE

Dear Doctor,

Thank you for seeing this 45-year old lady who complains of weight gain of more than 10kg over a year. She has a past medical history of hypertension treated with Lisinopril, and type 2 diabetes mellitus which has been difficult to control recently despite treatment with metformin, gliclazide and insulin. She is a non-smoker and drinks 12 units of alcohol per week

Many thanks for your opinion.

Acquiring the history

The differential diagnosis of weight gain is broad. The history should aim to differentiate adiposity from fluid retention, as well as to determine the underlying cause.

Causes of weight gain

Metabolic:
- Cushing's syndrome
- Hypothyroidism
- Polycystic ovarian syndrome
- Insulinoma
- Hypothalamic disease: trauma, infection, infiltration and neoplastic

Fluid retention:
- Congestive heart failure
- Ascites of any cause
- Nephrotic syndrome of any cause

Drugs:
- Insulin and sulphonylureas
- Oral contraceptive pill and hormonal depot injections
- Steroids
- Atypical antipsychotics, e.g. olanzapine, clozapine and risperidone
- Tricyclic antidepressants, e.g. amitriptylline
- Anti-epileptics, e.g. sodium valproate and carbemazepine

Other:
- Abdominal/pelvic mass
- Primary obesity
- Sedentary lifestyle
- Pregnancy
- Nicotine withdrawal

A. *History of presenting complaint:*
Age of onset
Characteristics of weight gain

- Determine the patient's baseline weight *'How much weight have you put on?'*
- Ask about the time course of the weight gain *'Over what period of time have you put on this weight?'* Weight gain over days to weeks is likely to be due to fluid retention whereas progression over months–years is suggestive of all other causes.
- *'Where have you put on the weight—abdomen? trunk? face? back of the neck? legs or ankles?'* *'Is the weight gain evenly distributed?'* Distribution of weight gain may give a clue to the underlying aetiology. For example, disproportionate truncal weight gain and facial fat is suggestive of Cushing's syndrome (see Vol 1, Case 101 Cushing's Syndrome). Abdominal weight gain is non-specific, but together with leg and ankle swelling may be due to fluid retention. Predominant abdominal weight gain should raise the suspicion of pregnancy in women of child-bearing age. Nephrotic syndrome is characterized by facial, periorbital and leg swelling (see Vol 1, Case 8 Nephrotic Syndrome).

Associated symptoms
- **Fluid retention**
  - **Congestive cardiac failure**—exertional dyspnoea, dyspnoea at rest, orthopnoea, paroxysmal nocturnal dyspnoea, ankle swelling and chest pain.
  - **Nephrotic syndrome** of any cause—frothy urine, haematuria, rash (SLE, HSP, vasculitis) and arthralgia.
  - **Renal failure** of any cause—most, but not all, patients become oligo-anuric when they approach end-stage renal failure.
  - **Chronic liver disease**—jaundice, previous ascites or liver disease.
  - **Metabolic diseases**
  - **Cushing's syndrome**—striae, easy bruising, acne, hirsutism, proximal muscle weakness, oligo/amenorrhoea in women and psychiatric symptoms such as low or elated mood, hallucinations and delusions.
  - **Hypothyroidism**—cold intolerance, dry skin, fatigue, neck swelling, menorrhagia in women, constipation, hoarse voice and cognitive impairment.
  - **Polycystic ovarian syndrome**—oligo/amenorrhoea, reduced fertility, acne and hirsutism/male pattern baldness.
  - **Insulinoma**—Ask about episodes of lightheadedness, blackouts, sweating, palpitations, and seizures. These symptoms occur during periods of fasting and on exercise.
  - **Hypothalamic disease**—headaches, vomiting, visual disturbance, polyuria, nocturia and polydipsia.
- **Pregnancy**—is there a chance that the patient might be pregnant? Ask about her last menstrual period.
- **Diet**—take a thorough dietary history. Begin with an open statement such as *'Tell me what you would eat in a typical day, starting with breakfast.'* Enquire specifically about
  - number of meals per day
  - frequency of snacks
  - type of food they eat including fast food and take-aways
  - size of portions
- Ask about attempts at weight reduction—diet, exercise, and previous dietetic consults.
- **Psychiatric symptoms**—stress, anxiety, depression and eating disorders all contribute to binge-eating.

B. Relevant medical and family history:

Past medical history

- A history of cardiac or pulmonary disease may indicate right heart failure.
- Chronic liver disease of any cause suggests ascites.
- Ask about a history of diabetes mellitus. Enquire about glycaemic control (recent $HbA1_c$), compliance with medication and the presence of complications. Diabetes mellitus may be a feature of Cushing's syndrome.
- Ask about a history of the following co-morbidities, which may also be due to underlying Cushing's syndrome
  - hypertension may also be the result of or worsened by Cushing's syndrome
  - fractures and osteoporosis
  - recurrent infections
  - cataracts
- Patients may be on treatment for conditions which contribute to weight gain. These are:
  - diabetes mellitus
  - inflammatory conditions for which steroids are required
  - epilepsy (valproate, carbamezapine and gabapentin)
  - schizophrenia and depression (atypical antipsychotics, tricyclic antidepressants)

Family history

A family history of obesity may suggest a genetic cause, however the aetiology of obesity is multifactoral.

C. Medications:

- Consider drugs that might be contributing to the weight gain. These include:
  - Insulin, sulphonylureas and glitazones.
  - Steroids including oral, topical and inhaled preparations.
  - Atypical antipsychotics, e.g. olanzapine, clozapine and risperidone.
  - Tricyclic antidepressants, e.g. amitriptylline, citalopram.
  - Anti-epileptics, e.g. sodium valproate and carbemazepine.
  - Non-steroidal anti-inflammatory drugs contribute to fluid retention.
- Ask about the use of hormonal contraceptive preparations—oral contraceptive pill, depots and implants.
- Enquire about the use of anabolic steroids.

D. Social issues:

- Ask the patient about participation in exercise *'Do you do take part in any physical activity? How many times a week?'.*
- Determine the impact of weight gain on their daily activities.
- Enquire about alcohol consumption as a cause of high calorie intake and pseudocushing's syndrome see Vol 1, Case 101 Cushing's Syndrome).
- Ask about cigarette smoking and any recent attempts at cessation, since nicotine withdrawal leads to weight gain.
- Elicit the patient's concerns about their symptoms.

Formulating a plan of action

*   Explain that a clinical examination will be required.
*   Reassure the patient that most causes of weight gain are not serious, but that investigations may be required to exclude secondary causes of weight gain. If a secondary cause is unlikely, then explain the health risks of obesity and suggest a further appointment to discuss diet and exercise as initial lifestyle modifications.
*   Consider the following investigtations:
    *   **Urinalysis** for protein, blood and glucose, protein:creatinine ratio or 24 hour urine collection to quantify protein
    *   **Blood tests**
*   **Urea, electrolytes and creatinine** may indicate renal failure, although severe nephrotic syndrome may occur without renal failure (e.g. minimal change disease). A low potassium level may occur in Cushing's syndrome.
*   **Serum albumin level** will be low in nephrotic syndrome or chronic liver disease.
*   **Thyroid function tests** low free T4 and high TSH suggests hypothyroidism.
*   **Tests for determining cortisol excess and Cushing's syndrome** (see examiner's questions)
*   **Tests for polycystic ovarian syndrome:**
    *   LH:FSH ratio is increased
    *   Testosterone levels are mildly elevated
    *   Reduced level of sex-hormone binding globulin (SHBG).
*   **Test for insulinoma:** Supervised 72 hours fast with plasma glucose, insulin and C-peptide levels. Glucose is low, and insulin and C-peptide levels are increased in insulinoma.
*   **Plain chest radiograph** may reveal appearances of congestive cardiac failure.
*   **Ultrasound of abdomen and pelvis/Transvaginal ultrasound scan of pelvis** for investigation of a suspected abdominal or pelvis mass and for polycystic ovaries.
*   **Echocardiography** for left ventricular function in cardiac failure.
*   **MRI scan of head** will show a hypothalamic or pituitary lesion as a cause of the weight gain.

Questions commonly asked by examiners

What are the causes of secondary obesity?

*   Neuroendocrine obesity—hypothalamic injury can cause hyperphagia and obesity. This may be due to trauma, tumour, inflammation, posterior fossa surgery or elevated intracranial pressure. Patients may have other neuroendocrine symptoms such as diabetes insipidus, impaired reproductive function and thyroid or adrenal insufficiency.
*   Cushing's syndrome—causing centripetal obesity (see Vol 1, Case 101 Cushing's Syndrome).
*   Hypothyroidism
*   Polycystic ovarian syndrome—is characterized by obesity and insulin resistance.
*   Genetic causes—leptin deficiency (see below) and Prader-Willi syndrome are genetic disorders causing obesity.

What is the genetic basis of obesity?

Obesity is influenced by genetic and environmental factors. Leptin, an adipose tissue derived hormone, is central in the regulation of appetite. High levels lead to an inhibition in neuropeptide Y and stimulation in the release of MSH (melanocyte-stimulating hormone) leading to suppression of appetite. Several mutations in the genes encoding leptin, hypothalamic leptin receptors, neuropeptide Y and MSH have been identified. These may contribute to inherited obesity syndromes accounting for approximately 20% of cases of obesity.

What is the approach to the management of obesity?

Secondary causes of weight gain should be treated if identified. The complications of obesity should be managed. These include: cardiovascular disease, diabetes mellitus, gastro-oesophageal reflux, gallstones, sleep apnoea and increased risk of gastrointestinal, breast and uterus malignancy.

A structured weight loss programme targeted at dietary changes, encouraging exercise and psychological support should be initiated.

Anti-obesity drugs include: orlistat (a competitive intestinal lipase inhibitor) and sibutramine (serotonin and noradrenaline re-uptake inhibitor). These may be indicated in patients with a BMI >30kg/m^2 *and* who have failed to lose weight with conservative management. Treatment is continued for 2 years if weight loss of at least 5% is achieved at 3 months of treatment. Rimonabant, a cannabinoid receptor antagonist, has recently been withdrawn due to psychiatric side-effects.

Bariatric surgery, either gastric banding or bypass, is considered in patients with a BMI greater than 35kg/m^2 *with* co-morbidites, or a BMI greater then 40kg/m^2.

Case 22 ♦ **Fever and Neck Stiffness**

INFORMATION FOR THE CANDIDATE

Dear Doctor,

Thank you for seeing this 25-year old gentleman who has had a fever and neck stiffness for the past three days. He has not vomited, but is unable to tolerate bright lights. He is otherwise well and there is no history of head injury. I am concerned he has meningitis. Please could you see and advise.

Many thanks for your opinion.

Acquiring the history

In clinical practice, if there is concern about bacterial meningitis following triage and initial evaluation, a detailed history should be acquired *after* management for bacterial meningitis has been commenced (see below). If antibiotics are administered prior to hospital admission blood cultures are less likely to be positive, however the microbiological diagnosis can still be made from nasopharyngeal and cerebrospinal fluid (CSF) cultures as well as PCR studies for meningococcus.

A. History of presenting complaint:

The classical triad of bacterial meningitis is fever, neck stiffness and altered conscious level. Up to one-third of patients do not present with all three features, but virtually all patients present with one of these features.[1]

Duration of illness:

The differential diagnosis of fever and neck stiffness includes infectious and neoplastic causes of meningitis. The onset and duration of illness helps to differentiate these:

*   Acute bacterial meningitis is usually of *acute* onset, with associated headache, photophobia and systemic symptoms.
*   Fungal, viral and tuberculous meningitis may have a longer history of greater than one week with less florid symptoms. Immunosuppressed patients with bacterial meningitis may also have an insidious onset of symptoms.
*   Metastatic malignancy or leukaemia may present with symptoms of meningitis rapidly or over weeks to months. There are often associated features of the underlying condition.

Associated symptoms:

*   **Headache**: occurs commonly in patients with meningitis. Nausea and vomiting strongly suggests elevated intracranial pressure (see Case 27 Headache). The presence of neck stiffness suggests meningeal inflammation, however several conditions may present with fever and headache in the absence of neck stiffness:
    *   systemic bacterial infection
    *   referred facial/ENT pain (see below)
    *   subarachnoid haemorrhage
    *   brain abscess/subdural empyema
*   **Rash:** a petechial or purpuric rash is suggestive of meningococcal sepsis requiring immedi-ate resuscitation and high-dependency care. In this context the rash is due to *disseminated intravascular coagulation*, which may also occur in systemic sepsis due to any bacterial infection. Viral causes of meningitis, particularly enteroviruses, may cause a maculo-papular viral 'exanthem'. However, the features of this rash are rarely distinctive enough to confirm the diagnosis. Lyme disease may occasionally present with meningitis, however the classical signs of erythema migrans and arthritis may be absent at this stage. Thrombotic thrombocy-topenic purpura may also cause fever, rash, and focal neurology, although neck stiffness is rare and there is usually associated renal failure and haemolysis.
*   **Confusion:** the presence of altered mental status suggests *meningo-encephalitis* rather than simply meningitis. Typical abnormalities are altered behaviour, personality change and confusion. However, isolated sensory and motor deficits may occur in association with fever in brain abscess and familial hemiplegic migraine.
*   **Neck stiffness/neck pain:** neck stiffness suggests meningeal inflammation. However, focal neck tenderness and fever suggests a focal lesion such as a spinal epidural abscess, osteomy-elitis, metastatic malignancy or lymphoma. Causes of spinal epidural abscesses include *Staphyloccus aureus*, tuberculosis and brucellosis.
*   **Visual disturbance, speech abnormalities, weakness**: Focal neurological lesions, such as a brain abscess, will cause specific neurological signs. Chronic 'basal' meningitis may also cause cranial nerve palsies, particularly affecting the nerves of eye movement and the facial nerve. The causes of basal meningitis are tuberculosis, carcinomatous meningitis, fungal meningitis (e.g. *Cryptococcus neoformans*) and sarcoidosis.

Systemic enquiry

Enquire about symptoms of extra-cranial infection, which may be a cause of systemic sepsis as well as a source of intracranial or meningeal infection (e.g. lung, paranasal or mastoid sinuses). Also enquire about symptoms suggestive of autoimmune disease causing aseptic meningitis.

*   **Respiratory**: dyspnoea, cough, purulent sputum, pleuritic pain?
*   **Ear, nose, and throat:** earache, headache, facial pain, sore throat?

- **Abdominal:** abdominal pain, nausea, vomiting, diarrhoea?
- **Dermatological:** rash, oral ulceration, alopecia, nail fold infarcts?
- **Genitourinary:** genital ulceration, genital discharge, rash, urinary symptoms?
- **Musculoskeletal:** joint pain, joint swelling, joint stiffness?

B. HIV risk factors:

Determining the risk of HIV infection is essential, since HIV seroconversion is an increasingly common cause of aseptic meningitis, and in established HIV infection there are many causes of fever and headache depending on the stage of illness (see below).

- Sexual history—ask sensitively about sexual contacts, type of encounter (heterosexual, homosexual), number of partners, and the use of barrier protection (see Case 17 Sexually Transmitted Infection).
- Needle and blood exposure—shared needles, tattoos, piercings, dental, or medical care abroad?
- If known HIV infection, ask about most recent CD4 count, current treatment, and previous OIs (see Case 18 HIV Treatment).

C. Travel history:

Travel history during the preceding few months is important for both HIV risk assessment, and for specific organisms causing meningitis (see Case 16 Fever in the Returning Traveller):

- Ask about travel to regions endemic for tuberculosis.
- Arthropod-borne viral infections causing encephalitis (such as St Louis virus, West Nile virus and eastern equine encephalitis virus) are present in eastern and central USA.
- Tick-borne rickettsial illnesses causing fever and headache can be confused with meningitis. These are also acquired in the eastern USA.
- Lyme disease is also tick-borne, and is acquired in forest areas such as the New Forest in the UK.
- Pilgrims undergoing the Hajj or Umrah pilgrimage are at risk of Meningococcus. Proof of immunisation is required to obtain a visa for Saudi Arabia.

D. Relevant medical and social history:

- Ask about other conditions which suggest immunosuppression, such as previous splenectomy or recurrent bacterial infections. Recurrent meningitis may also occur due to a defect in the cranial vault, specifically the cribiform, sphenoid, or temporal bones.
- Ask about unwell contacts, specifically those with 'flu', 'viral' infections or headache.
- Drinking unpasteurised milk is a risk factor for Listeria meningitis and neurobrucellosis.

E. Medications, vaccines, and chemoprophylaxis:

- Ask about medications which are immunosuppressive, such as corticosteroids.
- Ask about over-the-counter medications, and antipyretic use.
- Some medications may cause fever and CSF lymphocytosis, such as NSAIDs and sulphonamides.
- Vaccination history should be enquired about. The patient may not know specifics, but ask specifically about:
  - Haemophilus influenzae type b (Hib)—typically during infancy
  - BCG—previously during school age, but now targeted from infants to adults
  - Meningococcus C—anytime from infancy to adult.

Formulating a plan of action

- Explain that any concern of bacterial meningitis warrants urgent admission, treatment, and further investigation. However, emphasise that these measures do not necessarily mean a definitive diagnosis of meningitis and confirmatory tests are necessary.

- Suggest an initial workup of FBC, electrolytes, liver enzymes, blood cultures, throat swab, and CT imaging. Explain that a lumbar puncture may also be necessary.
- Explain that possible further investigations include HIV testing, which may need to be repeated in 3 months to exclude a seroconversion illness.
- If bacterial meningitis is likely, explain that household contacts may require post exposure prophylaxis.
- Consider early notification to the Health Protection Agency if a serious transmissible disease is possible (see Case 16 Fever in the Returning Traveller).

Questions commonly asked by examiners

What are the initial steps in the management of suspected meningitis?

The initial evaluation of a patient with suspected meningitis involves assessment of severity, essential history, and immediate intervention:[2]

- Assess airway, breathing and circulation
- Administer high flow oxygen and commence fluid resuscitation
- Assess Glasgow Coma Score, and for neck stiffness, focal neurology, and papilloedema
- Ask about serious drug allergies, recent antibiotics, and HIV status.

Which investigations should be a priority?

- FBC, electrolytes, LFTs, clotting, CRP.
- Arterial blood gases
- Microbiology:
    1. Blood cultures
    2. Throat swab for urgent gram stain
    3. Rash scraping for urgent gram stain
    4. Urine for pneumococcal antigen
    5. Blood (ethylenediaminetetraacetic acid (EDTA)) sample for meningococcal PCR

What about lumbar puncture?

If the syndrome is of *meningococcal septicaemia* (with rash, hypotension, delayed capillary refill time, or acidosis) lumbar puncture should *not be attempted*. These patients require high-dependency management for septic shock.

If the syndrome is of *meningitis* (with neck stiffness and fever) then lumbar puncture may be attempted:

- written consent must be obtained
- ensure platelets >80 and international normalized ratio (INR) <1.4
- other contraindications are local sepsis and elevated intracranial pressure

Because of the difficulty of excluding elevated intracranial pressure, and the risk of cerebral herniation (coning) following lumbar puncture (LP) in this circumstance, CT imaging is often performed prior to lumbar puncture. However, CT of the brain may not be adequate to exclude elevated intracranial pressure and is not necessary in all patients. A prospective study of 301 adults with suspected meningitis demonstrated three high risk groups requiring CT prior to LP:[3]

- abnormal neurology or altered mental status
- immunosuppressed
- age >60

If lumbar puncture will be delayed for more than 30 minutes following presentation then intravenous antibiotics should be administered first.

Which antibiotics should be used?

Third generation cephalosporins (cefotaxime/ceftriaxone) should be administered at the correct dose for bacterial meningitis. These drugs are active against most bacterial pathogens, although ampicillin should be added if Listeria infection is suspected and vancomycin should be added if penicillin-resistant Streptococci are present locally.

Is there a place for steroids in the management of bacterial meningitis?

Dexamethasone improves survival in bacterial meningitis and should be given with the first dose of antibiotic. Studies showing benefit have demonstrated decreased mortality in adults with Pneumococcal meningitis.[4] Corticosteroids are also of benefit in HIV- negative patients with tuberculosis meningitis[5].

What is the differential diagnosis of fever and headache in patients with HIV?

Unknown HIV status:	HIV seroconversion illness
Any CD4 count:	TB meningitis
CD4 <100:	Cryptococcal meningitis
Any stage including on HAART:	CNS lymphoma

References

1. Sigurdardottir B, Bjornsson OM, Jonsdottir KE et al. Acute bacterial meningitis in adults. A 20-year overview. Arch Intern Med. 1997; 157:425–30.

2. Heyderman RS, Lambert HP, O'Sullivan I et al. Early management of suspected bacterial meningitis and meningococcal septicaemia in adults. J Infect. 2003; 46:75–77.

3. Hasbun R, Abrahams J, Jekel J et al. Computed tomography of the head before lumbar puncture in adults with suspected meningitis. N Engl J Med. 2001; 345:1727–33.

4. de Gans J, van de Beek D. Dexamethasone in adults with bacterial meningitis. N Engl J Med. 2002; 347:1549–56.

5. Prasad K, Singh MB, Corticosteroids for managing tuberculosis meningitis. Cochrane database of systematic reviews 2008.

Case 23 ♦ Joint Pains

INFORMATION FOR THE CANDIDATE

Dear Doctor,

Thank you for seeing this 40-year old lady who has had painful hands and knees for the last 3 months. She is a secretary, but has been unable to work recently despite regular analgesia. Please could you see and advise.

Many thanks for your opinion.

Acquiring the history

A. History of presenting complaint:

The approach to patients with joint pains should be to establish the following:

1. *Is this a musculoskeletal emergency?* Musculoskeletal emergencies, such as septic arthritis, have an acute onset and are generally monoarticular. There may also be constitutional symptoms such as fever, weight loss, and malaise.
2. *Is the distribution of symptoms monoarticular or polyarticular?*
3. *Is there associated joint inflammation (arthritis or synovitis)?* Both the distribution and presence of inflammation influence differential diagnosis and management (see below).

Begin with open questions, such as *'How have you been recently?'*, or *'How have the joint pains been affecting you?'*. Since rheumatic diseases are chronic conditions associated with disability and psychological symptoms, it is important to use open questioning to allow the patient to volunteer non-rheumatic complaints before focusing on rheumatic symptoms (see Vol 1 Cases 108 Rheumatoid Arthritis, 109 Psoriatic Arthropathy, 110 Ankylosing Spondylitis, and 111 Gout).

Distribution of symptoms

• One or many joints involved?
• Symmetrical or Asymmetrical?
• Large or small joints?
• Involvement of ligament or tendon insertions (enthesitis)

Osteoarthritis (OA): may be asymmetrical and typically affects the hand, knee, hip and spine, and rarely affects the elbow, wrist and ankle. The distal interphalangeal (DIP) joints and the first metacarpophalangeal (MCP) joint at the base of the thumb are usually affected in the hands.

Rheumatoid arthritis (RA): causes a symmetrical peripheral polyarthritis typically affecting the MCP and proximal interphalangeal (PIP) joints of both hands. However, this presentation is not specific to RA, and other causes of inflammatory arthritis may also present in this way. The shoulders, knees, and cervical spine are also commonly affected.

Crystal arthritis: gout most commonly causes a monoarthritis affecting the first metatarsophalangeal joint, but may also affect the knees. Pseudogout most commonly affects the knees and shoulders.

Seronegative arthritis: is usually asymmetrical and affects large joints and the spine. They are also associated with enthesitis, or inflammation at tendon or ligament insertions (e.g. Achilles tendonitis).

Differential diagnosis of monoarthritis/oligoarthritis	Differential diagnosis of polyarthritis
Trauma	Rheumatoid arthritis
Infection (gonococcal, non-gonococcal)	Osteoarthritis
Crystal arthritis	Seronegative arthritis (reactive arthritis, ankylosing spondylitis, psoriatic arthritis, enteropathic arthritis)
Seronegative arthritis	Viral infection
Lyme disease	Systemic rheumatic condition (SLE, vasculitis)
Malignancy	Systemic illness (malignancy, sarcoid)

Joint symptoms

• *Pain:* 'Which joints are painful?', 'Are they most painful first thing in the morning or later in the day?', *'Tell me about the pain'*. Joint pain is typically described as a constant localized ache, which is worse on movement. Inflammatory arthritis causes joint pain that is worse in the mornings, whereas degenerative conditions progress throughout the day. *'Does the pain keep you awake at night?'*. Night pain suggests malignancy or very severe arthritis, and is a 'red-flag' symptom for further investigation. Neuropathic pain (burning, numbness or parasthesia) may also be present due to associated carpal tunnel syndrome, or acute myelopathy or radiculopathy, which are also musculoskeletal emergencies.

- *Swelling:'Do your joints swell?', 'Which ones?', 'Where is the swelling?'*. The presence of synovial swelling differentiates *arthritis* from *arthralgia*. Ask the patient about joint swelling and duration, and attempt to distinguish synovial swelling from a joint effusion (localized and large) and bony swelling (longstanding bone deformity, e.g. Heberden's node).

- *Stiffness: 'Are your joints stiff when you wake up in the mornings?', 'How long does it take you to get them going?'*. Joint stiffness differentiates inflammatory arthritis from degenerative conditions. Morning stiffness greater than one hour is typical of RA. Stiffness also occurs in OA after a period of inactivity, but rarely lasts longer than one hour and not always in the morning. This is termed 'gelling'.

Onset of symptoms
- Onset over *hours:* infection, gout, trauma, rheumatoid arthritis (can occasionally present with acute polyarthritis over 24–48 hours).
- Onset over *weeks:* inflammatory arthritis, osteoarthritis, pseudogout.

Duration of symptoms
Symptoms lasting longer than 6 weeks help to differentiate the cause of inflammatory arthritis. Inflammatory symptoms that have been present less than six weeks may be due to viral infection, whereas after six weeks RA is far more likely.

Associated feature
- **Rash:** The differential diagnosis of rash and arthritis is broad, but the presence of any rash should be documented and the relationship to joint symptoms and medications should be enquired about.
  - Psoriasis
  - SLE (malar rash, photosensitivity)
  - Infection (rheumatic fever, Lyme diseae, viral exanthem)
  - Drug reaction (NSAIDs, gold, penicillamine, sulphasalazine)
  - Vasculitis (including rheumatoid vasculitis)
  - Raynaud's phenomenon (see Vol 1, Case 127 Raynaud's Phenomenon).
- **Oro-genital ulceration:** Oral ulceration is common in SLE. Oro-genital ulceration may occur in Behcet's disease, which is associated with an asymmetrical non-erosive arthritis. *Reactive arthritis* (formerly termed Reiter's syndrome) occurs following bacterial infection causing enteritis or urethritis. The arthritis is asymmetrical and usually affects the lower limbs. The genital lesions include circinate balanitis, although they are a consequence of the genito-urinary infection and are not specific for reactive arthritis.
- **Alopecia:** is a feature of SLE.
- **Eye symptoms:** A red or painful eye may be a consequence of episcleritis or scleritis in RA. Episcleritis is a painless, acute red eye without discharge, whereas scleritis causes deep ocular pain. Ask about dry and gritty eyes suggesting keratoconjunctivitis sicca, which may represent secondary Sjogren's syndrome.
- **Recent infection:** Reactive arthritis may be caused by enteritis or urethritis:

Enteritis	Urethritis
Salmonella	Chlamydia trachomatis
Shigella	
Yersinia	
Campylobacter	
Clostridium difficile	

Rheumatic fever following streptococcal infection is a cause of post-infectious arthritis, but is not classified as a 'reactive' arthritis because of the different clinical features including cardiac involvement.

Gonococcus may also cause arthritis and urethritis, although this is usually a septic arthritis due to disseminated gonococcal infection.

- **Systemic features:** Fever, weight loss, anorexia, and night sweats raise the suspicion of sepsis, but may also be features of severe connective tissue disease.

Systemic enquiry

- Enquire about symptoms of extra-articular disease using a structured systemic enquiry.
- In patients presenting with other complaints, use the GALS screen (gait, arms, legs, spine) to screen for rheumatological conditions. Ask the following questions: *'Do you have pain or stiffness in your muscles, joints or back?'*, *'Can you dress yourself without difficulty?'*, *'Can you walk up and down stairs without difficulty?'*.
- Patients with rheumatic disease often have associated psychological symptoms and sexual dysfunction. Ask openly and sensitively about these: *'How are the joint pains affecting you?'*, *'Are the joint pains affecting your relationship?'*.

B. Relevant medical and family history:

Other relevant aspects of the medical history include previous fractures and orthopaedic procedures. Rheumatoid arthritis is also associated with an increased prevalence of infections, lymphoproliferative disease, renal disease, and cardiovascular disease.

Ask about a family history of rheumatoid arthritis and psoriasis.

C. Medications and interactions:

- Ask about current and previous use of NSAIDs, steroids and disease-modifying agents. Also ask about common side effects (NSAIDs—dyspepsia, GI bleeding; steroids—diabetes, osteoporosis; sulphasalazine- rash; azathioprine—pancreatitis, lymphopenia) (see Vol 1, Case 108 Rheumatoid Arthritis).
- Several drugs are associated with drug-induced lupus: diltiazem, procainamide, hydralazine, penicillamine, and isoniazid.

D. Social issues:

- Ask about occupation and leisure activities that may predispose to joint pains, e.g. kneeling causing prepatellar bursitis (housemaid's knee), repetitive joint use causing tenosynovitis, or tennis elbow.
- Determine the level of disability. Ask about activities of self-care (e.g. washing, dressing) and daily living (e.g. shopping, cooking). Ask about mobility, both within the home and driving outside.
- Ask about the use of aids and appliances to assist with mobility and activities of daily living.
- Enquire about their accommodation and whether it is modified for access.
- Ask about social services support and how the patient is supporting themselves financially. Also ask about the patient's social support network.

Formulating a plan of action

- Explain that further workup will involve a full clinical examination as well as blood tests and imaging, since joint pains may be the first signs of a systemic illness.
- Explain that polyarticular joint pains do not necessarily mean a diagnosis of rheumatoid arthritis, particularly if the duration of illness is less than six weeks.
- If the presentation is with monoarthritis or with constitutional symptoms of infection, explain that the initial test will be a joint aspirate to exclude septic arthritis.
- Other initial tests to consider include:
    - FBC, electrolytes, CRP, ESR
    - antinuclear autoantibody (ANA), extractable nuclear antigens (ENAs) (anti-DNA, Sm, ribonuclear protein (RNP), Jo1, Ro, La antibodies), ANCA, rheumatoid factor, anti-CCP antibodies
    - Serum urate
    - Plain radiographs of hands and feet (to look for joint erosions suggesting RA)
- Tell the patient that a follow-up appointment will be given to discuss the results of above tests.

Questions commonly asked by examiners

(See Vol 1 Cases 108 Rheumatoid Arthritis, 109 Psoriatic Arthropathy, 111 Gout)

Do you know of any diagnostic criteria for rheumatoid arthritis?

The American College of Rheumatology have developed diagnostic criteria, primarily for the purposes of categorizing research rather than clinical use. Indeed, most patients have an insidious onset of fever, malaise, and arthralgia before the onset of joint swelling, and do not fulfil these criteria until they have advanced disease. A small proportion of patients (approximately 10%) have rapidly progressive disease, with an acute onset of synovitis and extra-articular manifestations.

The American College of Rheumatology criteria (1987) require at least 4 of the following to be present for the classification of RA:

- Morning stiffness > 1 hour*
- Symmetrical joint involvement*
- Arthritis affecting ≥ 3 joints*
- Involvement of small joints of the hands*
- Positive rheumatoid factor
- Rheumatoid nodules
- Radiographic evidence

Which viral illnesses are associated with arthralgia?

Common	Rare
Hepatitis B and C	EBV
Rubella / rubella vaccine	HIV
Parvovirus B19	Mumps
	Coxsackie virus
	Chikungunya virus

---

* present for ≥ 6 weeks

What is the differential diagnosis of fever and arthritis?

- Infectious arthritis (bacterial or viral)
- Postinfectious or reactive arthritis
- Rheumatoid arthritis or Still's disease
- Systemic rheumatic illness (SLE, vasculitis)
- Crystal arthritis
- Other systemic conditions (e.g. sarcoidosis, cancer)

Case 24 ◆ **Back Pain**

INFORMATION FOR THE CANDIDATE

Dear Doctor,

Thank you for seeing this 25-year old gentleman who presents with a 4-month history of lower back pain and stiffness. He has no past medical history of note and does not take any regular medications.

Many thanks for your opinion.

Acquiring the history

Back pain is one of the most common reasons for attendance to primary and secondary care. The focus of the history should be to identify patients with systemic symptoms, neurological symptoms, and to engage the patient regarding their degree of physical and psychological disability.

A. History of presenting complaint:

Age of onset

Consider ankylosing spondylitis in patients presenting below the age of 40 years.

Onset, duration and progression

- **Onset.**
    - ◆ *'When did the pain first start? Did it come on suddenly?'* Sudden onset of back pain should alert the physician to the possibility of a serious mechanical cause, such as intervertebral disc prolaspe or fracture, and the physician should rule out neurological symptoms suggesting spinal cord compression or cauda equina syndrome (see below).
    - ◆ Ask about a history of recent injury to the back which can give rise to sudden onset back pain. Enquire specifically about trivial injury or falls which may cause vertebral fracture in patients with underlying osteoporosis.
    - ◆ Subacute and gradual onset back pain suggests degenerative, inflammatory, malignant, or metabolic causes.
- **Progression**
    - ◆ *'Has the pain changed over time—is it the same, getting better or worse?'* Progressive pain is suggestive of malignancy or ankylosing spondylitis.

◆ *'Do you usually suffer with back pain?'*; *'How is this pain different from previous episodes?'*
Determine any change in the nature, severity, and progression of pain and associated
symptoms in patients with chronic recurrent back pain.

Character of pain

* Determine the site of the pain.
* *'What is the pain like—dull, sharp, shooting, electric-shock like, stabbing, burning?'* A dull pain or
ache occurs with degenerative back pain, malignancy, and inflammatory causes. Sharp,
shooting, 'electric-shock' and burning pain is suggestive of nerve root compression
* Pain that comes in waves suggests renal or biliary colic.
* Establish if the pain is true back pain or referred pain by asking *'Where did the pain start?'*;
'Did it start in the back, or elsewhere then radiate to the back?' Acute pain *originating* in the
epigastrium with radiation to the back may suggest pancreatitis, ruptured abdominal aortic
aneurysm, or aortic dissection.
* Determine the severity of the pain on a scale of 1–10 (with 1 rated as no pain and 10 the
most severe pain experienced by the patient.)

Radiation

* *'Does the pain spread from the back to other areas?'*
* Radiation to the legs bilaterally can be due to cord compression or cauda equina syndrome.
* Thoracic back pain radiates to the anterior chest wall.
* Sciatic pain radiates down the thigh and leg, typically below the knee. The level to which the
pain reaches may suggest the level of nerve root compression: anterior thigh (L3/L4), lateral
aspect of the leg, dorsal foot, and great toe (L4/L5) and, posterior calf, heel, and little toe
(L5/S1).
* Radiation of pain from the loin to the groin is suggestive of renal colic, pyelonephritis or
osteoarthritis of the hip.

Exacerbating factors

* *'Is the pain precipitated or made worse by anything?'*
* Movement, coughing, sneezing, and straining exacerbates pain caused by disc prolapse and
cord compression.
* Pain that is caused by walking a fixed distance and is relieved by rest is typical of spinal
stenosis. This is called spinal claudication.

Relieving factors

* *'Does anything make the pain better?'*
* Sitting or bending forwards relieves the pain of spinal stenosis
* Pain that is *not* relieved by lying down suggests malignancy or infection.
* Has the patient tried any analgesics?

Alarm symptoms (red flags)

The following features suggest a systemic cause for back pain, which may require urgent
investigation:

* **History of malignancy, immunosuppression, HIV**
* **Age over 50 years**
* **Fever, night sweats**
* **Weight loss**
* **Duration greater than one month**
* **Lack of response to analgesia**

- **Night pain**
- **Thoracic pain**
- **Night pain**
- **Neurological symptoms.** Ask specifically about
  - Paraesthesiae and sensory loss in the perineum, limbs, trunk, and abdomen.
  - Lower limb weakness. *Unilateral* lower limb weakness may be due to nerve root compression with associated radicular back pain. *Bilateral* lower limb weakness may be due to flaccid paralysis of cauda equina syndrome or spastic paraparesis of cord compression (see Vol 1, Station 3 Neurology and Central Nervous System).
  - Urinary retention with subsequent incontinence, hesitancy, constipation, or faeceal incontinence suggests sphincter disturbance resulting from cord compression or cauda equina syndrome.
  - Gait disturbance may be a result of lower limb weakness.

Rheumatological symptoms

Enquire about symptoms associated with inflammatory arthritis: (see Vol 1, Cases 110 Ankylosing Spondylitis, 109 Psoriatic Arthropathy vol 2 Case 23 Joint Pains):

- Stiffness of the neck and back that is *worse* in the mornings and after rest, and *relieved* with exercise.
- Reduced range of movement of the spine
- Asymmetrical large joint pain and stiffness; hips, knees, ankles, and shoulders
- A painful eye, blurred vision, and photophobia are symptoms of anterior uveitis.
- Dyspnoea may be indicative of upper lobe pulmonary fibrosis.
- Ask about small joint pain, swelling and deformity, and any nail changes that may suggest psoriatic spondylitis.

Systems review

This may reveal symptoms suggestive of illness causing referred pain to the back. Ask specifically about:

- Urinary symptoms suggestive of renal colic or pyelonephritis.
- Gastrointestinal symptoms suggesting pancreatitis, biliary or peptic ulcer disease.
- Symptoms of hypercalcaemia suggesting myeloma or disseminated malignancy: abdominal pain, vomiting, polyuria, polydipsia, and constipation.

B. Relevant medical and family history:

Past medical history

- Malignancy—breast, lung, colorectal, renal, thyroid, and prostate cancers metastasise to bone.
- Tuberculosis or staphylococcal infection—these are common causes of bone and joint infection.
- Any recent hospital admission or venous cannulation? Staphylococcus aureus bacteraemia, including MRSA, may result from any form of venous cannulation. This often causes bone and joint infection by haematogenous spread. Haemodialysis through an indwelling dialysis catheter is also associated with this risk.
- Osteoporosis predisposes to vertebral fractures. Enquire about risk factors for osteoporosis: past history of fracture, maternal history of hip fracture or osteoporosis, steroid use, early menopause, oopherectomy, thyrotoxicosis, and cigarette smoking.
- Aortic aneurysm

Family history
- Osteoporosis
- Psoriasis and ankylosing spondylitis

C. Medications:
- Long term use of steroids as a risk factor for osteoporosis.

D. Social issues:
- Occupational history. Ask about the nature of the work—does it involve heavy lifting precipitating back injury. Ask about the impact of back pain on their work—has the patient had to take time off work? Are there any financial repercussions from this?
- Enquire about the functional status of the patient, particularly the impact on the activities of daily living such as self-care, cooking, shopping, and driving.
- Ask about participation in recreational and sporting activities. Is the pain a result of a sports injury? Has the patient had to give these activities up due to the back pain?
- Ask about cigarette smoking and alcohol consumption—both are risk factors for osteoporosis.
- Ask openly about mood and psychological stress—both depression and anxiety are independent risk factors for low back pain.

Formulating a plan of action

Explain to the patient that a clinical examination will be required—including a straight leg raise and a neurological examination.

If there are no alarm symptoms, reassure the patient that the cause is likely to be benign and investigations may not be helpful. Avoid phrases that imply 'damage' or 'deterioration' to the back, such as 'degenerative arthritis'. Phrases such as 'back strain' are less likely to have a negative psychological effect and promote somatization.

Consider the following investigations:
- **Blood tests**
  - **Blood count.** A normocytic normochromic anaemia is a feature of myeloma, whilst a pancytopenia suggests bone marrow infiltration. A leucocytosis points towards an infection.
  - **ESR.** Raised in inflammatory conditions such as ankylosing spondylitis, discitis, infection, and malignancy.
  - **Urea, electrolytes, and creatinine.** Renal function may be impaired in myeloma due to deposition of light chains and amyloid.
  - **Serum corrected calcium.** Hypercalcaemia occurs in myeloma and other malignancies.
  - **LFTs.** Alkaline phosphatase is raised in pathological fractures and bony metastases, however the alkaline phsophatase is typically *normal* in myeloma.
  - **Serum and urine protein electrophoresis** will reveal a paraproteinaemia in myeloma. The paraprotein is IgG in 60% of cases, IgA in 20% and light chains in the remainder, which are often not detected on serum electrophoresis but on urine electrophoresis.
  - **HLA-B27 typing.** This is not routinely performed but may be a useful 'rule out' test for ankylosing spondylitis, since it is positive in approximately 95% of patients with ankylosing spondylitis but also 10% of the general healthy population.
  - **PSA** to screen for prostate cancer in men.
- **Urine tests**
  - **Urinalysis.** A positive urine dipstick for leucocytes and nitrites indicates pyelonephritis.
  - **Bence Jones protein.** Urinary free light chains can be detected in myeloma.

- **Imaging**
  - **Plain radiograph of the spine** will reveal vertebral fractures, osteolytic lesions of myeloma, and typical features of ankylosing spondylitis. *However* plain radiographs are not indicated for mechanical back pain, in the absence of trauma, because X-ray features of osteoarthritis are common and not associated with clinical symptoms. Moreover, the presence of X-ray changes may divert the physician's attention from a more serious cause of back pain.
  - **Plain radiograph of sacroiliac joints**. Features of sacroiliitis may be seen in ankylosing spondylitis, although typically MRI is performed if ankylosing spondylitis is suspected due to the superior sensitivity.
  - **MRI of the spine** indicated in patients with suspected cord compression, cauda equina syndrome, malignany, or back pain unresponsive to conventional therapy.
  - **Radioisotope bone scan** is indicated in cases of suspected metastatic bone disease.
  - **DEXA scan** to determine bone mineral density in patients at high risk of osteoporosis to evaluate the degree of osteopenia and future fracture risk.

Questions commonly asked by examiners

How would you proceed to clinically evaluate this patient after acquiring the history?

Clinical examination:

- *Inspection of back and posture*—anatomical abnormalities such as kyphosis and scoliosis may be noted, as well as scars from previous surgery.
- *Range of motion of back*—limited lumbar flexion may suggest ankylosing spondylitis (see Vol 1, Case 110 Ankylosing Spondylitis—modified Schober's test), although this test is not specific for this disorder.
- *Palpation of vertebrae*—for focal tenderness suggesting infection or malignancy. Soft-tissue tenderness is non-specific.
- *Straight leg raise*—passive elevation of the straightened leg with the patient supine may reproduce radicular pain. The test is considered positive if pain occurs between 10 and 60 degrees of elevation. The *crossed straight leg raise* is positive if pain is elicited on elevation of the *unaffected* leg. This test is more specific for intervertebral disc herniation.
- *Neurological examination*—this is essential to differentiate disc herniation, cauda equina syndrome, and cord compression (see below and Vol 1, Case 49 Commom Peroneal Nerve Palsy and L5 Root Lesion). Most disc herniation occurs at L4–5 and L5–S1, hence examination should focus on the L5 and S1 nerve roots if disc disease is suspected.

How can cauda equina syndrome be differentiated from cord compression clinically?

The spinal cord terminates at the level of the first lumbar vertebra and the lumbosacral spinal roots descend as the cauda equina to reach their respective vertebral foramina to exit the spinal canal. Lesions to the cauda equina give rise to *lower* motor neurone signs, whereas lesions to the cord itself manifest as *upper* motor neurone signs.

Which patients require referral?[1]

- *Urgent* neurosurgical referral:
  - Cauda equina syndrome
  - Suspected cord compression
  - Progressive or severe neurological deficit
- *Urgent* specialist referral:
  - Any 'red flags' for cancer or infection

Clinical features	Cord compression	Cauda equina syndrome
Motor	Hypertonia (Spasticity) Bilateral, pyramidal weakness Brisk reflexes	Flaccid paralysis Absent/reduced reflexes
Sensory	Sensory spinal level with loss of sensation in all modalities below the level of the lesion	Dermatomal sensory impairment Saddle anaesthesia
Other	Sphincter disturbance (automatic bladder)	Sphincter disturbance (sensory bladder urinary retention, and incontinence)

- *Soon* specialist referral:
  - Radicular back pain that persists after four to six weeks of conservative therapy
  - Persistent radicular pain with other signs of nerve root compression (positive straight leg raise).
  - Risk factors for osteoporosis
- Pain clinic referral: Patients with pain that persists longer than 6 weeks should be assessed for markers of chronicity (yellow flags). These patients may benefit from referral to a multidisciplinary pain team.
  - Belief that back pain is harmful or disabling
  - Reduced activity levels pain avoidance behaviour
  - Tendency to low mood and social withdrawal
  - Expectation of passive treatment rather than active participation
  - Work-related psychological problems
  - Work-related disciplinary action or litigation
  - Over-protective family or lack of family support

Reference:

1. Airaksinen O, Brox JI, and Cedraschi C et al., European guidelines for the management of chronic non specific low back pain. European Commission, Research Directorate. Available at:www.backpaineurope.org, 2004.

Case 25 ◆ **Dizziness**

INFORMATION FOR THE CANDIDATE

Dear Doctor,

Thank you for seeing this 40-year old lady who presents with recurrent episodes of dizziness with associated nausea and vomiting. There is no past medical history of note and she does not take any regular medications. She is a dance teacher and complains that her symptoms are significantly affecting her job.

Many thanks for your opinion.

Acquiring the history

Dizziness is a term used by patients to describe presyncope, syncope, and vertigo, therefore the history should initially aim to differentiate these conditions and identify an underlying cause for the dizziness. Presyncope and syncope are discussed in Case 26 Collapse.

A. History of presenting complaint
Age of onset
Although age is not specific in narrowing the differential diagnosis of dizziness, vestibular dysfunction, stroke, and cardiac causes of dizziness are more common with increasing age, whereas presyncope is more prevalent in younger patients. Dizziness in the elderly is common and may have multiple causes including vertigo, cerebrovascular disease, neck disease, and medications. Additionally, visual impairment and physical deconditioning may exacerbate the disability from dizziness.

Description of symptoms
- As for collapse, the history for episodes of *dizziness* should be evaluated in three parts, determining the associated features *preceding*, *during* and *after* the event.
- Invite the patient to describe their symptoms by using open phrases such as *'Tell me about your symptoms'* followed by focused questioning aiming to differentiate presyncope, syncope, and vertigo.
- *'Do you experience light-headedness as if you're about to faint?*—suggests presyncope.
- *'Do you lose consciousness?'* History of any impairment in consciousness and associated features should be obtained from a witness.
- *'Do you experience the sensation of the room spinning around you or yourself spinning?'* Vertigo is an abnormal perception of movement of the surrounding environment or self. Patients may also use terms such as *'whirling'*, *'tilting'*, or *'moving'*.

Precipitants
- *'Is there anything that triggers the dizziness?'*
- Ask about the following common precipitants of vertigo:
  - Sudden head and neck movements, is associated with peripheral vestibular dysfunction, vertebrobasilar ischaemia, and carotid sinus hypersensitivity.
  - Rapid head movements may trigger benign paroxysmal positional vertigo (BPPV). This must be distinguished from postural presyncope which occurs on standing. BPPV also occurs during manoeuvres which alter head position *without* affecting blood pressure, such as rolling over in bed, or bending the neck upwards.
  - Coughing, sneezing, and straining raises intracranial pressure which precipitates vertigo caused by perilymphatic fistulae.
  - Recent viral illnesses suggest labyrinthitis or vestibular neuronitis.
  - Trauma: carotid or vertebral artery dissection and head injury can cause BPPV; barotrauma from flying and swimming are associated with a perilymphatic fistula.
- Exclude precipitants of presyncope/syncope (see Case 26 Collapse):
  - Standing from a sitting or lying position provoking orthostatic hypotension
  - Prolonged standing, large meal, and hot environment causes vasovagal syncope
  - Prolonged fasting causing dizziness due to hypoglycaemia
  - Situational syncope during micturition, defecation, and circumstances causing fear.

Relieving factors
'Is there anything that makes the dizziness better such as sitting down or keeping your head still?'
Presyncope is relieved by sitting down. Limiting head movements also improves vertigo in BPPV,

labyrinthitis, and vestibular neuronitis. Peripheral vestibular dysfunction is improved by fixation on a distance object.

Onset and duration

- **Onset.** *'Did the dizziness start suddenly or gradually?'* Consider cerebrovascular disease in patients presenting with acute vertigo. Note that *peripheral* vestibular dysfunction can also cause acute vertigo whereas vertigo secondary to *central* vestibular dysfunction is usually of insidious onset.

- **Duration.**
  - *'How long does the dizziness last—a few seconds, minutes, hours or longer?'* Dizziness lasting less than a minute, is most often due to presyncope or BPPV. Prolonged episodes of vertigo, lasting minutes to a few hours, are commonly due to labyrinthitis, vestibular neuronitis, TIAs, and migraine. Prolonged vertigo is suggestive of stroke, relapse of multiple sclerosis, and bilateral vestibular failure. However, persistent vertigo lasting months is rare since the central nervous system adapts to the defect over time. Persistent vertigo lasting months is usually psychogenic.
  - *'Have you had previous episodes of dizziness? Are the episodes similar?'* Recurrent vertigo is most often due to BPPV or Ménière's disease.

Associated symptoms

- **Nausea and vomiting** occurs frequently with vestibular dysfunction.
- **Otological symptoms:**
  - Otalgia, otorrhoea, and pruritis indicate otitis media or externa.
  - Deafness is suggestive of a peripheral cause of vertigo.
  - Tinnitus, deafness, and a sensation of fullness of the ear is characteristic of Ménière's disease.
  - An auricular rash of the vesicular type is pathognomonic of Ramsay-Hunt syndrome (herpes zoster virus infection). It is accompanied by hyperacusis and facial weakness.
- **Neurological symptoms:**
  - Headaches with features of raised intracranial pressure (nausea, vomiting, aggravated by postural changes, seizures, and blurred vision) point towards a space-occupying lesion. Take a detailed history of headache to exclude migraine.
  - Brainstem symptoms include diplopia, dysarthria, dysphagia, limb weakness, sensory disturbance, and loss of consciousness.
  - Cerebellar symptoms to identify in the history are tremor, ataxia of limb movements, gait and balance disturbance leading to falls.
  - Facial sensory loss and weakness are symptoms seen together with hearing loss, tinnitus, dysarthria, and signs of raised intracranial pressure in cerebellopontine angle tumours. Vertigo is often a late symptom.
  - Oscillopsia is an abnormal perception of objects moving side to side, or up and down, and is a symptom of impairment of the vestibulo-ocular reflex caused by peripheral vestibular dysfunction. Ask the patient *'Do you have difficulty seeing objects clearly or reading road signs whilst walking?'*
- **Cardiac symptoms.** Cardiac causes of dizziness may be accompanied by chest pain, dyspnoea, palpitations, orthopnoea, and paroxysmal nocturnal dyspnoea.
- **Psychiatric symptoms.** Ask about anxiety and panic attacks and aim to identify potential triggers.

B. Relevant medical history:

- Enquire about known cardiac conditions such as ischaemic heart disease, arrhythmias, valvular and other structural heart disease, and determine any recent deterioration in symptoms.
- Ask about known neurological disease such as migraine, epilepsy, and multiple sclerosis. Again, establish any recent deterioration in symptoms and their current management.
- Determine the presence of vascular risk factors (hypertension, diabetes mellitus, hyperlipidemia, previous vascular events) predisposing to vertebrobasilar ischaemia.
- Previous head injuries should be noted.
- Ask about a previous or current history of malignancy that may support a diagnosis of metastatic or paraneoplastic disease with a predilection for the cerebellum (breast, lung, and melanoma)?

C. Medications and allergies:

Patients may have a history of medical conditions treated by medications that cause dizziness as a side effect. Take note of:

- Anti-epileptics—phenytoin and carbemazepine may cause a cerebellar syndrome resulting in vertigo.
- Anti-hypertensives causing orthostatic hypotension.
- Ask specifically about previous administration of ototoxic drugs (aminoglycosides, salicylates, furosemide, and platinum-based chemotherapeutic agents).
- Has there been a recent increase in the doses or the frequency of current medications that can explain the dizziness?
- Insulin and oral hypoglycaemics.

D. Social issues:

- Chronic, excessive consumption of alcohol may support a diagnosis of cerebellar syndrome.
- Determine the impact of the patient's symptoms on their occupation and daily activities.

Formulating a plan of action

- Explain to the patient that a full clinical examination is required. This should include a full cardiovascular, neurological, and ENT examination, as well as postural blood pressure measurements. The integrity of the vestibulo-ocular reflex should be assessed in all cases to confirm or exclude peripheral vestibular dysfunction. In addition, the Hallpike test may be performed if BPPV is suspected.
- Explain the possible causes of dizziness as directed by the history and discuss the investigations necessary to determine the diagnosis.

Causes of vertigo

Consider the following investigations

- Blood count for anaemia. Excessive alcohol intake may cause a macrocytosis.
- Urea, creatinine, and electrolytes.
- 12-lead ECG for possible arrhythmias. Ambulatory ECG monitoring followed by echocardiography may be required for further evaluation of cardiac causes of dizziness.
- Audiometry is necessary for patients with hearing loss to define the type of deafness.
- CT/MRI scan of the head to exclude stroke, tumours, and traumatic injury to the petrous temporal bone. In addition, appearances consistent with demyelination suggest a possible diagnosis of multiple sclerosis. MRI scan is superior to CT for imaging the posterior fossa and brainstem.

Peripheral
- **Otological**
  - Otitis media/externa
  - perilymphatic fistula
- **Labyrinthine dysfunction**
  - Labyrinthitis
  - Vestibular neuronitis
  - Cerebrovascular disease (labyrinthine ischaemia/haemorrhage)
  - Trauma (fracture of petrous temporal bone, barotrauma)
- **Benign Paroxysmal Positional Vertigo (BPPV)**
- **Méniére's disease**
- **Bilateral vestibular failure**
  - Ototoxicity (see drug history)
- **Migrainous vertigo**

Central
- **Cerebellar and brainstem dysfunction**
  - Multiple sclerosis
  - Tumours: cerebellopontine angle (CPA), glioma, metastatic.
  - Basal meningitis
  - Cerebrovascular disease: vertebrobasilar ischaemia, Posterior fossa infarction, haemorrhage
  - Drugs (see drug history)
  - Migraine
- **Cerebrum**
  - Temporal lobe epilepsy
- **Hereditary**
  - Arnold-Chiari malformation
  - Friedreich's ataxia
  - Spinocerebellar ataxia

- Carotid duplex ultrasound and MRA (magnetic resonance angiogram)should be considered for suspected carotid or vertebrobasilar dissection.
- Caloric testing may be undertaken by specialists to assess vestibular dysfunction.

Questions commonly asked by examiners

What is Benign Paroxysmal Positional Vertigo (BPPV)?

Benign paroxymal positional vertigo (BPPV) is a condition associated with acute episodes of vertigo precipitated by rapid head movements in a particular direction thought to result from deposition of otoliths in the posterior semicircular canal. The condition is commonly idiopathic but can also be secondary to previous head injury or recent vestibular neuronitis.

How is BPPV distinguished from central vestibular lesions clinically?

- Nystagmus in BPPV is characteristically rotational and the fast phase is *away from* the affected side, occurring after a few seconds in the provoking position. Like other causes of peripheral vestibular dysfunction, the nystagmus fatigues with repeated testing. In contrast, nystagmus of a central cause persists for as long as the head remains in the position triggering it.
- The Hallpike manoeuvre confirms a diagnosis of BPPV. Vertigo is reproduced and a rotational nystagmus is observed when the head is suddenly turned to the affected side in the upright position and allowed to then hang off the edge of the examination couch.
- Patients with central disease will have other neurological symptoms and signs allowing localization of the lesion and differentiation from BPPV.

Clinical features of central and peripheral vertigo (see Volume 1 case 12: Nystagmus)

	Peripheral vertigo	Central vertigo
Nystagmus Direction	Unidirectional, fast phase *away from* the affected side	Bi-directional (can be unidirectional), fast component changes with direction of gaze
Type	Horizontal with a rotatory component	Horizontal, vertical, rotatory, mixed
Fatiguability	Fatigueable (continued gaze suppresses)	Non-fatigueable
Effect of lying still	Nystagmus improves	Nystagmus does not improve
Other neurological signs	Absent	Often present
Postural stability	Unidirectional tendency to fall (towards lesion)	Often multi-directional tendency to fall
Deafess/tinnitus	May be present	Absent

How is BPPV managed?

Physical manoeuvres such as the Epley and Semont manoeuvres, are effective in dispersing the otoliths. These strategies are therapeutic in 70–80% of patients. Recurrence is seen in approximately 20–30% and the Brandt-Daroff exercises are effective in controlling symptoms in such cases.

Drug therapy is of limited value in the treatment of BPPV.

Case 26 ◆ Collapse

INFORMATION FOR THE CANDIDATE

Dear Doctor,

Thank you for seeing this 24-year old gentleman whom I saw today accompanied by his friend. He has suffered with recurrent episodes of 'blackouts', each lasting a few seconds and preceded by 'lightheadedness'. He made complete recovery after each episode. There is no past medical or family history of note.

Many thanks for your opinion.

Acquiring the history

The history of any episodes of collapse should be evaluated in three parts: the events *preceding*, *during*, and *after* the event. Syncope must be differentiated from presyncope, dizziness, and vertigo. Presyncope refers to the prodromal symptoms prior to 'fainting'—these patients usually present with dizziness. A collateral history is *crucial* for an accurate account of the event.

A. History of presenting complaint:

Patients use various terms such as *collapse, funny turns, dizziness, passing out, faints*, and *fits* to describe syncope. It is important to determine exactly what the patient means, and if they lost consciousness (see below).

Age of onset

Most causes of collapse can present at any age, although cardiac syncope is more common in those with pre-existing cardiac disease.

Details of the event

(a) Symptoms preceding the collapse

*   Begin with an open statement such as *'Describe what happened'*, followed by focused questions to delineate the prodrome.
*   **Prodromal symptoms** *'How did you feel just before the collapse?'*; *'Did you experience any warning symptoms prior to the collapse?'* Ask specifically about:
    *   Nausea, abdominal pain, flushing, light-headedness, and blurred vision are premonitory symptoms associated with neurally mediated syncope.
    *   An aura may precede seizure activity. A general question may be *'Did you experience any strange sensations just before the episode?'* (Refer to Case 33 Seizures)
    *   Focal neurological symptoms suggest cerebrovascular disease. However, subsequent seizure activity may also represent secondary generalization of a partial seizure.
    *   Sudden onset of headache with meningism suggest subarachnoid haemorrhage.
    *   Headache, fever, meningism, and rash suggest meningitis.
    *   Chest pain, dyspnoea, or palpitations suggest a cardiac cause or palpitations. However, a sudden loss of consciousness without warning with rapid recovery is most likely to represent an arrhythmia.
*   **Precipitants** *'What were you doing just before the collapse?'* and *'Is there anything that triggers the episodes?'*. Ask specifically about precipitants of:
    *   Orthostatic hypotension—collapse occurring on standing, or during a change in posture, is most likely due to neurocardiogenic syncope. Syncope whilst supine suggests a cardiac cause.
    *   'Vasovagal'—triggered by a hot environment, prolonged standing or eating a large meal, is neurocardiogenic in origin.
    *   Situational syncope—during micturition, defecation, coughing, or sneezing, is also neurocardiogenic in aetiology.
    *   'Subclavian steal'—raising the arms above the head may precipitate collapse by a 'steal' phenomenon causing vertebrobasilar ischaemia.
    *   Seizure activity—triggers include stroboscopic/flashing lights, sleep deprivation, hunger, recent illness, illicit drugs, and alcohol.
    *   Carotid sinus hypersensitivity—neck movements, shaving, wearing a tight collar.
    *   Exertional syncope is cardiac in origin until proven otherwise, typically resulting from left ventricular outflow obstruction (e.g. aortic stenosis or hypertrophic obstructive cardiomyopathy) or arrhythmia.
    *   Hypoglycaemia—prolonged periods of fasting, during the night, or before mealtimes.
    *   Anxiety or fear leading to hyperventilation and consequent neurocardiogenic syncope.

(b) Determine the events during the episode. These questions are essential to distinguish seizures and epilepsy (see Case 33 seizures).

- *'Did you lose consciousness?'* Impairment in consciousness *always* occurs in generalized seizures, complex-partial seizures, and syncope, but not simple-partial seizures and pre-syncope.
- *'Do you remember falling to the floor?'* or *'Do you remember what happened during the collapse?'* may distinguish true syncope or seizures from presyncope, dizziness and falls.
- **Collateral history.** Establish the nature of the event from a witness. Ask specifically about:
- Colour of the patient during the event; pallor suggests syncope, cyanosis may occur with tonic-clonic seizures.
- Seizure activity.
  - ◆ *Tonic-clonic seizures:*
    - − *'Was there any stiffening followed by jerking of the limbs?*
    - − *'Tongue-biting?'*
    - − *'Frothing at the mouth?'*
    - − *'Loss of control of urine or faeces?'*
    - − *'Rolling of the eyes?'*
    - − *'Repeated head turning to one side?'*
  - ◆ *Absence seizures:*
    - − *'Did he/she appear vacant with repetitive eyeblinking?'*
- Duration of the episode. Syncope usually lasts a few seconds, whereas seizure activity may last several minutes.
- Presence of a pulse during the episode. This can be extremely useful, although unless the witness is medically trained to examine for a pulse the information may not be reliable.

(c) Ask about symptoms after the episode

- Ask about time to recovery, *'How long did it take for you to feel back to normal?'* Recovery is rapid in cardiogenic and vasovagal syncope and more prolonged after seizure activity.
- Determine if there was any confusion, headache, or limb weakness after the collapse suggestive of a post-ictal period and thus seizure activity.
- Evidence of injury sustained during the event either from the collapse itself or tonic-clonic movements.
- **Number of previous episodes** *'How many times has this happened before? Did you experience the same symptoms each time?'.* Benign causes of syncope are usually associated with a single episode, although the risk of a serious disorder increases with multiple episodes.

B. Relevant medical and family history:

Past medical history

- Previous history of structural or ischaemic cardiac disease strongly favours a cardiogenic syncope.
- Epilepsy.
- Diabetes mellitus can cause syncope through autonomic failure and orthostatic hypotension or as a result of hypoglycaemia caused by treatment. Enquire about symptoms of hypoglycaemia awareness.
- Parkinson's disease or multisystem atrophy similarly cause autonomic failure and syncope.
- Respiratory disease may cause cough syncope.
- Anxiety disorders may cause hyperventilation and syncope.
- Hypothyroidism may cause sinus bradycardia and collapse.

Family history:

• Sudden death suggesting hypertrophic cardiomyopathy and long QT syndrome.

C. Medications and interactions:

• Insulin and oral hypoglycaemics. Ask about frequency and dose. Is there possibility of overdose?

• β-blockers (including eye drops) can cause symptomatic bradycardia.

• Diuretics, ACE inhibitors, and angiotensin receptor blockers cause postural hypotension.

• Calcium channels blockers and nitrates cause vasodilatation.

• Anticonvulsants. Ask about frequency, dose and compliance with medications.

D. Social issues:

• Enquire about the nature of the patient's current occupation, and establish the risk for the patient and others from recurrent collapse (e.g. if the patient operates heavy machinery).

• Ask the patient if they drive, and the type of vehicle. Ask if they are aware of DVLA regulations.

• Ask about recreational activities which may be hazardous.

• Ask about the patient's alcohol consumption.

Formulating a plan of action

• Explain to the patient that a clinical examination and ECG will be required.

• Reassure the patient that a single episode of collapse is likely to be benign, but further investigations may be necessary as suggested by the history.

• Consider the following investigations

◆ **Capillary blood glucose** for hypoglycaemia.

◆ **ECG** for arrhythmias (bradycardia, second degree and complete heart block, prolonged QT syndrome, and sustained ventricular tachycardia) and ischaemic changes.

◆ **Blood tests**

– Blood count. Anaemia may cause dizziness and pre-syncope.

– U&Es.

– Serum corrected calcium and magnesium. Electrolyte imbalances precipitate arrhythmias and seizures.

– Serum glucose.

– Cardiac enzymes and troponin for cardiac ischaemia.

◆ **Echocardiography** for diagnosis of aortic stenosis, features of hypertrophic obstructive cardiomyopathy, and left ventricular function.

◆ **24-hour ambulatory ECG monitoring**, although this will only be of value during symptomatic periods.

Further investigations:

• **Prolonged ambulatory ECG monitoring** such as event recorders or implantable loop recorders.

• **Imaging**

• CT of the brain will not usually be adequate to fully assess the posterior circulation, therefore a subsequent MRI may be required.

• Carotid doppler for carotid stenosis or dissection

• MRA of the vertebral vessels for suspected vertebrobasilar ischaemia.

• **Electrophysiological studies (EPS)** for evaluation of tachyarrhythmias.

• **Tilt table test** for diagnosis of neurally mediated syncope.

- **Carotid sinus massage** for definitive diagnosis of carotid sinus hypersensitivity.
- **Electroencephalogram** may be indicated in patients with seizures when no other cause is identified.

Questions commonly asked by examiners

How can syncope and seizures be differentiated clinically?

FEATURES	SYNCOPE	SEIZURES
Prodromal features	• Usually warning, unless cardiac cause. • Often external triggers, e.g. anxiety, meals. • 'Pre-syncopal symptoms', e.g. flushing, nausea, sweating, pallor, blurred vision	• Aura or no warning. • Duration of few seconds
Loss of consciousness	• Short duration— few minutes	• Longer duration— few minutes
Features during episode	• Usually motionless • Incontinence and myoclonic jerks may occur • Possible injury	• Automatisms • Tonic-clonic movements (stiffening then jerking of limbs) • Cyanosis • Tongue biting • Incontinence
Recovery	• Rapid and complete recovery in a few seconds	• Slow recovery with possible confusion, headache and post-ictal weakness (Todd's paralysis)

What is the mechanism of neurocardiogenic (vasovagal) syncope?

Patients with neurocardiogenic syncope are usually young and otherwise healthy, and typically have a prodrome of nausea, sweating, warmth, pallor, and light-headedness. The mechanism is autonomic activation resulting in:

- a cardioinhibitory response due to increased parasympathetic tone, causing bradycardia and AV block.
- a vasodepressor response due to decreased sympathetic activity causing hypotension.

How is neurally mediated syncope diagnosed?

The tilt-table test is indicated in patients with suspected neurocardiogenic syncope. Baseline heart rate and blood pressure are measured, and ECG monitoring performed in the supine position. The patient is then tilted upright to 60 degrees. The onset of syncope and a cardioinhibitory, vasodepressor, or mixed response, upon tilting the patient from a supine to upright position, confirms the diagnosis of neurally mediated syncope.

If the initial response is negative, a glycerine trinitrate or isoprenaline infusion is administered and the procedure is repeated. The tilt test may also reveal other forms of neurally mediated responses: postural hypotension (hypotension with no drop in heart rate) and postural orthostatic tachycardia syndrome (hypotension with tachycardia).

Table 26.1 Causes of syncope

Cardiac
- Arrhythmias: Sinus bradycardia, sick sinus syndrome, heart block, sustained ventricular tachycardia, prolonged QT syndrome
- Aortic stenosis
- Hypertrophic obstructive cardiomyopathy
- Myocardial infarction

Neurological
- Epilepsy
- Autonomic failure: diabetes mellitus, Parkinson's disease, multisystem atrophy
- Neurally mediated syncope: vasovagal, situational (cough, micturition, defecation)
- Carotid sinus hypersensitivity
- Vertebrobasilar ischaemia

Metabolic
- Hypoglycaemia

Other
- Orthostatic hypotension: drugs, haemorrhage, dehydration
- Hyperventilation syndrome

What is carotid sinus hypersensitivity?

Carotid sinus hypersensitivity is an inappropriate cardioinhibitory and vasodepressor response initiated by increased baroreceptor sensitivity, triggered by neck movements and pressure to the neck. The diagnosis is made when there is a ventricular pause of at least 3 seconds and a fall in blood pressure of more than 50 mmHg during carotid sinus massage. Cardiac pacing is indicated for symptomatic bradycardia.

Case 27 ◆ Headache

INFORMATION FOR THE CANDIDATE

Dear Doctor,

Thank you for seeing this 28-year old lady presenting with a 3-day history of sudden onset headache with nausea and vomiting. She has a background of frequent episodes of headache different to this headache. She uses the combined oral contraceptive pill only.

Many thanks for your opinion.

Acquiring the history

Headache is a common presentation and a detailed history must be obtained to guide investigation and treatment. The diagnostic approach is to exclude serious causes of headache before a diagnosis of a benign primary headache type is made.

A. History of presenting complaint
Age of onset
Characteristics of the headache:

- **Onset of headache.** Determine if the headache was sudden or gradual in onset. Sudden-onset headache and vomiting is characteristic of subarachnoid haemorrhage (SAH), and warrants urgent investigation and management.
- **Site** *'Where did the pain first start?'*
  - Tension headache is a bilateral pain across the forehead
  - Migraine is usually unilateral and frontoparietal (60-70%), although can be bilateral or global.
  - Cluster headache is always unilateral and retrorbital.
  - Temporal arteritis is usually temporal in location.
  - Subarachnoid haemorrhage and meningitis are usually occipital, although they can present in any location and are therefore differentiated by onset (e.g. sudden onset for SAH), and associated features (e.g. meningism).
- **Radiation** *'Did the pain spread anywhere?'.* Pain which radiates into the neck and shoulders may represent meningism, and should be investigated further.
- **Character** Begin with an open statement such as *'Describe the pain to me'* and give examples if necessary: *'Is it throbbing? Tight? Shooting? Stabbing?'*

Alarm symptoms
- *Sudden onset headache*, reaching maximal intensity within a few minutes, suggests SAH.
- *Change in nature of headache*—patients with recurrent, severe headache are likely to have migraine, although a severe headache out of keeping with severe episodes may be SAH.
- *Progressive increase in severity of headache* suggests space-occupying lesion, subdural haemorrhage or analgesia-overuse headache.
- *Focal neurological symptoms, other than typical visual or sensory aura,* suggest a space-occupying or vascular lesion.
- *Any change in conscious level* suggests a serious cause of headache.
- *New headache in high risk groups,* such as patients with malignancy (cerebral metastases), pregnancy (venous sinus thrombosis, pituitary apoplexy) and HIV (opportunistic infection or cerebral lymphoma).

Frequency and analgesia. The 'brief headache screen' has been proposed by the American Academy of Neurology to differentiate causes of chronic headache.
1. *How often do you get severe headaches (severe enough to impair daily function)?*
2. *How often do you get milder headaches?*
3. *How often do you take painkillers for headaches?*

The first question has a high sensitivity and moderate specificity for patients with migraine. The second and third questions are useful to identify patients with medication overuse for mild headache (daily headache or medication use more than three times per week).

- **Duration.** Migraine usually lasts 12–24 hours and may persist up to 72 hours. Cluster headache typically lasts minutes to hours.
- **Temporal pattern**
  - *'Is the pain worse on waking up in the morning?'.* This suggests raised intracranial pressure.
  - *'Is the pain worse at the end of the day?'.* This is characteristic of tension type headache.
  - *'Does the pain wake you up from sleep?'* and *'Does it occur at the same time each day?'.* These are typical features of a cluster headache.

Associated symptoms:

- *Aura* is a feature of migraine in approximately 30% of patients. Patients usually experience prodromal visual aura in the form of fortification spectra (ziz-zag lines and flashing lines) and scintillating scotoma (areas of loss of vision with bright edges). Patients may also experience positive sensory or motor aura, as well as olfactory and gustatory hallucinations.
- *Photophobia, phonophobia, osmophobia* (sensitivity to light, sounds, and movements respectively) are features of migraine.
- *Limb weakness* suggests cerebrovascular disease, but can also be a feature of migraine.
- *Sensory disturbance*—positive sensory symptoms occur in migraine with aura.
- *Visual disturbance*—as well as visual aura, ask about sudden loss of vision due to amaurosis fugax or giant cell arteritis, and diplopia in pituitary masses and apoplexy. Visual disorders may also cause headache—refractive errors may cause frontal headache, acute angle closure glaucoma may cause a red eye and severe unilateral headache.
- *Fever, neck stiffness, photophobia, and rash* suggest meningitis
- *Scalp tenderness and jaw claudication* are indicative of giant cell arteritis,
- *Lacrimation, rhinorrhoea, sweating, drooping of the eyelid, and conjunctival suffusion* are all features of a cluster headache.
- *Ear, tooth, facial, and neck pain* are causes of referred pain to the head.
- *Nausea and vomiting* are symptoms of migraine and elevated intracranial pressure. The vomiting is profuse, projectile, and unprovoked in space-occupying lesions.
- *Confusion, behavioural change, and seizures* suggest space occupying lesions in particular brain tumours and encephalitis.
- *Constitutional symptoms*: weight loss and anorexia suggesting neoplastic disease, fever suggests infection, proximal muscle weakness occurs with polymyalgia rheumatica/giant cell arteritis.

Precipitating factors

- Certain foods and drink can trigger a migraine: red wine, cheese and chocolate
- Hunger
- Sleep deprivation
- Sounds and bright lights
- Menstruation
- Sexual activity

Aggravating factors

- Ask the patient specifically about features of raised intracranial pressure; *'Is the headache made worse by coughing, sneezing, or bending forwards?'* Note that a benign cough headache is also a recognized primary headache type therefore can be a non-specific symptom.
- *'Does light, noise, certain smells, and movement make the headache worse?'* This is typical of migraine.
- *'Does alcohol make the headache worse?'* This is a feature *during* a cluster headache and ceases as the headache subsides.

Relieving factors

- Sleep, quiet darkened room
- Analgesia

Severity and progression

- Assess the severity of the pain on a scale; *'Where do you rate your pain on a scale of 1 to 10, 1 being mild pain and 10 the worst headache ever experienced?'*
- Assess the progression; *'Is the headache the same when it first started, getting better or worse?'*

Other factors

- Is there a history of recent head injury, trauma, a fall or neck injury? Headaches caused by intra and extracranial haemorrhage can arise from head injuries and neck trauma is a cause of extracranial arterial dissection.
- Enquire about recent illnesses: ear, eye infection, and sinusitis as a cause of the headache. An intracerebral abscess can result from spread of a middle ear infection to the CNS.

B. Relevant medical and family history:

- Enquire about personal history of:
  - Migraine
  - Autosomal dominant polycystic renal disease is associated with berry aneurysms and therefore subarachnoid haemorrhage
  - Previous malignancy
  - HIV and immunosuppression. Such patients are at risk of toxoplasmosis, cerebral abscesses, and meningitis.
  - Depression or anxiety as a trigger
  - Bleeding disorders or coagulopathies that can cause haemorrhage or venous sinus thrombosis
- Enquire about family history of:
  - Subarachnoid haemorrhage
  - Migraine
  - Thromboses

C. Medications:

- Enquire about medications that the patient takes that cause a headache as a side effect:
  - Nitrates
  - Calcium channel blockers
  - Dipyridamole
  - Others: Tetracycline, vitamin A derivatives and steroids are associated with idiopathic intracranial hypertension
- Anticoagulant and antiplatelet agents can cause cerebral haemorrhage subtherapeutic anticoagulation is a risk factor for cerebral venous sinus thrombosis in patients with a thrombophilia
- Ask about what analgesics the patient takes for headache relief: ask specifically about type, dose, frequency, and efficacy. Headaches despite the use of regular analgesics may suggest medication overuse headache. This is confirmed if the headaches subside within a two month period after discontinuing analgesics.
- In women, ask about the use of the oral contraceptive pill which increases the risk of cerebral venous sinus thrombosis. This risk is further increased in patients with migraine with aura and idiopathic intracranial hypertension.
- Ask about recreational drug use and withdrawal. Cocaine abuse is a risk factor for subarachnoid haemorrhage.

Social issues:

- Ask about the patient's occupation and enquire about any particular stresses at work which may be a trigger for headaches. Also ask about the impact of frequent headaches on attendance at work.

- Ask about financial problems and about any difficulties at home as precipitants.
- Ask about any recent travel abroad (meningitis, cerebral TB, and malaria) and ill contacts (meningitis).
- Smoking history and any recent attempts at cessation as nicotine withdrawal can result in headache.
- Elicit the patient's ideas and concerns about the nature and cause of their symptoms.

Formulating a plan of action

- Explain to the patient that a *new, sudden onset* or a *change in the character* of headache from previous episodes will require a full clinical examination and investigation for the cause.
- Investigations will be determined by the history
- Blood tests:

Diagnoses to consider in acute onset headache	Primary headache types	Secondary headache types
Subarachnoid haemorrhage	Migraine with or without aura	Infection: meningitis, abscess
Meningitis	Tension type	Neoplastic: primary brain tumour and metastases
Carotid or vertebral dissection	Trigeminal autonomic cephalgias: Cluster headache	Vascular: subarchanoid haemorrhage, giant cell arteritis, extracranial arterial dissection, venous sinus thrombosis
Cerebral venous sinus thrombosis	Exertional	Trauma: head or neck injury
Pituitary apoplexy	Medication over use	Referred pain; ear, teeth, sinuses, face

- Blood count. A raised white cell count will indicate an infection
- ESR and CRP will be raised in giant cell arteritis and infection
- Consider pituitary hormone profiles in cases of pituitary adenoma or apoplexy for hypopituitarism. Tests will include serum prolactin, thyroid function tests, growth hormone (GH), luteinizing hormone/follicle stimulating hormone (LH/FSH), and a short synacthen test.
- Consider a thrombophilia screen in patients with cerebral venous sinus thrombosis. Tests will include assays for activated protein C resistance, protein C and S, factor V leiden PCR, antithrombin, anti-cardiolipin antibody, lupus anticoagulant.
- **Imaging:**
  - Plain x-rays of the skull and the cervical spine are indicated in patients with a history of head and neck trauma to exclude these as a cause for a headache.
  - CT scan of the head is indicated in any patient presenting with:
    - New, sudden onset, or a change in the character of headache
    - Clinical suspicion of intracerebral space-occupying lesion: postural headache, seizures and focal neurological signs, papilloedema on examination
    - Confusion, behavioural change, and impaired consciousness
  - MRI head is considered in patients with suspected pituitary disease. Magnetic resonance venography (MRV) is performed in patients with suspected cerebral venous thrombosis.

- Angiography (CT, MRI, or digital subtraction) is performed to determine the integrity of the extracranial vasculature. It will detect a carotid or vertebral dissection, and is performed after a positive CT scan for a subarachnoid haemorrhage or the presence of CSF xanthochromia to detect the presence and site of intracranial aneurysms amenable to neurosurgical intervention.

- **Lumbar puncture:** Opening pressure is raised in intracranial pressure of any cause and idiopathic intracranial hypertension
  - Appearance of fluid: turbid indicates infection
  - Cell count: red cell, white cell count, and differential
  - Biochemistry: protein, glucose
  - Microbiology: gram stain, India ink for Cryptococcus, and Cryptococcal antigen
  - Ziehl-Nielson stain for tuberculosis
  - Xanthochromia for subarachnoid haemorrhage in patients with no evidence of haemorrhage on CT head
  - Note to take a simultaneous blood sample for serum glucose, total protein, and bilirubin at the time of LP.

- **Other investigations:** these are requested according to the history
  - Temporal artery biopsy is done ideally within 7 days of commencing steroid therapy for a definitive diagnosis of giant cell arteritis.
  - Throat swab, stool culture, and viral PCR for bacterial and viral meningitis.

Questions commonly asked by examiners

What is the aetiology of a subarachnoid haemorrhage?

The causes of a subarachnoid haemorrhage are can be subdivided into aneurysmal and non-aneurysmal:

- **Aneurysms:** Berry, traumatic and mycotic
- **Non-aneurysmal:** perimesencephalic, arteriovenous malformation, clotting dysfunction, trauma, cocaine abuse

80% of cases are the result of a ruptured aneurysm.

How is a suspected subarachnoid haemorrhage investigated and managed?

All patients with a suspected subarachnoid haemorrhage should undergo a CT scan of the head as soon as possible. The sensitivity of CT in detecting subarachnoid blood is 95% within 12 hours of symptom onset and decreases with time (50% on day 7 and 30% on day 14).

A lumbar puncture for the detection of xanthochromia is mandatory if the CT scan is negative and the clinical suspicion of a subarachnoid haemorrhage is high. It should be performed at least 12 hours after symptom onset and xanthochromia is sensitive for a subarachnoid bleed up to two weeks post-haemorrhage: sensitivity is 70% at 3 weeks and 40% at 4 weeks post-haemorrhage. Spectrophotometry is performed to calculate the net bilirubin and oxyhaemoglobin, both of which will be present in a subarachnoid haemorrhage. False positive results occur with hyperbilirubinaemia and high CSF protein, therefore results should be interpreted in conjunction with serum bilirubin.

Once a subarachnoid haemorrhage has been confirmed, either CT angiography or digital subtraction angiography is required for the identification of an aneurysm as the source of the bleed.

Management of a subarachnoid haemorrhage involves:

- Symptom relief with adequate analgesia
- Prevention of vasospasm induced ischaemia with hydration and nimodipine

- Maintenance of normal blood pressure with nimodipine or labetalol
- Prevention of re-bleeding with neurosurgical intervention. Options include early microvascular clipping or endovascular coiling of the aneurysm.

What is the medical management of migraine?

The medical management of migraine is twofold:

- **Prevention of attacks** (considered in patients with 3 or more migraine attacks per month, severe disability or those unresponsive to acute attack treatment)
    - First-line agents are propanolol and atenolol
    - Second-line agents include amitriptylline, topiramate, and sodium valproate
- **Treatment of acute attacks**
    - Simple analgesia: paracetamol and non-steroidal anti-inflammatory agents
    - Anti-emetics
    - Triptans: rapid onset triptans include sumatriptan and zolmitriptan. Delayed onset with longer duration triptans in use are naratriptan and frovatriptan.
    - Ergot derivatives such as ergotamine are used in patients with contraindications to triptans.

Further reading

1. Goadsby PJ et al., Migraine—Current understanding and treatment, New Engl J Med. 2002; 346:257–69.

2. Suarez JI et al, Aneurysmal Subarachnoid Hemorrhage, New Engl J Med. 2006; 354:4: 387396.

3. Dodick D, Chronic daily headache, New Engl J Med. 2006; 354:2: 158–65.

4. Cruickshank A et al, Revised national guidelines for analysis of CSF for bilirubin in suspected subarachnoid haemorrhage, Annals of Clinical Biochemistry. 2008; 45:238–44.

5. Bederson JB et al. Guidelines for the Management of Aneurysmal Subarachnoid Hemorrhage. A Statement for Healthcare Professionals From a Special Writing Group of the Stroke Council, American Heart Association. Stroke 2009; 40(3):994–1025.

Case 28 ◆ **Visual Disturbance**

INFORMATION FOR THE CANDIDATE

Dear Doctor,

Thank you for seeing this 32-year old lady who complains of 'blindness in the right eye' over last 2 days. She reports a similar episode a few months ago which resolved spontaneously within 2 weeks of onset. There are no associated symptoms. Her medical history included type 1 diabetes with good glycaemic control. She is a non smoker and drinks alcohol occasionally. She works as a medical secretary and is concerned about her symptoms affecting her work.

Many thanks for your opinion.

Acquiring the history

Obtaining a history about visual disturbance involves enquiry about a range of visual symptoms which may be of an ocular or neuro-ophthalmic cause. Symptoms include: visual loss, blurring, diplopia, reduced coloured vision, and positive symptoms such as scintillations, fortification spectra, floaters, and illusions.

A. History of presenting complaint:

Begin with an open statement such as *'Tell me about your symptoms'* to determine the type of visual disturbance the patient is experiencing, followed by detailed questioning to establish a likely cause for the patient's symptoms.

Age of onset
Type of visual disturbance

(1) Visual loss. A detailed history about visual loss is important to avoid missing causes that may lead to progressive and permanent visual loss if left untreated. Patients will often use the term 'visual loss', or 'blindness' to describe reduced visual acuity, blurred vision, and reduced coloured vision and it is vital to probe further to reveal the exact nature of the visual disturbance for possible clues to the underlying aetiology.

- **Onset.** *'When did you first notice the loss of vision? Did it come on suddenly or gradually?'* The speed of onset of the visual loss can be helpful in determining the underlying cause. Occasionally conditions causing progressive visual loss may only be noticed incidentally when one is closed and therefore the time of onset may be inaccurate.

Acute onset visual loss	Gradual onset visual loss
Ocular	**Ocular**
Acute closed angle glaucoma*	Retinitis Pigmentosa
Retinal detachment	Open angle glaucoma
Vitreous haemorrhage	Cataracts
Central retinal artery/vein occlusion	Diabetic/hypertensive retinopathy
Anterior uveitis*	Macular degeneration
Endophthalmitis*	
Neuro-ophthalmic	**Neuro-ophthalmic**
Demyelinating optic neuritis#	Optic nerve compression of any cause
Anterior ischaemic optic neuropathy (Giant cell arteritis)	Nutritional and toxic optic neuropathies
Non-arteritic anterior ischaemic optic neuropathy	Papilloedema of any cause
Leber's hereditary optic neuropathy	
Amaurosis fugax	
Stroke	
Migraine	

* Common cause of acute painful visual loss.
# Demyelinating optic neuritis is characterized by subacute onset of painful visual loss over a period of hours to days with recovery within two to four weeks of onset.

- **Unilateral vs. bilateral.** *'Is the visual loss affecting one eye or both?'* Unilateral visual loss is highly suggestive of ocular and optic nerve pathology. However, patients with visual field defects such as homonymous hemianopias will also complain of unilateral visual loss which is detected objectively on clinical examination. Bilateral visual loss suggests pathology posterior to the optic chiasm, and the patient will complain of visual loss when both eyes are closed in turn.

- **Extent of visual loss.** *'Which part of the vision is affected? All? Top half? Bottom half? Sides? Central?'; 'Is this the same in both eyes?'* The extent of visual loss is difficult to determine in the history alone but can give important clues to the type of visual field loss present and the possible underlying cause. It may be useful to ask the patient to map out the area(s) of visual loss.

    ◆ Monocular visual field defect is complete visual loss in one eye that results from optic nerve lesions anterior to the optic chiasm in the affected eye.

    ◆ Central scotomas occur with optic neuropathies and age-related macular degeneration.

    ◆ Altitudinal visual loss suggests anterior ischaemic optic neuropathy in which patients experience visual loss in the upper or lower half of the visual field.

    ◆ Peripheral visual field defects, for example retinal detachment, bitemporal, and homonymous hemianopias, may go unnoticed by patients. In advanced cases of bitemporal visual field loss, patients may complain of colliding into peripheral objects on both sides and with homonymous hemianopia patients may have difficulty reading lines across a page.

- *'Did the visual loss begin on the outside and extend to the centre?'* This is characteristic of rhegmatogenous retinal detachment. Floaters and flashing lights are associated symptoms.

- **Progression and recovery.** *'Is it getting better, staying the same or getting worse over time?'* If visual loss is transient, determine the frequency of episodes of visual loss, duration and aggravating factors.

Monocular transient visual loss is seen with:

- **Amaurosis fugax.** Patients often describe this as a 'curtain coming down' in their field of vision in one eye which resolves completely within minutes to hours. It is a result of thromboembolism.

- **Demyelinating optic neuritis.** Visual loss improves gradually over a period of two to four weeks.

- **Papilloedema.** Patients with papilloedema can experience unilateral or bilateral transient visual obscurations (TVO) that include symptoms of transient blurring or loss of vision lasting a few seconds with complete recovery between episodes. TVOs are aggravated by changes in intracranial pressure such as postural changes and straining.

- **Giant cell arteritis.** Transient and intermittent episodes of visual loss can precede permanent visual loss in some cases.

Binocular transient visual loss is caused by: papilloedema, migraine, optic chiasmal compression, and postural hypotension and vertebrobasilar ischaemia.

Demyelinating optic neuropathy characteristically resolves within a few weeks of onset. Causes of gradually progressive visual loss are listed above.

(2) Eye pain.

- *'Do you have any pain in or around the eye?' 'Describe the type of pain you have?'* Localized eye or periorbital pain is suggestive of orbital pathology. Optic neuritis is associated with a deep, dull, retrobulbar pain which is characteristically worse on moving the eye. Acute closed angle glaucoma, iritis, and thyroid ophthalmopathy are other causes of such pain. Cluster headache is also associated with retrobulbar pain and may be mistaken for ocular pathology.

- Gritty or burning type pain is suggestive of dry eyes, keratitis, conjunctivitis, blepharitis, corneal ulceration, and thyroid ophthalmopathy.

- *'Is the pain worse on moving the eye?'* A number of conditions are associated with pain on movement of the eyes. The causes for painful ophthalmoplegia are listed in the section in examiner's questions for Case 29 Double Vision.

(3) Diplopia
Ask about double vision, and follow with focused questions about the double vision if necessary (Case 29 Double Vision).

(4) Reduced colour vision
- *'Have you noticed any greying of the vision or loss of colour vision?'* Disturbance of colour vision is a typical feature of optic nerve disorders.

(5) Positive visual symptoms
- *'Do you experience flashing lights, zig-zag, or other patterns in your field of vision?'* Positive visual symptoms such as scintillating scotomas (flashing lights and zig-zag patterns) are associated with migraine, retinal lesions (posterior vitreous detachment, retinal detachment), occipital lobe space-occupying lesions, and occipital epilepsy.
- *'Do you see haloes around lights?'* Haloes typically occur with acute glaucoma and cataracts.

(6) Other eye symptoms. Ask about ptosis and redness of the eye.
- **Associated neurological symptoms** Headache has a wide differential diagnosis and may be associated with ocular, orbital and intracranial pathology therefore a detailed history about headache is necessary. Ask about:
  - Site of headache—generalized headache may result from a wide range of causes such as space-occupying lesions, trauma, and tension type headache. Localized frontal and facial pain may be associated with refractive errors, sinus disease, ocular, and intraocular pathology. Facial pain, paraesthesiae, and numbness particularly in the territory of the ophthalmic and maxillary divisions of the trigeminal nerve and in the context of cranial nerve palsies suggest a lesion in the cavernous sinus. Temporal headache with scalp tenderness suggests giant cell arteritis.
  - Sudden onset headache occurs with giant cell arteritis, intracranial haemorrhage, and meningitis.
  - Headache that is typically aggravated by postural changes, straining, and coughing suggests raised intracranial pressure. Vomiting is also a symptom.
- Ask about other neurological symptoms: limb weakness, facial weakness, sensory disturbance, gait difficulty, hearing impairment, tinnitus, bulbar symptoms, and bladder dysfunction are useful in localizing intracranial lesions.
- **Trauma** to the eye, face, head, and neck can result in various visual disturbances.

B. Relevant medical and family history:
Past medical history
- The presence of vascular risk factors, ischaemic heart disease, atrial fibrillation or cerebrovascular disease suggests a cardioembolic mechanism of disease causing visual disturbance (amaurosis fugax).
- Visual complications of diabetes mellitus include: retinopathy, maculopathy, and ischaemic cranial nerve palsies.
- Optic neuritis can occur in patients with a history of multiple sclerosis.
- Previous history of malignancy may suggest intracranial metastatic disease.
- Vitamin B12 and folate deficiency can give rise to optic neuropathy.
- Graves disease with eye involvement can give rise to diplopia due to extraocular restrictive myopathy.

- Upward lens dislocation leading to diplopia is a feature of Marfan syndrome.
- Childhood strabismus and congenital fourth nerve palsy are potential causes of diplopia in adulthood.

Family history

Enquiry about family history of Leber's hereditary optic neuropathy, other congenital optic neuropathies, and retinitis pigmentosa can be useful for future genetic counselling.

C. Medications:

- Medications causing optic neuropathy include: isoniazid, ethambutol, vincristine, cisplatin, ciclosporin, disulfiram, sidenafil, and amiodarone.
- Antiepileptics (phenytoin, topiramate, and carbamazepine) can cause diplopia as a side effect.

D. Social issues:

- Ask the patient about smoking which is a risk factor for atherosclerosis and Graves ophthalmopathy.
- Take a detailed dietary and alcohol consumption history since thiamine, folate, and vitamin B12 deficiencies all lead to nutritional optic neuropathies.
- Enquire about previous exposure to toxins such as lead and carbon monoxide that are associated with optic nerve disease.
- Determine the impact of the patient's visual disturbance on occupation, daily, and recreational activities.

Formulating a plan of action

Explain the likely diagnosis or differential diagnoses to the patient based on the history. Also explain that a definitive diagnosis can only be made based on the history together with a clinical examination and appropriate investigations. Consider the following investigations:

- Blood count: a leucocytosis and raised inflammatory markers suggest infective or inflammatory cause.
- Vitamin B12 and folate levels. Consider anti-intrinsic factor antibodies in suspected cases of pernicious anaemia.
- Thyroid function tests for Graves disease. TSH receptor antibodies may be measured to confirm the diagnosis of Grave's disease.
- ACE and C-ANCA titres for suspected inflammatory and granulomatous disease (sarcoidosis and Wegener's granulomatosis respectively).
- Syphilis serology.
- Mitochondrial DNA analysis may be considered if there is a family history of Leber's hereditary optic neuropathy.
- Consider temporal artery biopsy in giant cell arteritis.
- Acetylcholine receptor antibody titres for the diagnosis of myasthenia gravis. A tensilon test is rarely required.
- Neuroimaging (CT head, MRI brain, MRA) is undertaken if intracranial and orbital pathology is suspected and in multiple sclerosis.

Questions commonly asked by examiners

What are the causes of optic neuropathies?

- Demyelinating optic neuritis (multiple sclerosis)
- Anterior ischaemic optic neuropathy (caused by giant cell arteritis)

- Non-arteritic anterior ischaemic optic neuropathy (associated with vascular risks factors, anaemia, hypotension, and collagen vascular disorders).
- Compressive optic neuropathies: meningioma, optic nerve gliomas, and metastases (lymphoma, leukaemia, and solid tumours)
- Nutritional: thiamine, vitamin B12, and folate deficiency
- Drugs and toxins: ethambutol, amiodarone, isoniazid, vincristine, cisplatin, sildenafil, disulfiram, ciclosporin, lead, carbon monoxide, and ethylene glycol.
- Orbital trauma.
- Infection: syphilis and Lyme disease
- Hereditary: Leber's hereditary optic neuropathy and congenital.

What is the treatment of demyelinating optic neuritis?

Optic Neuritis Treatment Trial, a randomized controlled trial that evaluated the effect of treatment with corticosteroids for acute optic neuritis revealed that a 3-day course of intravenous methylprednisolone followed by a two week course of oral prednisolone at 1mg/kg/day for 11 days then tapered over the remaining 4 days, accelerated the recovery of visual disturbance in comparison to a two week course of oral prednisolone alone and placebo. However, corticosteroids only speed recovery from symptoms and do not modify disease progression in multiple sclerosis.

NICE guidance recommends the use of intravenous methylprednisolone at a dose of 500mg–1g for 3–5 days or high dose oral methylprednisolone 500mg–2g daily for 3–5 days for an acute relapse of multiple sclerosis.

Further reading

1. The Optic Neuritis Study Group. Multiple Sclerosis Risk after Optic Neuritis: Final Optic Neuritis Treatment Trial Follow-Up. Arch Neurol. 2008; 65(6):727–32.

2. National Institute for Health and Clinical Excellence Multiple Sclerosis: Management of multiple sclerosis in primary and secondary care. London: NICE, November 2003.

Case 29 ◆ Double Vision

INFORMATION FOR THE CANDIDATE

Dear Doctor,

Thank you for seeing this 50-year old gentleman who complains of 'double vision' and drooping of the right eyelid. He has no previous history of any ophthalmic problems. He was recently diagnosed with hypertension for which he is taking ramipril and bendroflumethiazide. He is smoker and works as a taxi driver.

Many thanks for your opinion.

Acquiring the history

Diplopia is a symptom with a wide differential diagnosis that includes both ophthalmic and neurological causes. A comprehensive history alongside a thorough clinical examination leads to the diagnosis with minimal investigation in most cases. In addition, a thorough history is important to elicit symptoms which may warrant immediate investigation and/or specialist input to exclude serious pathology. Consider the following differential diagnoses when evaluating a patient presenting with diplopia.

Monocular diplopia	Binocular diplopia
Cataract	**Orbital lesions**
Corneal disease	• Acute orbitopathy
Lens dislocation	• Orbital fractures
Refractive errors	• Cellulitis
Macular disease	• Tumours
Visual cortex disease (rare)	
	Muscle disease
	• Graves ophthalmopathy
	• Orbital myositis
	• Genetic myopathy: chronic progressive external ophthalmoplegia (CPEO), Kearns-sayre syndrome (triad of CPEO, pigmentary retinopathy and onset before age 20).
	Neuromuscular junction
	• Myasthenia Gravis
	• Botulism
	Nerve
	• Third, fourth, and sixth cranial nerve palsies
	• Unilateral multiple cranial nerve palsies: orbital apex syndrome and cavernous sinus syndrome
	• Bilateral multiple cranial nerve palsies: meningitis, Miller Fisher variant of Guillain Barre syndrome, and Wernicke's encephalopathy
	Brain
	• Internuclear ophthalmoplegia: multiple sclerosis, stroke, tumour, Wernicke's encephalopathy.
	• Skew deviation: brainstem disease (stroke, infection, tumour, and multiple sclerosis)
	Other
	• Decompensated phoria (ocular deviation)

A. History of presenting complaint:
Determine whether the patient has true diplopia (two distinct images of the same object)
'Describe what you mean by double vision?'; 'Do you see two clear images of the same object? Is there any blurring of the images?'

Patients often use the term 'double vision' to describe blurring or 'ghosting' of an image. Therefore it is necessary to ask the patient what exactly they mean by the term double vision and to differentiate true diplopia from other symptoms.

Is the diplopia monocular or binocular?
'Does the double vision disappear if either eye is closed?'

The importance of distinguishing monocular from binocular diplopia is the significant difference in aetiology. Determining the type of diplopia present will allow the clinician to focus the remainder of the history and direct the clinical examination towards the possible underlying cause. Diplopia resolves when *either* eye is occluded in binocular diplopia since the false image is the result of misalignment of the eyes most often caused by extraocular muscle paresis or restriction. In contrast, monocular diplopia persists when the unaffected eye is occluded.

Alignment of images in diplopia

'Are the two images side by side, one on top of the other, or at an angle and tilted?'

In horizontal diplopia the images appear parallel as a result of impairment of the horizontal recti muscles (lateral and medial recti). Vertical diplopia is characterized by one image on top of the other and in some cases at an angle (oblique displacement). It is caused by disease affecting the superior rectus, inferior rectus, superior or inferior oblique muscles.

Torsional diplopia (tilting of the false image) results from dysfunction of the oblique muscles and often occurs with a fourth nerve palsy.

'Is the double vision always the same?'

Variable diplopia is typical of Myasthenia gravis.

Separation of the images

'In which direction is the distance between the two images the greatest? Left? Right? Up? Down? All directions?' . This is to say in which direction is the diplopia the worst?

The direction in which the separation of the images is maximal gives a clue to which nerve and/ or muscle is involved. Image separation and hence diplopia is maximal when gaze is in the direction of action of the affected muscle. This is paretic myopathy. However, in restrictive myopathy, the diplopia is maximal in the opposite direction of action of the affected muscle, e.g. diplopia is worse on the left in left medial rectus restrictive myopathy.

Diplopia in multiple directions should raise the suspicion of myasthenia gravis, multiple unilateral cranial palsies (cavernous sinus and orbital apex syndrome), and Graves ophthalmopathy.

Onset

'Did it start suddenly or gradually?'

Acute onset of diplopia is highly indicative of vascular and most orbital causes. Pituitary apoplexy should be borne in mind in patients presenting with sudden onset of diplopia in multiple directions.

Duration, progression, and recovery

'How long have you had double vision?'; 'Is the double vision getting worse? That is, has the distance between the images increased over time?'; 'Over what period of time has this occurred?'

Increasing distance between the images is an indicator of progressive diplopia.

'Do you have double vision all the time, or does it come and go?'

Myasthenia gravis can cause variable and intermittent diplopia, particularly worse at the end of the day. Other causes of intermittent diplopia include Graves ophthalmopathy and decompensated phoria.

'Is the double vision getting better?'

Spontaneous recovery within weeks of onset can occur with ischaemic cranial nerve palsies.

Aggravating factors

'Is the double vision worse when looking at near or distant objects?'

Diplopia worse at a distance is characteristic of lateral rectus muscle dysfunction, whilst diplopia that is worse when looking at near objects is typical of medial rectus muscle involvement.

'Is there anything that makes the double vision worse?'

Diplopia is typically worse with fatigue in myasthenia gravis. Decompensated phoria can be precipitated by intercurrent illness and stress.

Associated symptoms

- **Pain.**
  - Pain localized to the eye is suggestive of orbital lesions. Acute orbitopathy is associated with deep retrobulbar and periorbital pain. Pain on eye movements is also typical of orbital lesions, cavernous sinus and orbital apex syndromes and extraocular myopathy. Note that painful eye movements, *without* diplopia is characteristic of optic neuritis.
  - Facial pain, numbness, and paraesthesiae in the territory of the ophthalmic and maxillary divisions of the trigeminal nerve are associated with cavernous sinus lesions.
- **Headache.** The presence of headache in the context of diplopia should raise the suspicion of serious intracranial pathology and must be thoroughly enquired about. Ask about:
  - Onset: sudden onset of severe headache may represent rupture of an intracranial aneurysm and associated haemorrhage. It may be associated with neck stiffness, photophobia, and limb weakness.
  - Site of headache: Although not specific for certain aetiologies, occipital headache with neck stiffness occurs in subarachnoid haemorrhage and meningitis. A temporal headache with jaw claudication, scalp tenderness, fever, and malaise is suggestive of giant cell arteritis.
  - Headaches that are typically worse in the morning and on bending forwards or straining are features of raised intracranial pressure. Vomiting is also a symptom of raised intracranial pressure.
- **Ptosis.** *'Have you noticed any drooping of your eyelids or difficulty in opening your eyes?'*. A partial unilateral ptosis may be the result of a third nerve palsy. Bilateral ptosis which worsens with fatigue is a feature of myasthenia gravis. (see vol 1, Case PTDSIS)
- **Associated neurological symptoms.** Make a detailed enquiry about other neurological symptoms such as limb and facial weakness, sensory impairment, speech disturbance, hearing impairment, gait difficulty, and dysphagia which will be useful in localizing a brain-stem or intracerebral lesion.
- **Associated eye symptoms**
  - Loss of colour vision and reduced visual acuity in association with diplopia are features suggestive of optic nerve involvement in orbital apex syndrome. Blurred vision, red eye, conjunctival chemosis, and proptosis can occur with any cause of acute orbitopathy.
  - Both intermittent visual loss and diplopia can be one of the presenting features of giant cell arteritis prior to permanent visual loss as the disease process progresses.
- **Symptoms of myasthenia gravis.** Systemic features of myasthenia gravis include: fatigue, proximal muscle weakness, dysphagia, dysarthria, dysphonia, and dyspnoea.
- **Symptoms of thyroid disease.** Features of Graves ophthalmopathy include: proptosis, periorbital oedema, chemosis, irritation, and dry eyes. There may also be associated symptoms of thyrotoxicosis.
- **Trauma.** Diplopia may be a result of direct trauma to the eye, face or head.
- **Systemic symptoms.** Fever occurs with a range of infective and inflammatory conditions of the eye, orbit, and central nervous system. Weight loss and anorexia may point towards malignancy.

B. Relevant medical and family history:

Past medical history

- The presence of vascular risk factors may suggest atherosclerosis as the disease mechanism leading to ischaemia.
- Ischaemic third and sixth nerve palsies are recognized complications of diabetes mellitus.
- Previously known intracranial aneurysm should alert the physician to the possibility of rapid expansion or aneurysmal rupture.
- Consider internuclear ophthalmoplegia in a patient with multiple sclerosis.
- Consider upward lens dislocation as a cause of monocular diplopia in a patient with Marfan syndrome.
- A history of previous malignancy should raise the suspicion of metastatic disease.
- Childhood history of latent strabismus may point towards decompensated phoria. Congenital fourth nerve palsy may present as 'new' diplopia in adulthood when compensatory mechanisms fail.

Family history

Ask about:

- Strabismus
- Autosomal dominant polycystic kidney disease and intracranial aneurysms

C. Medications:

Drugs that cause diplopia as a side effect include: phenytoin, carbamazepine, topiramate, and SSRIs.

D. Social issues:

- Ask about smoking history as a risk factor for atherosclerotic and Graves ophthalmopathy.
- Enquire about occupation and recreational activities and determine the impact of the patient's symptoms on daily activities.

Formulating a plan of action

Explain to the patient that a definitive diagnosis for the diplopia is achieved by a thorough neurological, ophthalmic, and systemic examination in conjunction with investigations. Consider the following investigations and select the most appropriate investigations guided by the history and examination

- A leucocytosis and raised inflammatory markers are consistent with an infective and/or inflammatory process. A particularly raised ESR without a raised white cell count occurs with giant cell arteritis.
- Neuroimaging of the orbit and brain is necessary in most patients presenting with sudden onset diplopia with neurological symptoms and signs suggestive of a space occupying lesion, aneurysms, cavernous sinus, and orbital apex syndromes, trauma and in patients who do not meet the criteria for ischaemic cranial nerve palsies. CT is widely available, however an MRI with angiography is more sensitive for detection of aneurysms, orbital, and cavernous sinus disease. MRI is also useful in the diagnosis of multiple sclerosis.
- Consider a temporal biopsy prior to or within 7 days of starting high dose steroid therapy in cases of suspected giant cell arteritis.
- Acetylcholine receptor autoantibody titres are raised in 90% of patients with myasthenia gravis but only in approximately 50% of patients with ophthalmic features. A tensilon test may be performed if the clinical features are suggestive of the diagnosis and autoantibodies are negative. Those patient s diagnosed with myasthenia gravis should have a thoracic CT scan to exclude a thymoma which is present in 10% of patients.
- Thyroid function tests in patients with Graves disease.

Questions commonly asked by examiners

What do you understand by the term acute orbitopathy?

Acute orbitopathy is a syndrome of acute onset proptosis, ocular injection, and diplopia. The causes include:

- **Infection:** herpes zoster ophthalmicus, fungal infection
- **Inflammation:** sarcoidosis, Wegener's granulomatosis
- **Vascular:** cavernous sinus thrombosis, carotico-cavernous fistula, and giant cell arteritis
- **Neoplastic:** primary orbital tumour, meningioma, metastases (lymphoma).

What are the causes of a painful ophthalmoplegia?

- **Vascular**
  - Cavernous sinus syndrome, posterior communicating artery aneurysm, ischaemic third nerve palsy, giant cell arteritis.
- **Neoplastic**
  - Pituitary adenoma, pituitary apoplexy, orbital tumours, metastatic nasopharyngeal tumour.
- **Infective and inflammatory disease**
  - Sinusitis, herpes zoster ophthalmicus, mucocele, mucormycosis, sarcoidosis, and orbital pseudotumour.

What are the structures of the cavernous sinus?

- Intercavernous internal carotid artery
- Cranial nerves II, III, IV, VI, and V (ophthalmic and maxillary divisions)
- Sympathetic nervous plexus

What are the clinical differences between cavernous sinus and orbital apex syndromes?

Orbital apex syndrome has the same clinical features of cavernous sinus syndrome with additional features of ipsilateral optic nerve involvement (reduced visual acuity, reduced colour vision, and relative afferent papillary defect). The causes for orbital apex and cavernous sinus syndrome are the same and are investigated in the same manner.

What clinical features are associated with a cavernous sinus syndrome?

- Diplopia
- Painful ophthalmoplegia
- Visual loss
- Sensory loss in the ophthalmic and maxillary divisions of the trigeminal nerves and loss of corneal reflex
- Proptosis
- Pulsating exophthalmos if carotid-cavernous fistula
- Ipsilateral third, fourth, and sixth cranial nerve palsies

What are the causes of a cavernous sinus syndrome?

- **Vascular**
  - cavernous sinus thrombosis
  - intracavernous carotid artery aneurysm
  - posterior communicating artery aneurysm
  - carotico-cavernous fistula

- **Neoplastic**
  - Primary: meningioma, local extension of nasopharyngeal carcinoma
  - Secondary: lymphoma, breast and lung
- **Infective and inflammatory disease**
  - sinusitis
  - herpes zoster ophthalmicus
  - mucormycosis of sphenoid sinus
  - Wegner's granulomatosis
  - sarcoidosis

Case 30 ◆ Limb Weakness

INFORMATION FOR THE CANDIDATE

Dear Doctor,

This 60-year old gentleman presents with right arm weakness which has progressed to involve the right leg over a few days with difficulty walking. He finds it difficult to write and grip objects. There are no other neurological symptoms. His past medical history includes a TIA four years ago, hypertension, and hyperlipidaemia for which he takes ramipril and atorvastatin. On examination, power is reduced in the right upper and lower limbs graded 4/5 on the MRC scale, dysmetria of the right upper limb and ataxic gait. There is no sensory deficit.

He is an ex smoker. He works as a dentist and is worried that his symptoms are interfering with his work.

Many thanks for your opinion.

Acquiring the history

Limb weakness is a common presentation and the wide differential includes disease of the nervous and musculoskeletal system. Weakness caused by neuromuscular junction and muscle disorders is discussed in Case 35 Muscle weakness.

The history for limb weakness should be focused on differentiating true weakness, that is, reduced muscle power caused by neurological or muscle disease, from motor impairment of other causes such as systemic illness. In addition the history in conjunction with the clinical examination should aim to localize the lesion and determine the underlying aetiology.

A. History of presenting complaint:
Establishing true limb weakness
Patients may use the term 'weakness' to denote tiredness and malaise or to describe extrapyramidal features such as incoordination and rigidity that leads to functional motor impairment but without loss of muscle power. Therefore it is important to establish

what the patient means and establish whether there is true loss of muscle strength.
Use questions such as:

- 'What exactly do you mean by weakness?'
- 'Is there loss of strength of your arm or leg?'
- 'Are you unable to coordinate movement of the arm or leg?'
- 'Does the arm or leg feel stiff?'

Distribution of weakness

Patterns of weakness are helpful in localizing the lesion within the neuromuscular system.
Determine which areas are affected and if this is asymmetrical or symmetrical weakness.
Asymmetrical weakness can be caused by disease affecting both the central and peripheral
nervous systems. Other causes are peripheral neuropathies. Symmetrical limb weakness is typical
of muscle disease. Ask the patient:

- 'What parts of the body feel weak?
- 'Is it the same on both sides?'

Onset

'When did it start? Did it come on suddenly or has it been developing over a period of time?' Sudden
onset of limb weakness is highly indicative of a vascular event. Establish the exact timing of the
weakness since it will in part inform your decision about management with thrombolysis in the
setting of an ischaemic cerebrovascular event.

Infective, inflammatory, and traumatic causes of weakness develop in a subacute manner
whereas, neoplastic, degenerative, and metabolic disorders develop insidiously over a period of
months to years.

Duration, progression, and recovery

Determine the duration and progression of symptoms. By definition the symptoms of transient
ischaemic attacks (TIA) resolve within 24 hours of onset. However, if patients present within this
timeframe, be aware of evolving symptoms as persistence and progression of symptoms over
24 hours constitutes a stroke:

- 'How long have you had the weakness?'
- 'Is the weakness the same it was when it first started, getting worse or improving?'

Weakness arising from other causes may be progressive over a number of days, months or years;

- 'Over what period of time has the weakness been getting worse?'
- 'Where did the weakness first start? Has it progressed to involve other areas?'

Ask about periods of resolution of symptoms and any relapses. Pyramidal weakness may occur
with multiple sclerosis and can take a primary progressive, relapsing/remitting, secondary
progressive course:

- 'Have there been times where the weakness partially or completely resolves?'

Associated neurological symptoms

Enquiring specifically about associated neurological symptoms helps to narrow the differential
diagnosis to the most likely cause and localize the lesion. Ask about:

- Dysphasia (a 'cortical' sign).
- Facial weakness and sensory loss.
- Sensory disturbance. Ask about sensory loss 'Do you have any numbness or loss of feeling to
  pain, cold or warmth?'. Also determine the presence of positive symptoms such as tingling,
  pins and needles, pain, and allodynia. (Refer to Case 34 Paraesthesiae). Cerebrovascular

disease is typically associated with negative sensory symptoms, but other causes of weakness and sensory disturbance may have negative or positive symptoms.

- Visual disturbance. Transient episodic loss of vision (amaurosis fugax) is the result of thromboembolism or vertebrobasilar ischaemia.
- Bulbar symptoms include dysphagia, dysarthria, dysphonia, diplopia, oscillopsia, vertigo, vomiting, and hearing impairment suggests brainstem involvement.
- Ask about gait disturbance (Case 31 Gait Disturbance).
- Cerebellar symptoms include ataxia, dysarthria, tremor, and incoordination.
- Sphincter disturbance is suggestive of distal spinal cord disease and warrants urgent attention to exclude cord compression.
- Headaches may be associated with space occupying lesions and subarachnoid haemorrhage. Weakness and other focal neurological deficits rarely develop as a result of subarachnoid haemorrhage, however if present it suggests extension of bleed into the intracerebral matter. Elicit symptoms suggestive of raised intracranial pressure: vomiting, and headaches aggravated by postural changes, straining, and coughing.
- Seizures in the context of limb weakness suggest a space occupying lesion (Case 33 Seizures). In addition Todd's paresis can cause focal weakness.

Other symptoms

It is useful to ask about the presence of the following non-neurological symptoms to help determine the cause of the lesion:

- Fever suggests an infective or inflammatory process.
- Neck pain is often the result of trauma and is associated with carotid dissection.
- Back pain in the context of limb weakness and sphincter disturbance is an emergency as it indicates spinal cord pathology (Case 24 Back Pain).
- Constitutional symptoms such as malaise and weight loss suggest either a systemic illness or metastatic malignancy with spread to either the vertebrae or brain in the context of limb weakness.

Functional impairment

Enquire about the impact of the symptoms on the patient's ability to perform motor acts. It is easier to ask the patient *'What activities or physical tasks can you no longer do because of your weakness?'* as an opening question to establish the degree of functional impairment present. Follow up by specifically asking about the patient's ability to perform certain motor tasks such as raising arms above the head, climbing stairs, writing, etc.

B. Relevant medical and family history:

Past medical history

Ask about

- Vascular risk factors: hypertension, diabetes mellitus, hyperlipidaemia, and previous ischaemic events (angina, peripheral vascular disease, myocardial infarction, previous stroke, and/or TIAs).
- Atrial fibrillation is a strong risk factor for stroke.
- A previous history of multiple sclerosis may suggest demyelination as a cause for new, recurrent, or progressive episodes of limb weakness.
- Malignancy.
- Epilepsy. Todd's paresis is a cause of weakness in patients who experience tonic-clonic seizures.
- A history of known arteriovenous malformation suggests intracerebral haemorrhage a cause

Family history
- Ischaemic heart disease
- Stroke

C. Medications:

A thorough drug history will enable you to gather information about current treatment for co-morbidities and whether the patient is taking the correct medications for secondary prevention for cerebrovascular disease if this is the suspected diagnosis for the patient's symptoms.

Some medications may cause muscle weakness as a side effect (Case 35 Muscle Weakness).

Ask specifically about antiplatelet and anticoagulation therapy. Over-anticoagulation may be the precipitant for a haemorrhagic stroke whereas subtherapeutic anticoagulation could be the cause of a thrombotic stroke.

D. Social issues:

- Ask about current and previous history of smoking.
- Enquire about the patient's occupation and recreational activities and advise the patient to discontinue certain high risk activities if affected by the patient's symptoms.
- Ask the patient if he/she drives as driving regulations apply to patients who have had a TIA or stroke in the past or have chronic neurological conditions that cause limb weakness, for example multiple sclerosis, motor neurone disease, and muscle disorders.
- Determine any use of recreational drugs. Cocaine and amphetamine use are recognized causes of cerebrovascular disease.
- Establish the social circumstances in the view of functional disability. Does that patient have adequate support from family, friends, or carers for the daily activities of living? Ask specifically about the physical characteristics and layout of the patient's home—does the patient have adequate physical support at home? Consider an occupational therapy assessment for further support for the patient at home.

Formulating a plan of action

- Explain the possible causes of the patient's symptoms and explain that a clinical examination together with appropriate investigations will be required to establish a definitive diagnosis.
- Consider the following investigations for the evaluation of patients presenting with limb weakness:
  - ECG may reveal AF, a risk factor for thromboembolic stroke.
  - Blood count—A leucocytosis and raised inflammatory markers may indicate an infective or inflammatory process.
  - Serum glucose—hypoglycaemia can cause transient, weakness mimicking a stroke. Hyperglycaemia may occur as a stress response to a stroke, but may also indicate undiagnosed diabetes mellitus.
  - Urea, creatinine, and electrolytes—electrolyte imbalance can lead to certain myopathies (eg. hypokalemic periodic paralysis)or indicate renal failure as a cause of peripheral neuropathy.
  - ESR will be raised in infective and inflammatory muscle disorders and giant cell arteritis.
  - creatine kinase (CK) will be raised in muscle disease.
  - Neuroimaging to exclude central and peripheral nervous system pathology.
- The following investigations should be done as part of a routine work up of TIA and stroke:
  - ECG for AF.
  - Consider ambulatory ECG for paroxysmal AF

- Blood tests—blood count, ESR, glucose, lipids, thyroid function tests, clotting, urea, creatinine, and electrolytes
- Carotid dopplers to exclude carotid artery stenosis and dissection
- Neuroimaging—CT, MRI, MRA/MRV according to clinical indication, but a CT is essential to exclude at least a haemorrhage and space occupying lesion if MR is not available immediately.
- Echocardiography is considered in patients with AF, recent MI, new onset murmurs to assess for atrial and/or mural thrombus formation and endocarditis as embolic sources. A bubble echocardiogram is indicated in young patients with confirmed deep vein thrombosis and central neurological symptoms to exclude a patent foramen ovale causing a paradoxical stroke.
- Consider a vasculitic, autoimmune, and thrombophilia screen in young patients presenting with cerebrovascular disease or patients of any age with a history suggestive of a rare cause of stroke.
- Consider temporal artery biopsy in patients presenting with a clinical picture suggestive of giant cell arteritis as a cause for stroke.
- Consider TTP in patients with recurrent TIAS- UREs, creatinine, platelets, blood film for schistocytes and adamts 13 assay.

Questions commonly asked by examiners

How can the stroke syndromes be classified?

Stroke can be broadly classified into ischaemic and haemorrhagic strokes.

Ischaemic stroke can be further classified into four types according to the Oxfordshire Community Stroke Project anatomical classification system that categorizes stroke anatomically based on clinical features and underlying mechanism.

1. **Total anterior circulation infarct (TACI): thromboembolic**
   - Contralateral hemiparesis and/or sensory deficit involving at least two of face, arm, and leg
   - Contralateral homonymous hemianopia
   - Cortical dysfunction (aphasia, apraxia, agnosia, acalculia, visuospatial problems)
   - In the presence of impaired consciousness, then cortical dysfunction and visual problems are assumed.
2. **Partial anterior circulation infarct (PACI): embolic**
   - Requires two of the three criteria of TACI or:
   - Cortical dysfunction alone or contralateral hemiparesis and/or hemisensory deficit
3. **Posterior circulation infarct (POCI): 80% thrombotic, 20% embolic**
   - Cranial nerve dysfunction with contralateral hemiparesis and/or hemisensory loss
   - Bilateral infarcts
   - Conjugate gaze disorder
   - Isolated cerebellar stroke
   - Isolated homonymous hemianopia
4. **Lacunar circulation infarct (LACI): thrombosis of deep penetrating end-arteries**
   - See below.

What types of lacunar stroke syndromes do you know about?

There are five lacunar stroke syndromes. Occlusion of the deep penetrating end arteries lead to small areas of subcortical infarcts termed lacunes resulting in significant neurological deficits.

1. **Pure motor lacunar stroke** is the most common lacunar syndrome presenting as hemiparesis without cortical signs. Partial lacunar syndrome involves weakness of either the

face *and* arm or arm *and* leg. Infarcts occur in the internal capsule, corona radiata, and corticospinal tract.

2. **Pure sensory lacunar stroke** presents with hemisensory loss of the face, arm, and leg without motor and cortical signs. Thalamic infarcts are responsible for this syndrome.

3. **Sensorimotor lacunar stroke** is the second most common lacunar syndrome presenting with hemisensory loss and hemiparesis without cortical signs. Lesions occur in the posterior limb of the internal capsule, corona radiata, and occasionally elsewhere in the internal capsule or thalamus.

4. **Ataxic hemiparesis** consists of ataxia and hemiparesis resulting form lesions in the posterior limb of the internal capsule or pons.

5. **Dysarthria and clumsy hand syndrome** is a variant of the ataxic hemiparesis lacunar syndrome in which the patient presents with dysarthria and weakness of a hand.

Other lacunar presentations occur with infarction of the basal ganglia that leads to hemiballismus and hemichoreiform movement disorders.

How can the risk of stroke be assessed in patients presenting with a TIA?

The ABCD$_2$ score is a prognostic score that predicts the risk of stroke within a week in a patient presenting with a TIA based on five independent clinical parameters on presentation:

*   A Age ≥60 years (1 point)
*   B Blood pressure: systolic >140 mm Hg or diastolic ≥90 mm Hg (1 point)
*   C Clinical features: unilateral weakness (2 points), speech impairment without weakness (1point)
*   D Duration ≥60 min (2 points) or 10–59 min (1 point)
*   D Diabetes (1 point).

NICE guidance recommends that patients with a moderate to high score (score greater than 4 points) should have neuroimaging alongside other assessments and investigations within 24 hours of presentation. These patients are admitted to hospital and undergo endarterectomy within two weeks if criteria are met. All other patients should be reviewed in the rapid access TIA clinic within two weeks with the view to investigate and initiate secondary prevention management.

What advice about driving would you give to a patient after a TIA or stroke?

For group 1 licenses patients presenting with TIA or stroke must refrain from driving for least one month after onset and can resume driving provided the patient is symptom free. This also applies to patients who have seizures at or within 24 hours of onset of the cerebrovascular event.

Patients do not need to notify the DVLA of their diagnosis unless there is residual neurological deficit (visual field defect, residual weakness, and cognitive impairment) after this period has lapsed. In this case the patient should be advised to stop driving. In addition, patients with crescendo TIA or multiple TIAs within a short period of time must be advised to inform the DVLA and are not permitted to drive unless they have been symptom free for at least three months.

Patients who experience seizures in the context of cerebral vein thrombosis must be symptom free for at least 6 months before they resume driving. In this case the patient must notify the DVLA.

Case 31 ◆ **Gait Disturbance**

INFORMATION FOR THE CANDIDATE

Dear Doctor,

Thank you for seeing this 62-year old gentleman who presents with a 1-month history of difficulty walking. He complains of his feet dragging whilst walking, and has to deliberately lift his feet off the ground. He has a past medical history of type 2 diabetes mellitus for which he takes Novorapid and Glargine insulin, and is awaiting cataracts surgery. He has had several falls over the last month resulting in minor injuries and his wife reports that he is now reluctant to leave the house because of his symptoms.

Many thanks for your opinion.

Acquiring the history

The *type* of gait disorder present may be best determined by clinical examination. However, the history remains a vital part of establishing the underlying *aetiology* for optimal management. A collateral history may also be useful.

Causes of gait disturbance

Neurological causes	Non-neurological causes
Frontal lobe disease (including dementia, normal pressure hydrocephalus)	**Musculoskeletal disease / arthritis**
Cerebellar ataxia	**Intermittent claudication**
Parkinsonism	**Postural hypotension**
Spasticity	**Fear of falling**
• Hemipareisis / hemiplegia	
• Paraparesis / paraplegia	
Peripheral sensory	**Alcohol**
• Sensory ataxia	
• Vestibular ataxia	
• Visual ataxia (eg parietal lobe disease)	
Peripheral motor	**Medications** (eg. benzodiazepines,
• Myopathy / neuropathy (weakness)	antidepressants, antipsychotics)

A. History of presenting complaint:
Age of onset
Gait disorders are typically due to chronic diseases or congenital conditions. Acute onset of gait disturbance is rare, and is an alarm symptom (see below). Hereditary neurological conditions such as Friedreich's ataxia, spinocerebellar ataxias, and hereditary spastic paraparesis present in childhood or adolescence. Multiple sclerosis and HIV infection are other conditions to consider in young adults.

Onset, duration and progression

Sudden onset and rapid progression (over hours to days) of gait disorder is an alarm symptom (see below), and raises the suspicion of spinal cord compression, stroke, or trauma, requiring immediate radiological imaging and appropriate management. Progression over several months to years is consistent with a systemic disease, Parkinsonism, peripheral neuropathy, or cerebellar disease.

Identify alarm symptoms.

The key alarm symptoms are (i) *acute onset*; (ii) *associated sphincter disturbance*; (iii) *systemic symptoms (see below)*.

The serious causes of gait disturbance that must be excluded are:

- **Spinal cord impingement**
  - Onset over hours/days?
  - Associated urinary incontinence/constipation?
  - Associated numbness in buttock / groin area (*'Does it feel normal when you wipe yourself with a toilet tissue?'*)
  - History of cancer (suggesting spinal cord compression by metastatic malignancy)?
  - History of fever, bacterial infection or intravenous drug use (suggesting spinal cord compression by an epidural or subdural abscess)?
- **Stroke**
  - Onset over minutes/hours?
  - Associated loss of vision or limb weakness?
  - Past history of stroke?
  - Risk factors for stroke—AF, hypertension, cardiovascular disease, peripheral vascular disease, diabetes mellitus, cigarette smoking?
- **Spinal cord ischaemia**
  - Acute onset over minutes?
  - Associated severe back pain (present in over 80% of cases and may suggest underlying aortic dissection)
  - Past history of vasculitis (e.g. SLE, polyarteritis nodosa)
  - Associated urinary incontinence/constipation?
- **Guillain-Barré Syndrome (acute inflammatory demyelinating polyradiculopathy (AIDP)—see Case 35 Muscle Weakness)**
  - Onset over hours/days
  - Sensory symptoms precede weakness?
  - Ascending paralysis?
  - Typically *no* loss of sphincter function at presentation (unlike spinal cord lesions—although urinary retention may subsequently occur due autonomic dysfunction).
- **Normal pressure hydrocephalus**
  - Onset over weeks/months?
  - Associated urinary incontinence?
  - Associated decline in cognitive function (collateral history)?

Nature of gait disturbance

Determine the type of gait disturbance present (see Examiner's Questions below). Begin with an open question: *'Describe the problem you have when walking?'* Follow-up with focused questions to establish the type of gait disorder that might be present.

- **Spastic gait.** *'Do you have to drag both feet at the side to walk?'*; *'Does your foot cross over the other when you walk?'*
- **Hemiparetic gait.** *'Do you drag one foot at the side to walk?'*
- **Stepping gait.** *'Do you have to lift your feet high off the ground to walk?'*; *'Does it feel as if you are walking up steps when you walk' on flat ground?*[11]
- **Ataxic gait.** *'Do you have trouble maintaining your balance when you walk?'*; *'Do you fall towards one side when you walk?'*; *'Do you have to look at your feet to see where you are walking?'*; *'Are you unsteady on your feet with your eyes closed?'*
- **Parkinsonian gait.** *'Do your feet shuffle along the ground?'*; *'Do you sometimes have difficulty starting to walk or stopping suddenly?'*
- **Waddling gait.** *'Do you feel as if you are waddling from side to side when you walk?'*

Pain on walking

Ask the patient if they have pain when they walk. Determine the site, character, radiation, aggravating, and relieving factors.

- **Arthritis.** *'Do you have any joint pain when you walk?'* If so go on to enquire about which joints are affected, presence of stiffness, swelling and other extraarticular features of musculoskeletal disease (see Case 23 Joint Pains).
- **Intermittent claudication.** *'Do you have pain in the back of your legs when you walk?'*;;*'Does the pain get better when you rest?'*; *'How far can you walk before you experience this pain?'*
- **Radiculopathies, disc herniation, spinal stenosis.** *'Do you have back pain?'*; *'Describe the pain to me—is it a sharp, shooting, stabbing pain?'*; *'Does the pain travel down the back of your leg?'*; *'Is the pain better when you rest?'* Spinal stenosis mimics intermittent claudication, however patients with spinal stenosis have other neurological symptoms and signs on examination to allow differentiation from peripheral vascular disease.

Walking capacity

Determine the patient's walking capacity in terms of distance and speed, and ask specifically about what stops the patient from walking further (e.g. leg pain, chest pain, or shortness of breath).

Falls or injuries

Ask about any falls and injuries sustained as a result of the abnormal gait. Ask if the patient requires assistance to walk or uses any walking aids. Is there a history of trauma to the lower limbs, back or neck?

Associated symptoms

- **Neurological**—limb weakness, paraesthesiae, visual disturbance, urinary incontinence and retention, facial weakness, tremor, speech disturbance, memory impairment, and visual hallucinations.
- **Muscle disease**—weakness, difficulty climbing stairs or combing hair (proximal myopathy), fever, arthralgia, rash (dermatomyositis), ptosis, and fatigability.
- **Psychiatric**—low mood, early morning wakening, insomnia, and reduced appetite, neight loss.
- **Systemic illness causing generalized weakness**—weight loss, loss of appetite, night sweats.
- **Recent infection**—bacterial or viral infection suggesting Guillan-Barré syndrome (especially *Campylobacter jejuni* or HIV).

B. Relevant medical and family history:

Past medical history

- Causes of peripheral neuropathy—diabetes mellitus, thyroid disease, chronic renal disease, sarcoidosis, rheumatoid arthritis, SLE, Sjogren's disease (see Case 34 Parasthesiae).
- Vascular risk factors—hypertension, hypercholesterolaemia, ischaemic heart disease, diabetes mellitus, previous vascular events including previous stroke, and/or TIAs.
- Active malignancy or previous malignancy (causing metastatic cord compression or a paraneoplastic peripheral neuropathy).
- Known Parkinson's disease or Parkinson plus syndrome
- Previous syphilis
- Multiple sclerosis
- Depression

Family history

- Muscular dystrophy
- Neurodegenerative condtions—Parkinson's disease, Huntington's disease, spinocerebellar ataxias, and Charcot-Marie-Tooth.
- Hereditary spastic paraparesis

C. Medications:

- Peripheral neuropathies may be the result of side effects of certain drugs (see Case 34 Parasthesiae).
- Antipsychotics may cause Parkinsonism, and dopamine agonists may give rise to dyskinesias interfering with mobility.
- Chronic corticosteroid use causes myopathy (see Case 35 Muscle Weakness).
- Ask specifically about recreational drug use, in particular intravenous drug use.

D. Social issues:

- Enquire about the patient's alcohol consumption as a cause of peripheral neuropathy.
- Take a careful dietary history. Vegan and vegetarian diets may predispose to vitamin B12 deficiency.
- Take an occupational history and determine the impact of the patient's symptoms on their job.
- Ask about the patient's accommodation specifically about stairs, hands rails, etc. Determine whether the patient is able to mobilize safely at home.
- Take a sexual history and determine risk factors for HIV and syphilis if suspected.
- Ask specifically about the patient's own concerns regarding their symptoms.

Formulating a plan of action

- Explain to the patient that a clinical examination and investigations will be required to establish a diagnosis.
- Consider the following investigations:
  - Peripheral neuropathy screen see Case 34 Parasthesiae): blood count, vitamin B12, folate, urea, creatinine, electrolytes, thyroid function tests, fasting glucose, autoimmune profile inculding ANCA.
  - Serum CK and ESR will be raised in myopathies, followed by electromyography (EMG) and muscle biopsy.
  - Syphilis serology will be indicated if there is suggestion of past infection.
  - HIV test should be considered in young adults presenting with spastic paraparesis.

- CT or MRI head/spinal cord may reveal characteristic features of cerebrovascular disease, primary brain tumours, metastases, multiple sclerosis, syringomyelia, and cord compression.
- Lumbar puncture is indicated in normal pressure hydrocephalus and in multiple sclerosis for oligoclonal bands.
- Plain radiographs of limbs and joints may be needed if musculoskeletal pathology is suspected.
- An ophthalmic review may be necessary if visual impairment is contributing to the gait disturbance.
- Arrange a physiotherapy and occupational therapy assessment for rehabilitation assessment, walking aids, and assessment of safety at home.

Questions commonly asked by examiners

What types of gait disturbance do you know about?

Hemiparetic. The patient walks with a characteristic posture of flexion of the upper limb and extension of the lower limb. The extended limb is circumducted, moving in an arc at the side, with an upward tilt of the pelvis on the affected side. The foot is dragged along the floor and the tip of the sole of the shoe is worn out. This is caused by upper motor neuron lesions of the cortex and brainstem, such as stroke, multiple sclerosis or space-occupying lesion.

Spastic or 'scissoring' gait. This type of gait is seen in patients with spastic paraparesis and is characterized by bilateral circumduction resulting in one foot crossing over the other with each stride.

Parkinsonian gait. Patients with Parkinsonism have a narrow based gait and walk with a stooped posture and take small, shuffling steps. The patient appears to run forward in order to maintain their centre of gravity, described as *festination*. The patient takes small steps to turn around and may have difficulty in initiating gait (hesitancy) or may suddenly stop and be unable to walk (freezing). Loss of arm swing, a unilateral tremor, and masked facies are other typical features.

Marche à petits pas. This is a broad based gait with small shuffling steps that resembles a Parkinsonian gait with loss of arm swing. However, the patient maintains an upright posture. Because the feet appeared to be stuck to the ground, it is also referred to as a 'magnetic gait'. Common causes include normal pressure hydrocephalus and multi lacunar infarcts.

High steppage gait. This is a broad based gait. The patient lifts the foot up off the ground with each stride to prevent dragging of the foot and stamps it down on the ground. This may be unilateral due to a common peroneal nerve lesion causing a foot drop, or bilateral. Causes of bilateral high steppage gait include peripheral motor neurpathies such as Charcot-Marie-Tooth, chronic inflammatory demyelinating polyneuropathy (CIDP), lead poisoning, bilateral radiculopathies, and bilateral common peroneal nerve palsy. Patients also have difficulty walking on their toes and heels.

Sensory ataxia. This is a broad based high steppage gait caused by peripheral sensory neuropathies, subacute combined degeneration of the cord, tabes dorsalis, and multiple sclerosis. Since the patients have impaired joint position sense, they rely on visual clues to maintain balance. Therefore, they look down at their feet whilst walking and are unable to walk with eyes closed. Romberg's test is positive.

Cerebellar ataxic gait. This is a broad based, unsteady gait with the patient leaning or falling over towards the affected side and the patient appears to have a 'drunken gait'. Tandem gait is impaired. Other cerebellar signs may be present.

Waddling gait. A waddling gait is characteristic of proximal pelvic girdle weakness of any cause. Normally, to begin walking the hip is raised by contraction of the gluteals and quadriceps to lift the leg off the ground. If either muscle group is weak, the patient swings the leg laterally to keep it from dragging. The gait is broad based and resembles the waddling of a duck. Trendelenburg's test is positive when the pelvis is tilted upwards on the *opposite* side of the leg that is being raised, consistent with proximal weakness.

Antalgic gait. This is a painful gait in which the patient limps on the affected side. It is caused by lower limb arthritis.

Choreic gait. Patients with Huntington's disease or other causes of chorea are seen to walk with jerking of the limbs, abnormal posturing, and lurching.

What are the causes of spastic paraparesis?
*   Multiple sclerosis
*   Spinal cord tumours
*   Parasagittal meningioma
*   Disc herniation
*   Trauma
*   Syringomyelia
*   Subacute combined degeneration of the cord
*   Transverse myelitis
*   Tabes dorsalis
*   Infection: TB, brucellosis, human T-lymphotropic virus-1 (HTLV-1), HIV
*   Hereditary spastic paraparesis

What are the features of normal pressure hydrocephalus?
Normal pressure hydrocephalus occurs due to impaired absorption of CSF from the subarachnoid space leading to intermittently *increased* CSF pressure. It is idiopathic in many cases but can arise secondarily to subarachnoid haemorrhage, trauma, and infection. The disorder is slowly progressive and is characterized by a triad of *dementia, marche à petits pas* gait, and *urinary incontinence*. MRI scan shows dilated temporal horns of the lateral ventricles *without* atrophy. The opening pressure at lumbar puncture is normal. Treatment is with a ventriculoperitoneal, ventriculopleural, or ventriculoatrial shunt to reduce the intracranial pressure with marked improvement of symptoms. Shunt complications include infection, blockage, seizures, and haematoma.

What are the features of spinal cord infarction?
The vascular supply of the anterior 2/3 of the spinal cord is the anterior spinal arteries, and the posterior spinal arteries supply the posterior 1/3 of the cord. The anterior spinal arteries are in turn supplied by feeder arteries which originate in the aorta. The largest of these feeder arteries, the artery of Adamkiewic, is vulnerable to ischaemia in the thoracic region (T2–T4). Hypotension, atherosclerosis, aortic dissection, clamping during surgery, and vasculitis are causes of anterior thoracic spinal cord infarction. Typically patients develop sudden back pain, bilateral flaccid weakness, and loss of pain and temperature sensation (since the anterior spinal tracts are affected). Treatment is usually supportive, although the underlying cause may occasionally be treated (e.g. polyarteritis nodosa) and neurological deficits may partially resolve after the first few days.

Case 32 ◆ **Tremor**

INFORMATION FOR THE CANDIDATE

Dear Doctor,

Thank you for seeing this 40-year old lady who complains of progressive 'shaking' of her hands first noticed several years ago. Her father suffered from Parkinson's disease and she is worried that she may have it. She previously worked as a waitress and has had to give up her job because of her symptoms.

Many thanks for your opinion.

Acquiring the history

A. History of presenting complaint

Age of onset

Essential Tremor has a bimodal age of onset: adolescence and late adulthood. Patients with neuropsychiatric symptoms of Wilson's disease and familial movement disorders present at 20–30 years of age.

Onset, duration and time course

- Acute or insidious onset
- Ask when the patient first noticed the tremor

Distribution

- Is the tremor unilateral or bilateral? Gradually progressive, asymmetrical tremor favours Parkinson's disease.
- Which body parts are affected—hands, arms, legs, head, jaw, chin, voice? The laryngeal muscles and tongue may be involved in essential tremor causing a tremulous voice. A head tremor is also associated with essential tremor.
- Has the tremor progressed over time to involve other body parts?
- Determine the relationship of tremor to voluntary movement. Ask *'When do you notice the tremor?'* Ask specifically when the tremor is at its *worst*:
    - at rest suggesting a Parkinsonian resting tremor?
    - during voluntary movement, suggesting an intention tremor?
    - during a maintained posture suggesting a postural or exaggerated physiological tremor?
- *'Does anything make the tremor worse?'* All types of tremor, but especially essential and exaggerated physiological tremors are aggravated by emotional stress, anxiety, and caffeine.
- *'Does anything, for example alcohol or sleep make the tremor better?'* A small amount of alcohol relieves an essential tremor. Essential and Parkinsonian tremors disappear during REM (rapid eye movement) sleep. In Parkinsonism, patients may exhibit violent movements during REM sleep; this would be obtained from a collateral history.
- Are there any symptoms of an underlying condition causing the tremor:

Resting tremor (see Vol 1, Case 43 Parkinson's Disease)

- **Parkinson's Disease**
  - ◆ Bradykinesia: slow voluntary movements, micrographia
  - ◆ Rigidity: manifests as limb stiffness, pain, and difficulty turning in bed suggesting truncal rigidity
  - ◆ Gait disturbance: freezing, failure of gait ignition
  - ◆ Postural instability: anterograde falls. Patients fall forwards as a result of a stooped posture.
  - ◆ Autonomic failure: sialorrhoea, dysphagia
  - ◆ Cognitive impairment: onset of cognitive impairment before or within one year of developing Parkinsonism suggests Dementia with Lewy Bodies.
- **Parkinson Plus Syndromes:** Ask about symptoms suggestive of Parkinson Plus Syndromes:
  - **(a) Multisystem Atrophy:** autonomic features are characteristic of this condition, together with cerebellar and extrapyramidal symptoms and signs. These include:
    - ◆ Presyncope and syncope
    - ◆ Urinary symptoms: frequency, hesitancy, and incontinence
    - ◆ Constipation
    - ◆ Sialorrhoea
    - ◆ Impotence
    - ◆ Dysphonia and stridor
  - **(b) Progressive Supranuclear Palsy:**
    - ◆ Unsteadiness
    - ◆ Retrograde falls: falls tend to occur backwards due to impaired 'righting' reflexes
    - ◆ Dysphagia
    - ◆ Slurred speech
    - ◆ Visual disturbance
    - ◆ Emotional lability
  - **(c) Dementia with Lewy Bodies:**
    - ◆ Visual hallucinations *'Do you see images that other people cannot see?'*
    - ◆ Fluctuating cognition

Intention tremor Cerebellar Syndrome (of any cause):

- Ataxia
- Nausea, vomiting, and vertigo
- Stacatto speech—a slow scanning dysarthria where words are spoken as distinct syllables.
- Falls to the side

Exaggerated Physiological tremor

- **Hyperthyroidism**
  - ◆ Weight loss
  - ◆ Heat intolerance
  - ◆ Diarrhoea
  - ◆ Palpitations
  - ◆ Excessive sweating
  - ◆ Oligo/amenorrhoea in women
  - ◆ Neck swelling

- **Phaeochromocytoma**
  - Palpitations
  - Excessive sweating
  - Postural dizziness

Other

- **Wilson's disease:** Patients present with an akinetic rigid or cerebellar syndrome. Other features to ask about are:
  - Bulbar symptoms: speech difficulty, drooling, and dysphagia
  - Dystonia of limbs
  - Psychiatric symptoms: psychosis, depression, impairment in cognition
  - Previous episodes of hepatitis
- **Dystonic tremor:** Stiffness and 'twisting' of limbs, neck, writer's cramp
  - Are there any features of anxiety or depression? Opening questions may be *'Do you get anxious or worry about things?'* and *'How have you been feeling within yourself recently?'* Explore this further if there is indication of anxiety or depressive features.
  - Is the tremor causing functional impairment—difficulty writing or holding a glass of water?

B. Relevant medical and family history:

- Ask about medical conditions can cause a tremor directly—hyperthyroidism.
- Ask about conditions which are treated with medications that cause a tremor as a side effect—hypothyroidism, asthma, epilepsy, schizophrenia, bipolar disorder, depression.
- Is there a previous history of stroke or TIAs? Are there any vascular risk factors suggesting vascular parkinsonism?
- Is there a family history of tremor or other movement disorders? Approximately 60% of patients with essential tremor have a positive family history with an autosomal dominant mode of inheritance. Wilson's disease is inherited in an autosomal-recessive manner.

C. Medications:

- **Drugs inducing a resting tremor:**
  - Anti-emetics: Metoclopramide, Prochlorperazine
  - Neuroleptics: Chlorpromazine, Haloperidol
- **Drugs inducing intentional tremor:**
  - Anti-epileptics: Phenytoin (long-term use causes a cerebellar syndrome), sodium valproate
  - Lithium toxicity
- **Drugs causing an exaggerated physiological tremor:**
  - Sympathomimetics: salbutamol, salmeterol, Theophylline
  - Tricyclic Antidepressants
  - Corticosteroids
  - Levothyroxine
- **Recreational drugs**: cocaine, amphetamines, and anabolic steroids all cause an exaggerated physiological postural tremor.

D. Social issues:

- Occupational history—has the patient been exposed to any toxins: heavy metals, organophosphates, solvents?

- Alcohol consumption:
  - ◆ Does a small amount of alcohol consumption *relieve* the tremor as in essential tremor?
  - ◆ Is there a history of chronic excess alcohol consumption leading to a cerebellar syndrome? Is the tremor the result of alcohol withdrawal?
- Determine the impact of tremor on the patient's quality of life: has the patient had to give up recreational activities or a job? Does the patient need assistance with daily activities and personal care?

Formulating a plan of action

- Explain to the patient that tremor is a symptom of an underlying condition, which may not necessarily be Parkinson's disease.
- Explain that a full clinical examination is necessary to determine the type of tremor present, and to decide upon further investigations and management.
- Consider the following investigations:
  - ◆ **Thyroid function tests:** to exclude hyper/hypothyroidism
  - ◆ **Copper studies:** Wilson's disease must be excluded in young patients presenting with a movement disorder. Serum caeruloplasmin are low and 24-hour urinary copper is high. A slit lamp examination will detect Kayser-Fleischer rings.
  - ◆ **Drug levels:** lithium, phenytoin, and sodium valproate levels in patients taking these for toxicity.
  - ◆ **Imaging studies:** Imaging is only recommended in patients presenting with atypical features, for example with a bilateral resting tremor which is difficult to differentiate from a postural tremor.

Single Photon Emission Computed Tomography (SPECT) imaging is indicated when it is difficult to distinguish an Essential Tremor from a Parkinsonian tremor clinically. A reduction in the density of dopaminergic neurones is seen in Parkinsonism, however Parkinson's disease cannot be differentiated from Parkinson Plus syndromes.

Investigations may be indicated to exclude Parkinson Plus Syndromes:

- Autonomic dysfunction:
  1. Postural BP
  2. Tilt-table testing
  3. ECG-Holter monitoring
  4. Urodynamic studies and urethral sphincter electromyography
- MRI brain: specific appearance may be present in Progressive Supranuclear Palsy and Multiple System Atrophy.

Questions commonly asked by examiners

How are tremors classified?

A tremor is a movement disorder characterized by rhythmical, involuntary, oscillatory movements of body part(s). Tremors can be classified by:

1. *Amplitude*: coarse *vs* fine
2. *Frequency*: the number of waveforms per second (Hertz)
3. *Anatomical distribution*: affected body part and symmetry of tremor
4. *Voluntary*: relationship to voluntary movement.

The relationship of a tremor to voluntary movement is the most common way to classify a tremor and therefore a tremor may be a:

- **Resting tremor**—present at rest and disappears during voluntary actions, characteristic of Parkinsonism. In Parkinson's Disease the tremor is classically observed as asymmetrical, low frequency (4–6Hz) rhythmical circular movements of the thumb and index finger ('pill-rolling').

- **Action tremor**—tremor present during voluntary movement. This can be further subdivided into

    (a) **Intention tremor**—a low frequency <5Hz tremor, present during voluntary movement and gets worse as a target is reached. Commonly caused by cerebellar disease.

    (b) **Postural**—tremor present during a sustained posture. Postural tremors can be physiological or exaggerated physiological tremors. Physiological tremors are benign with a frequency of 8–12 Hz, detectable on EMG. Physiological tremors may be enhanced by factors such as drugs, stress, and enhanced metabolic states such as hyperthyroidism and fever.

- **Others:**

    - **Holmes tremor**—a low frequency (4–5Hz) mixed tremor present at rest and during a sustained posture which worsens with voluntary movement.

    - **Primary Orthostatic tremor**—this is a postural tremor of high frequency 13–18Hz present in the lower limbs on standing and relieved upon walking.

    - **Dystonic tremor**—present in a body part that is affected by dystonia. Characteristically it is a postural tremor and is relieved by tapping the affected site.

Further reading

1. National Institute for Health and Clinical Excellence Parkinson's Disease: Diagnosis and Management in Primary and Secondary Care. London: NICE, 2006.

2. Elan L. Essential Tremor. New Engl J Med. 2001; 345:887–91

3. Nutt J et al. Diagnosis and Initial Management of Parkinson's Disease. New Engl J Med. 2005; 353:1021–7.

Case 33 ◆ Seizures

INFORMATION FOR THE CANDIDATE

Dear Doctor,

Thank you for seeing this 22-year old female university student who presents with two episodes of 'fitting' involving the whole body, witnessed by a friend. She does not take any regular medication apart from the oral contraceptive pill, and has no relevant medical history. She has recently passed her driving test and is a keen swimmer.

Many thanks for your opinion.

Acquiring the history

A. History of presenting complaint:

The history of the presenting complaint should be evaluated in three parts, recording the events *preceding*, *during*, and *after* the seizure activity.

The aim is to differentiate true seizure activity from conditions that mimic seizures. These are: syncope, TIAs, migraines, and non-epileptic attack disorders (includes pseudoseizures, panic attacks, breath holding attacks, and hyperventilation).

A collateral history should be obtained for an accurate account of the event.

- Determine from the patient if this is a first presentation of seizure activity or if the patient is known to have epilepsy.
- Age of onset
- Ask about the total number of events the patient has experienced. Note the following:
  - time of onset
  - duration of each episode
  - time interval between each episode
  - pattern of symptoms of each episode
- Details of event:

1. **Ask about symptoms preceding the episode**
- **Prodromal symptoms:** lightheadedness, dizziness, palpitations, chest pain, and shortness of breath which suggest syncope rather than seizure activity.
- **Precipitants:**
  - Bright/flashing/stroboscopic lights
  - Fatigue, sleep deprivation
  - Recent illness
  - Alcohol withdrawal. Seizures typically occur within 48 hours of withdrawal or reduction in alcohol consumption.
  - Drug withdrawal, most commonly benzodiazepines.
  - Drug overdose (prescription and illicit drugs).
  - Non-compliance with medications in a known epileptic.
- **Associated symptoms for aetiology:**
  - Fever, rash, neck stiffness, or photophobia suggesting meningitis
  - Limb weakness, sensory or visual disturbance, or dysphasia, suggestive of cerebrovascular disease
  - Postural headache, nausea, and vomiting suggesting raised intracranial pressure
  - Recent ear or upper respiratory tract infections suggesting spread of infection to CNS
  - Recent history of head trauma
- **Aura:** Does the patient experience warning of an impending seizure? Auras can be motor, sensory, autonomic, or cognitive, and can help localize the epileptic focus. A general question may be *'Did you experience any strange smells, tastes, or other sensations before you lost consciousness?'*. Each of these sensations do *not* need to be asked about specifically:
  - Rising sensation in epigastrium
  - Hallucinations: unpleasant olfactory and gustatory, auditory
  - Autonomic: pallor, sweating, nausea, and vomiting
  - Affective: unexplained fear or anger
  - Dyscognitive states: déjà vu, jamais vu, depersonalization and derealization
  - Forced head and/or eye turning

2. Determine the events during the episode

- Ask about impairment in consciousness (*always* the case in generalized and complex-partial seizures, although not in simple-partial seizures) '*Did you lose consciousness?*'
- Determine the nature of the seizure. Use open questioning '*Do you know what happened during the event?*' The patient may not be aware of the events during the episode if there was loss of consciousness, and each of these symptoms do not need to asked about specifically. In such cases a collateral history should be obtained.

(a) Partial (simple vs. complex determined by altered consciousness)

- **Temporal lobe seizures**:
    - Automatisms: lip-smacking, grimacing, chewing, ineffectual movements.
    - Vocalizations
- **Frontal lobe seizures**:
    - Focal involuntary convulsions of a body part
    - Jacksonian seizures: convulsions beginning in one body part and spreading to adjacent ipsilateral body parts due to spread of electrical discharge to adjacent cortical regions.
    - Violent movements: kicking, punching, cycling
    - Forced head and eye turning, 'fencing' posture
    - Dysphasia
- **Parietal lobe seizures:** Positive sensory symptoms and pain
- **Occipital lobe seizures:** Visual hallucinations: lights, colours

(b) Generalized (primary vs. secondary)

- **Tonic-clonic seizures:**
    - Stiffening *followed by* jerking of the limbs
    - Rolling of eyes
    - Cyanosis and frothing at the mouth
    - Urinary and/or faecal incontinence
    - Loss of consciousness
- **Absence seizures:** Vacant stare and eyeblinking
- **Myoclonic seizures:** Sudden onset involuntary movement of body parts, usually in the morning.

3. Ask about symptoms after the episode

- Limb weakness (Todd's paresis)
- Confusion and headache
- Injury
- Time to full recovery
- Recollection of event

Could this event be a non-epileptic attack disorder? Determine any atypical features suggestive of pseudoseizures from an eye witness:

- atypical limb and trunk movements; pelvic thrusting, kicking
- retained awareness during the event
- vocalizations and response to commands during the attack
- rapid recovery with no post-ictal confusion
- atypical injuries

B. Relevant medical and family history:

- Enquire about:
    - Previous head injury/trauma
    - Stroke

- Meningitis/encephalitis
- Previous or current malignant disease which would suggest cerebral metastases
- Birth injuries and childhood febrile convulsions. 1% of patients with a history of febrile convulsions develop epilepsy, risk is greater with prolonged and recurrent febrile seizures.
- Psychiatric illness
- Is there any family history of epilepsy?

C. Medications and interactions:
- **Anti-epileptic medications in a known epileptic:** determine the dose, frequency, formulation, frequency of seizures since starting the medication and any side-effects. Enquire about compliance and missed doses that are commonly triggers for seizures.
- **Drugs that induce seizures:**
  - Lithium toxicity
  - Ciprofloxacin, flucloxacillin
  - Neuroleptics: clozapine, haloperiodol
  - Antidepressants: Imipramine
- **Drug interactions:** Antiepileptic medications affect the hepatic cytochrome P450 enzyme activity. The effects of this are twofold:
  1. Antiepileptic drugs can interact with each other when used in combination, thus resulting in either subtherapeutic levels and inadequate seizure control, or toxicity.
  2. Interactions with other drugs with a narrow therapeutic index have implications on their efficacy. These drugs often require monitoring and dose adjustment to achieve efficacy.
- **Cytochrome P450 enzyme inducers and inhibitors:** can alter the plasma levels of narrow therapeutic index drugs.

Enzyme inducers	Enzyme inhibitors	Narrow therapeutic index drugs
Alcohol (chronic use)	Isoniazid	Phenytoin
Rifampicin	Erythromycin	Oral Contraceptive Pill
Griseofulvin	Sulphonamides	Warfarin
Sulphonylureas	Ciprofloxacin	Digoxin
Barbiturates	Omeprazole	Theophylline
Carbemazepine	Protease inhibitors	Lithium
	Ketoconazole, Fluconazole	Ciclosporin tacrolimus
	Sodium valproate	

- **Drugs causing syncope:** Anti-hypertensives
- **Illicit drug use:** cocaine, amphetamines, ecstasy.

D. Social Issues:
- Enquire about the nature of the patient's current occupation and establish the risk of seizures for the patient and others. Ask about night shifts and lack of sleep as a trigger for seizures.
- Ask the patient if they drive and the type of vehicle.
- Ask about recreational activities which may be hazardous in epileptics
- Ask about the patient's alcohol consumption which may be a trigger for seizures.

Formulating a plan of action

- Reassure the patient that seizures do not necessarily mean a diagnosis of epilepsy.
- Explain to the patient presenting with a first seizure that a full clinical examination and investigations will be required to identify a cause. These are also necessary in a known epileptic in order to determine the trigger for recurrent seizures.
- Investigations to consider in all patients;
  - Blood tests:
    - FBC
    - U&Es: including magnesium and calcium
    - LFTs
    - Glucose
    - Serum Prolactin in suspected cases of pseudoseizures. Prolactin levels are increased to 2–3 times the upper limit of normal in true tonic-clonic seizures, but are only mildly elevated in syncope.
    - Drug levels: lithium, phenytoin, carbemazepine, and sodium valproate
  - Toxicology screen
  - ECG, 24 hour holter monitoring to exclude cardiac causes of syncope.
  - Imaging:
    - CT head: useful in the acute setting when it is necessary to exclude acute stroke or other lesion
    - MRI brain is the imaging modality of choice in:[1]
      1. adult-onset seizures
      2. patients with recurrent unprovoked seizures
      3. focal seizures or neurological signs
      4. known epileptics in whom first line medical therapy has failed
  - Electroencephalogram (EEG). An inter-ictal EEG is only indicated to support a diagnosis of epilepsy, determine the epileptic focus, seizure type, and the epilepsy syndrome. Video or ambulatory EEG recordings may be useful when the diagnosis is unclear or when a non-epileptic attack disorder is suspected. It should not be used in isolation to diagnose epilepsy.[1]
  - CSF analysis should be performed when meningitis or encephalitis is suspected from the clinical history and examination.
- Tell the patient that a follow up appointment will be arranged to discuss the results of the investigations.

Questions commonly asked by examiners

How are seizures classified?

Seizure type

Seizures can be classified according to seizure type: partial, generalized, or secondary generalized. *Simple partial seizures* originate from a focal area of the brain and are *not* associated with a loss of consciousness. *Complex partial seizures* are *always* associated with impairment in consciousness, although do not exhibit tonic-clonic movements. Instead, patients either remain motionless or engage in repetitive behaviour (automatisms). *Generalized* seizures involve both cerebral hemispheres at onset, and also cause loss of consciousness. Several types are recognized: absences, myoclonic, tonic-clonic and atonic. In addition partial seizures can evolve into generalized seizures.

What are the causes of a seizure?

Seizures can be:

*   Primary/unprovoked when other causes have been excluded.
*   Secondary/provoked to an underlying cause. The causes include:
    *   **INFECTION:** Acute meningitis, post meningitis, encephalitis, cerebral malaria, brain abscess, tuberculosis
    *   **NEOPLASTIC:** Primary or secondary (lung, breast, melanoma, and gastrointestinal malignancies metastasise to the brain)
    *   **VASCULAR:** Acute stroke and post-stroke, arteriovenous malformations
    *   **TRAUMA:** Head injury, birth trauma (Cerebral Palsy)
    *   **METABOLIC:** Hypoglycaemia, hyponatraemia hypocalcaemia, uraemia, porphyria
    *   **DRUGS:**
        *   Subtherapeutic levels of antiepileptic medications
        *   Lithium toxicity
        *   Neuroleptics: clozapine, phenothiazines, and butyrophenones
        *   Antidepressants: Imipramine
        *   Recreational: ecstasy, amphetamines, cocaine
        *   Drug withdrawal: alcohol, barbiturates, and benzodiazepines
        *   Ciprofloxacin, Imipenem, flucloxacillin
        *   Flumazenil
    *   **SYNDROMES ASSOCIATED WITH SEIZURES:** Tuberous Sclerosis, Sturge-Weber, Down's Syndrome

What lifestyle advice would you give a patient with a new diagnosis of epilepsy?

*   Patient education about epilepsy and its management is important for compliance and adequate seizure control. All patients and/or their carers should have a comprehensive care plan and be provided with written information for reference.
    *   **Avoidance of precipitants:** Advise the patient to drink alcohol in moderation and establish a regular sleeping pattern as alcohol and sleep deprivation lower seizure threshold. Advise the patient to avoid recreational drug use.
    *   **Driving:** Explain the risk of driving and operating machinery with a diagnosis of epilepsy. Encourage the patient to disclose their medical condition to the DVLA. The medical practitioner is obliged to notify the DVLA if the patient continues to drive with this advice.
    *   Patients should be seizure free for at least a year in order to drive an ordinary motor vehicle. This is extended to 10 years without medication in order to hold a licence for HGVs and buses.
    *   **Recreational activities:** Patients should be advised not to swim, cycle, and participate in isolation sporting activities unsupervised.
    *   **Pregnancy:** Women of child-bearing age must be given advice about contraception and pregnancy. The efficacy of the oral contraceptive pill may be reduced with the use of anti-epileptic medications therefore, the dose should be increased and barrier methods encouraged.
    *   The first-line anti-epileptics are teratogenic and so women should be made aware to discuss family planning with their doctor for alternative drug therapy to avoid congenital malformations and neural tube defects in advance of conception. Folate supplementation is important in pregnancy to prevent neural tube defects.

What is the medical management of epilepsy and what advice would you give to the patient about medical therapy?

Initiation of medical therapy is considered in patients presenting with;

- First unprovoked seizure with neurological deficit, structural brain lesion, or a high risk of recurrence.
- Second epileptic seizure

The need for compliance and follow up with routine blood tests for levels and side-effects should be discussed with the patient as well as informing the patient about the possible side-effects, drug interactions, and effects on pregnancy.

The choice of drug depends on the seizure type:[2]

Seizure type	1st line anti-epileptic drugs	2nd line anti-epileptic drugs
Partial +/− secondary generalized tonic-clonic	Sodium Valproate Carbamazepine Lamotrigine	Phenytoin Levetiracetam Gabapentin
Generalized tonic-clonic	Sodium Valproate Carbamazepine Lamotrigine	Levetiracetam

What is the prognosis in epilepsy?

Approximately 70% of epileptics will become seizure free requiring no further medical treatment. The risk of recurrent seizures is increased with a first unprovoked seizure, structural lesion, and associated learning disability. Mortality is greater in epileptics in comparison to the general population and the causes of death include:

- status epilepticus
- seizure associated accidents: commonly drowning and trauma
- underlying structural brain lesion, e.g. tumour
- Sudden Unexpected Death in EPilepsy (SUDEP).[3] This is the sudden unexpected, unwitnessed, and non-traumatic death in epilepsy without an identifiable cause.

References

1. National Institute for Clinical Excellence, The Epilepsies: Diagnosis and management of the epilepsies in adults in primary and secondary care. London: NICE, October 2004.

2. French JA et al. Initial Management of Epilepsy. New Engl J Med. 2008; 359:166–76

3. Kloster R et al. Sudden unexpected death in epilepsy (SUDEP): a clinical perspective and a search for risk factors. J Neurol Neurosurg Psychiatry 1999; 67:439–44

Case 34 ◆ **Paraesthesiae**

INFORMATION FOR THE CANDIDATE

Dear Doctor,

Thank you for seeing this 53-year old gentleman who has burning pains and tingling in his hands and feet for the last 4 months. He has a past medical history of epilepsy for which he has been taking phenytoin for many years. He is an electrician and is finding work difficult because of his symptoms.

Many thanks for your opinion.

Acquiring the history

Sensory disturbance can arise from lesions anywhere in the nervous system. The diagnostic approach should aim to determine four features:

*   *Is the lesion within the peripheral nervous system?*—exclude cortical, spinal, and neuromuscular junction lesions, as well as non-neurological causes.
*   *What part of the peripheral nervous system?*—Nerve root, plexus, single nerve, multiple nerves, or polyneuropathy.
*   *Which nerve fibres are involved?*—sensory, motor, or mixed.
*   *What is the primary pathology?*—demyelination, axonal, mixed.

A detailed history of the onset of symptoms, epidemiological and clinical features will help distinguish between central and peripheral lesions and determine the need for electrophysiological studies.

A. History of presenting complaint:

Age of onset

Consider hereditary neuropathies presenting in childhood and early adulthood.

Description of sensory disturbance

Patients use various terms to describe sensory disturbances. Symptoms may be positive: parasthesiae, pain, hyperalgesia, and allodynia (pain in response to a non-painful stimulus), or negative (numbness and sensory loss).

Invite the patient to tell you about their symptoms using open questioning such as *'Tell me about the problem with your hands and feet'* followed by focused questions if necessary to establish the exact symptoms.

*   **Ask about positive symptoms**
    *   *'Do you feel strange sensations such as pins and needles or tingling?'*
    *   *'Do you have pain? If so, what is the pain like—burning? electric-shock like? shooting? stabbing?'* These terms are typical descriptions of neuropathic pain. Other phrases used to describe sensations in the hands and feet are feeling *tight, wooden,* or *dead.* Remember that there are other causes of hand and foot pain, such as palmar/plantar fasciitis, arthritis, bursitis, tendonitis, and polymyalgia rheumatica.
    *   *'Do harmless sensations, such as a light touch, feel abnormally painful or unpleasant?'* indicates allodynia.

- **Ask about negative symptoms**
  - *'Do you have any numbness or loss of feeling to pain, cold or warmth?'* suggesting sensory loss.
- **Distribution of sensory impairment**
  - *'Where do you feel the abnormal sensations and/or pain?'* The distribution of sensory impairment is important in determining the location of the lesion. Common patterns include:
    1. *Dermatomal* sensory impairment suggestive of a mononeuropathy or radiculopathy.
    2. *Symmetrical*, *distal*, and *generalized* symptoms indicative of a polyneuropathy.
    3. *Asymmetrical* involvement of an entire limb, for example one arm or leg, suggests cervical or lumbar spinal nerve root compression respectively.
    4. *Isolated sensory disturbance* affecting one side of the body is due to a central nervous system lesion.
    5. Involvement of *both legs* suggests a spinal cord lesion—there will be sensory level.
    6. *Multifocal* involvement is characteristic of mononeuritis multiplex.
  - Ask about sensory level *'Where on your body does sensation feel normal again?'*
- **Radiation and progression of sensory impairment.** Establish whether the symptoms radiate and how the symptoms have progressed over time:
  - *'Where did the symptoms first start?'*
  - *'Have the symptoms spread to involve other areas of the body?'* Polyneuropathies typically affect the longest axons first, therefore symptoms first appear in the feet, progressing proximally, followed by the hands. Radiculopathies and mononeuropathies radiate in the distribution of the nerves involved.

Aggravating and relieving factors

- *'Is there anything that makes the symptoms better or worse?'* Neuropathic pain of a radiculopathy is exacerbated by coughing, sneezing, and straining.
- *'Is the pain worse at night?'* Most cases of neuropathic pain are worse at night.

Onset, duration, and temporal pattern of symptoms

- **Onset.** Sudden onset of symptoms suggests acute peripheral neuropathies or cerebrovascular disease.
- **Duration.** Neuropathies can be classified according to the duration of the symptoms:
  - Acute onset (<4 weeks). Guillain-Barré syndrome (GBS) must be excluded in all patients presenting with an acute neuropathy. Other causes are toxin exposure or porphyria.
  - Subacute neuropathies (4–8 weeks).
  - Chronic neuropathies (>8 weeks) such as hereditary, demyelinating and metabolic neuropathies.
- **Progression.**
  - Rapid progression of symptoms suggests acute polyneuropathy.
  - Gradual, persistent progression of symptoms is seen with most chronic polyneuropathies, myelopathies, and tumours. Patients with hereditary neuropathies generally do not complain of positive symptoms such as pain or parasthesiae, and may not come to medical attention for many years because disease progression is slow and insidious.
  - Transient symptoms, with resolution between episodes, occur with multiple sclerosis, TIAs, epilepsy, migraine with aura, anxiety, and hypoglycaemic attacks.

Associated symptoms

Questioning about associated symptoms is helpful in determining the underlying aetiology. Begin with an open question, such as *'Have you noticed any other problems apart from the numbness and tingling?'*. Further closed questioning covering the symptoms listed below may be indicated if abnormalities arise during systemic enquiry.

- **Neurological symptoms**
    - Motor symptoms—weakness in the distribution of the sensory disturbance. Determine where the weakness started and if it has progressed to involve other areas. In GBS, motor weakness is ascending and progresses to involve the respiratory muscles. Enquire about any associated muscle wasting by asking *'Have you noticed any loss in muscle bulk in the affected area?'*
    - Autonomic symptoms—dizziness, urinary retention or incontinence, constipation, abnormal sweating, and impotence
    - Headaches—may suggest migraine or a space-occupying lesion.
    - Pre-existing cerebrovascular disease—visual disturbance, facial weakness, sensory disturbance, dysphagia, or impaired speech.
    - Gait disturbance *'Do you have difficulty with balance or walking?'* can occur with weakness secondary to sensorimotor peripheral neuropathies as well as myelopathies, multiple sclerosis, cerebrovascular disease, and central nervous system tumours.
- **Other symptoms**
    - Hypothyroidism—weight gain, tiredness, cold intolerance, neck swelling, and menorrhagia in women.
    - Uncontrolled diabetes mellitus with complications—polyuria, nocturia, polydipsia, visual disturbance, and recurrent infections. Transient sensory disturbances also occur with hypoglycaemic attacks therefore ask about associated palpitations, sweating, and confusion.
    - Symptoms of chronic renal disease—lethargy, anorexia, nausea, and vomiting.
    - Recent respiratory tract or gastrointestinal infection preceding neurological symptoms may suggest GBS
    - Weight loss, loss of appetite, or night sweats may suggest malignancy.
    - Fever, rash, and joint pains occur with connective tissue and vasculitic conditions such as SLE, polyarteritis nodosa (PAN), and sarcoidosis.
    - History of trauma may suggest direct injury to the nervous system.
    - Ask about symptoms of anxiety—precipitants, hyperventilation, and palpitations.

B. Relevant medical and family history:

Past medical history

- Sensory disturbances are direct complications of the following conditions:
    - Diabetes mellitus
    - Chronic renal disease of any cause
    - Hypothyroidism
    - Connective tissue diseases—rheumatoid arthritis, SLE, sarcoidosis
    - HIV/AIDs (various neurological complications of HIV infection can give rise to sensory disturbance. In addition, peripheral neuropathy is a complication of many anti-retroviral agents)
    - Amyloidosis
    - Pernicious anaemia
- Enquire about conditions that may have previously been treated with medications causing a peripheral neuropathy:
    - Arrhythmias (amiodarone)
    - Tuberculosis (isoniazid)

- Malignancies (chemotherapeutic agents)
- Epilepsy (phenytoin)
- HIV/AIDs
- Rheumatoid arthritis (gold, hydroxychloroquine, leflunomide)
- Infections treated with metronidazole and nitrofurantoin

Family history
- Hereditary sensorimotor neuropathies.

C. Medications:

Take a thorough drug history, since sensory disturbance may be a side effect of medications.

Drugs causing peripheral neuropathies

Sensory	Motor	Mixed sensorimotor
Phenytoin	Dapsone	Amiodarone
Metronidazole		Isoniazid
Pyridoxine		Chemotherapeutic agents: vinblastine, vincristine, cisplatin, oxaliplatin
Hydroxychloroquine		Nitrofurantoin
Haart		Gold
		Leflunomide

D. Social issues:

- Enquire in detail about alcohol consumption.
- Dietary history is important in establishing vitamin deficiencies that can cause peripheral neuropathies.
- Take a detailed occupation history. Ask specifically about exposure to potential toxins such as organophosphates, heavy metals, and thallium. Work involving operation of vibrating tools can cause carpal tunnel syndrome.
- A sexual history for HIV risk factors is necessary if there is a clinical suspicion of HIV infection.
- Determine the impact of the patient's symptoms on function, mobility, and daily activities. If their ability to work is affected, ensure to ask about the social and financial implications of this.

Formulating a plan of action

- Explain to the patient that a full clinical examination will be required.
- Discuss with the patient the possible causes of the symptoms as suggested by the history and explain that a definite diagnosis will require investigations.

Central lesions causing sensory disturbance	Peripheral lesions causing sensory disturbance	Other causes of sensory disturbance
Multiple sclerosis	Mononeuropathy	Migraine with aura
Myelopathy of any cause	Mononeuritis multiplex	Anxiety/panic attacks
Stroke/ TIA	Polyneuropathy	Hypoglycaemia
Epilepsy	Radiculopathy	
Tumours		

- Consider the following investigations in all patients as first line investigations for suspected peripheral neuropathies.
  - **Urinalysis.** Detection of glucose and ketones indicates diabetes mellitus. Formal diagnosis is then required with either an elevated fasting glucose level or abnormal oral glucose tolerance test.
  - **Blood count and haematinics.** A macrocytic anaemia with a low cell folate and vitamin B_{12} indicates vitamin B_{12} deficiency and further testing for pernicious anaemia autoantibodies may be necessary. Chronic alcohol consumption is a further cause of macrocytosis. A normochromic normocytic anaemia is seen with chronic renal disease.
  - **Serum protein electrophoresis and urinary Bence-Jones protein** for multiple myeloma.
  - **ESR.** A raised ESR occurs with malignancy, connective tissue diseases, and vasculitis.
  - **Urea and creatinine** will be raised in chronic renal disease.
  - **Electrolytes:** sodium, potassium, serum corrected calcium, phosphate, and magnesium. Electrolyte imbalance can cause acute peripheral neuropathies.
  - **Serum glucose.** A raised fasting glucose confirms a diagnosis of diabetes mellitus.
  - **Thyroid function tests**. Low fT_4 and high TSH confirms a diagnosis of hypothyroidism.
  - **LFTs**
  - **Autoantibody screen:** Rheumatoid factor (RhF), ANA, anti-dsDNA, and ENA: anti-Ro and anti-La.
  - **Vasculitic screen:** cANCA, pANCA and cryoglobulins.
  - **Plain chest radiograph.** A chest radiograph may reveal conditions leading to peripheral neuropathy such as bronchogenic carcinoma, metastatic nodules, and sarcoidosis.
- Second-line investigations include:
  - **Serum ACE.** Levels may be raised in sarcoidosis.
  - **Serology:** Borrelia serology (Lyme disease) and HIV testing.
  - **Antineuronal autoantibodies (e.g. anti-Hu, anti-Yo, anti-Ri, anti-Tr).** Titres are raised in paraneoplastic syndromes indicating occult malignancy. Subsequently investigations may be undertaken to establish the primary malignancy.
  - **Electromyography (EMG) and nerve conduction studies.** Electrodiagnostic studies will distinguish primary nerve disorders (neuropathy) from muscle disorders (myopathy). They will also differentiate multiple mononeuropathy (characteristic of peripheral nerve vasculitis) from polyneuropathy (which is symmetrical), and axonal neuropathies (such as diabetic neuropathy) from demyelinating neuropathies. Normal studies are consistent with pure small-fibre neuropathy (see below).
- Third-line investigations for determining the cause of an underlying peripheral neuropathy:
  - **CSF analysis.** A lumbar puncture is considered in patients with progressive neuropathy of an uncertain aetiology. Raised protein and the presence of oligoclonal bands is suggestive of demyelinating conditions and CIDP
  - **Nerve biopsy.** Nerve biopsies may be necessary when the cause is not apparent from other investigations and is diagnostic in determining the cause of the neuropathy and facilitating appropriate management. Tissue is obtained from sural, peroneal, or radial nerves.
  - **Genetic testing.** Consider genetic testing for hereditary motor and sensory neuropathy (HSMN) and hereditary neuropathy with pressure palsies in patients with a strong family history of peripheral neuropathy.

- **Other investigations to consider as directed by the history**
  - CT/MRI head for space-occupying lesion, cerebrovascular disease.
  - MRI spine for spinal cord pathology.
  - EEG if epilepsy is suspected.

Questions commonly asked by examiners (see Vol 1, Case 48 Peripheral Neuropathy)

What types of peripheral neuropathy do you know about?

- Peripheral neuropathy is a general term ascribed to disorders of the peripheral nerves. There are several types of peripheral neuropathies:
  - Mononeuropathy involves a single peripheral nerve.
  - Mononeuritis multiplex affects several different peripheral nerves.
  - Polyneuropathy is a diffuse, distal, and symmetrical neuropathy affecting several peripheral nerve axons.
  - Radiculopathy is a disease process affecting the nerve roots.
- Peripheral neuropathies can be further subdivided according to the type of nerve fibre affected; sensory, motor, autonomic, or mixed:
  - **Sensory-motor axonal pattern (glove-stocking):** Diabetes, drugs, toxins, metabolic disorders, hereditary neuropathies, critical illness polyneuropathy
  - **Sensory-motor demyelinating pattern (proximal and distal):** GBS, CIDP.
  - **Sensory-motor asymmetric nerve/plexus pattern:** Diabetic amyotrophy, vasculitic mononeuritis multiplex.
  - **Sensory-motor asymmetric:** Leprosy, porphyria.
  - **Sensory symmetric or asymmetric:** Paraneoplastic neuropathy, Sjogren's syndrome, vitamin B6 toxicity, leprosy.
  - **Motor symmetric or asymmetric:** Motor neuron disease, poliomyelitis.
  - **Autonomic symmetric or asymmetric:** Diabetes, amyloid, HIV, GBS.

What are the causes of a sensory neuropathy and carpal tunnel syndrome?

- Diabetes mellitus, hypothyroidism, uraemia, and amyloidosis.

What is the cause of atrophic weakness without sensory loss?

- Radicular or mononeuropathy pattern: poliomyelitis
- No clear anatomical pattern: motor neuron disease

Outline the management of peripheral neuropathy

Treatment of the underlying process

- Axonal polyneuropathies: Treatment is directed at removing the toxin (e.g. alcohol, drugs) or treating the causative disease process (e.g. diabetes control, immunosuppression of autoimmune disease).
- Demyelinating polyneuropathy: Idiopathic GBS or CIDP may respond to intravenous immunoglobulin, plasmapharesis, or immunosuppression. CIDP secondary to multiple myeloma or Waldenstrom's macroglobulinaemia may respond to treatment of the underlying condition.

Treatment of symptoms and prevention of complications

- Neuropathic pain: Tricylic antidepressants or gabapentin are considered effective. Carbamezapine and pregabalin are second-line agents.
- Physiotherapy: walking devices and orthotics may improve mobility and prevent disability.
- Foot care: Foot and nail care, with the assistance of a podiatrist, is essential due to the increased risk of foot ulceration.

Case 35 ◆ **Muscle Weakness**

INFORMATION FOR THE CANDIDATE

Dear Doctor,

Thank you for seeing this 50-year old lady who presents with progressive weakness of the shoulders and legs. She has also recently had difficulty in swallowing liquids and solids. There is a past history of breast cancer, and of hypertension treated with bendroflumethiazide. She is concerned about her symptoms as she is no longer able to continue work as a housekeeper.

Many thanks for your opinion.

Acquiring the history

Muscle weakness is a common complaint with a wide differential. Aetiologies can be classified according to the site of the lesion responsible for causing weakness. It is important to distinguish *functional* weakness arising from pain, chronic illness, and depression from *true* muscle weakness of neuromuscular origin. A thorough history should also aim to localize and determine the cause of the lesion giving rise to muscle weakness.

Neuromuscular junction and muscular causes of weakness are discussed in this section.

A. History of presenting complaint:
Age of onset
Hereditary myopathies and peripheral neuropathies present in childhood.

Onset and progression of weakness
*   Begin with an open question such as *'Tell me about your weakness'*. Follow up with more focussed questions:
    *   *'When did the weakness start?'*; *'Did it come on suddenly?'*
    *   *'Is the weakness getting better, worse or staying the same?'*
    *   *'Over what period of time has the weakness been getting worse?'*
    *   *'Does the weakness come and go in waves?'*
*   *Acute onset* within hours to days and *rapidly progressive* weakness requires immediate management due to pending ventilatory failure. Causes of acute muscle weakness are: Guillain-Barré syndrome, stroke, botulism, organophosphate poisoning, lead poisoning, transverse myelitis, and myasthenia gravis crisis.
*   *Chronic* weakness with slow progression over several months to years is characteristic of central nervous system space-occupying lesions, myasthenia gravis, and most myopathies.
*   *Episodic* weakness with sudden onset of generalized weakness with full resolution between episodes favours hypokalaemic and hyperkalaemic periodic paralysis.

Distribution of weakness
The distribution of weakness may give clues to the underlying aetiology. *'Which muscles feel weak?'* If the weakness is localized, determine whether this is asymmetrical or symmetrical.

*   *Generalized* weakness is seen with myasthenia gravis, Guillain-Barré syndrome, hypokalaemic periodic paralysis, and cachexia.

Causes of muscle weakness

Upper motor neuron lesions	Lower motor neuron lesions	Neuromuscular junction	Muscle
Brain and brainstem	**Peripheral nerves**	**Hereditary muscle disease**	**Acquired muscle disease**
• Stroke	• Polyneuropathies	• Myasthenia Gravis	**Hereditary**
• Multiple Sclerosis	• Mononeuropathies	• Drug induced myasthenia	
• Space-occupying lesions	• Mononeuritis multiplex	• Lambert-Eaton syndrome	• Muscular dystrophies (Duchenne, Becker, Fascioscapulohumeral, Emery-Dreifuss, Limb-girdle and oculopharyngeal)
• Seizures causing Todd's paralysis		• Botulism	• Myotonic dystrophy
Spinal cord		• Organophosphate poisoning	• Hypo/hyperkalaemic periodic paralysis
• Trauma			**Acquired**
• Tumours			• Polymyositis/
• Myelitis (multiple sclerosis)			• Dermatomyositis
• Infections			• Inclusion body myositis
• Haematoma			• Electrolyte imbalances
• Arteriovenous malformations			• Endocrine disease (hypothyroidism, Cushing's syndrome, Addison's disease)
Anterior horn cell lesions			• Infection (viral, toxoplasmosis, trichinosis and cysticercosis)
• Motor neuron disease			• Drug induced myopathy
• Poliomyelitis and post-polio syndrome			• Rhabdomyolysis
• Lead poisoning			

- *Localized* weakness may be *asymmetrical* as commonly caused by central and peripheral nervous lesions, with the exception of polyneuropathies and symmetrical mononeuritis multiplex. *Symmetrical* weakness is characteristic of the neuromuscular junction disorders and myopathies.

- *Distal symmetrical* weakness, affecting the small muscles of the hands and feet, occurs with sensorimotor polyneuropathies, and motor neuron disease.

- *Proximal symmetrical* weakness affecting the deltoids, hip flexors, and axial muscles is seen in muscular dystrophies, and most causes of myopathy.

Myasthenia gravis causes a specific pattern of weakness affecting the proximal upper limb, oculomotor, levator palpebrae superioris (causing bilateral ptosis), bulbar, respiratory, and facial muscles.

Progression of weakness

'Where did the weakness first start? Has it progressed to involve other areas?'

- *Ascending* weakness begins in the distal muscles of the lower limbs and progresses up the body. Causes include: Guillain-Barré syndrome and spinal cord disorders. These warrant urgent investigation and treatment (see below).

- *Descending* weakness is characterized by weakness beginning in the facial muscles and progressing down the body. Causes include: organophosphate and lead poisoning, botulism, and the descending variant of Guillain-Barré syndrome.

Precipitating/aggravating and relieving factors

'Is there anything that brings on the weakness or makes it worse? Exercise? Meals?'

- Exercise and meals rich in carbohydrates and sodium precipitate attacks of hypokalaemic periodic paralysis, whereas potassium ingestion triggers hyperkalaemic periodic paralysis. Attacks usually occur upon awakening in the morning. Hypokalaemic attacks persist for several hours whereas hyperkalaemic attacks last for approximately one hour.

- Muscle weakness which progresses throughout the day, and fatigability with exercise, is classically seen with myasthenia gravis. *'Does your weakness / double vision get worse as the day goes on? Are your muscles weaker after a period of exercise, such as walking or cooking?'*. By contrast, the Eaton-Lambert syndrome may improve following exercise.

Associated symptoms.

- **Muscle cramps and stiffness** often described by patients with myotonic dystrophies.

- **Respiratory muscle weakness.** Ask about shortness of breath.

- **Bulbar symptoms.**
  - ♦ *'Do you have difficulty swallowing solids, liquids or saliva?'*
  - ♦ *'Have you or others noticed a change in the pitch of your voice'*
  - ♦ *'Are you still able to produce a forceful cough?'*

- **Neurological symptoms.** Ask about visual disturbances, in particular diplopia caused by oculomotor muscle weakness, ptosis, speech disturbance, paraesthesiae, and seizures. Back pain, gait, and sphincter disturbance should raise the suspicion of spinal cord disease. Visual loss, cerebellar symptoms, or spinal cord symptoms, disseminated in time, may indicate multiple sclerosis.

- **Thyroid disease.** Hypothyroidism may cause generalized weakness. Ask about weight gain, constipation, cold intolerance, neck swelling, and menorrhagia in women. Additionally, hyperthyroidism may cause proximal myopathy. Ask about heat intolerance, diarrhoea, and weight loss.

- **Cushing's syndrome.** Proximal myopathy is a feature of Cushing's syndrome. Ask about disproportional weight gain, striae, thinning of skin, easy bruising, acne, hirsutism, oligo/amenorrhoea in women, and psychiatric symptoms such as low or elated mood, hallucinations, and delusions.
- **Addison's disease.** Adrenocortical insufficiency may cause generalizsed weakness. Ask about buccal and palmer crease pigmentation, weight loss, and dizziness.
- **Rash.** An erythematous macular rash over the shoulders and back (shawl's sign) and a purple periorbital rash and oedema (heliotrope rash) are seen in patients with dermatomyositis. Gottron's papules, a purple-red rash over the MCP and PIP joints, is pathognomonic of dermatomyositis.
- **Constitutional symptoms.** Ask about recent viral illnesses. Weight loss may indicate underlying malignancy. A thorough systems review is indicated if malignancy is suspected.
- **Depressive symptoms.** Ask about low mood, early morning wakening, insomnia, reduced appetite, self-harm, and suicidal ideation.

Functional status

It is important to enquire about the functional status of patients with muscle weakness. Inability to perform certain activities may also give clues to the type of myopathy present. For example, ask the patient: *'Do you find climbing stairs, getting up from a seated position, or combing your hair difficult?'* This indicates proximal muscle weakness.

Patients with functional weakness find *all* types of daily activities difficult to perform.

B. Relevant medical and family history:

Past medical history

- Endocrinopathies: diabetes mellitus, thyroid disease, Cushing's syndrome.
- Vascular risk factors; hypertension, hyperlipidaemia, ischaemic heart disease, peripheral vascular disease, and previous cerebrovascular events may suggest cerebrovascular disease.
- Previous malignancy; breast, lung, colorectal, haematological, and gynaecological may point towards metastatic disease or paraneoplastic syndrome.
- Poliomyelitis

Family history

- Hereditary causes of muscle weakness include muscular dystrophies, myotonic dystrophy, periodic paralysis, and Charcot-Marie Tooth.

C. Medications:

- Drugs inducing myopathy include: corticosteroids, statins, fibrates penicillamine, anti-malarials, and zidovudine.
- Drugs that impair neuromuscular junction transmission and precipitate a myasthenic crisis are: aminoglycoside antibiotics, macrolides, benzodiazepines, β-blockers, and calcium channels blockers.
- Several drugs may induce peripheral neuropathy (see Case 34 Parasthesiae).
- Diuretics may cause hypokalaemia.

D. Social Issues:

- Enquire about smoking habits, alcohol consumption, and recreational drug use. Cocaine and heroin can induce myopathy. In addition consider heroin contamination with botulism toxin in intravenous drug users presenting with descending weakness.
- Take an occupational history and enquire about the impact of the patient's symptoms on their job. Farmers are at risk of organophosphate poisoning.

- Ask the patient if close contacts have similar symptoms suggesting botulism, lead or organophosphate poisoning.
- Ask specifically about the patient's concerns about their own symptoms.

Formulating a plan of action

- Explain the possible causes of the patient's symptoms as directed by the history and inform them that a thorough clinical examination followed by investigations will be required to determine the diagnosis.
- Consider the following investigations:
  - Blood count may indicate a leucocytosis in infection.
  - ESR will be raised in inflammatory myopathies such as polymyositis, dermatomyositis, and inclusion body myositis.
  - Urea, electrolytes, and creatinine for electrolyte imbalances causing myopathy or renal failure as a cause for peripheral neuropathy.
  - Thyroid function tests for hyper-/hypo-thyroidism.
  - Elevated fasting glucose indicates diabetes mellitus.
  - CK will be raised in muscular dystrophies, inflammatory myopathies, rhabdomyolysis, and drug-induced myopathies, but typically normal in metabolic myopathies.
  - ANA and anti-acetylcholine receptor antibody titres are raised in myasthenia gravis since these antibodies are highly sensitive and specific, the tensilon test is rarely required.
  - Dexamethasone suppression testing for confirmation of Cushing's syndrome.
  - Synacthen test for diagnosis of Addison's disease.
  - Spirometry must be performed in rapidly progressive muscular weakness to determine respiratory failure and need for mechanical ventilation.
  - CT/MRI head or spinal cord will reveal ischaemic or haemorrhagic strokes, space occupying and demyelinating lesions.
  - CSF analysis is necessary for detection of oligoclonocal bands for multiple sclerosis and may reveal raised protein in Guillain-Barre syndrome.
  - CT thorax may be indicated if there is suspicion of thymoma in myasthenia gravis.
  - EMG may reveal characteristic electrical activity of certain myopathies. For example, fibrillations or increased spontaneous activity are seen with inflammatory myopathies; reduced amplitude of compound motor action potential on repeated nerve stimulation demonstrates the fatiguability of myasthenia gravis. Myotonias produce complex discharges and a 'dive bomber' sound on stimulation.
  - Muscle biopsy is the gold standard test for determining the type of muscle disease present.

Questions commonly asked by examiners

What types of muscular dystrophies do you know about?

- *Duchenne's muscular dystrophy* is an X-linked recessive disorder caused by a mutation in the dystrophin gene on Xp21.1 locus. It is the commonest hereditary muscular dystrophy presenting in childhood with delayed motor milestones and symmetrical proximal muscle weakness. On examination patients have proximal muscle wasting and patients perform the Gower's manoeuvre in order to rise from a seated position, a waddling gait, pseudohypertrophy of the calf muscles, absent tendon reflexes although ankle jerks are present. Cardiac involvement is invariable leading to cardiac failure. Involvement of the spinal muscles leads to severe kyphoscoliosis and together with respiratory muscle weakness leads to ventilatory failure. Most patients die before the age of 20 years.

- *Becker's muscular dystrophy* is also an X-linked recessive disorder clinically similar to Duchenne's muscular dystrophy, but onset is in adolescence with a slower rate of progression.
- *Fascioscapulohumeral dystrophy* is an autosomal dominant muscular dystrophy. Patients present in childhood and adolescence with facial and shoulder muscle weakness and a winged scapula. Weakness can progress to involve the pelvic girdle.
- *Limb girdle muscular dystrophies* are a genetically heterogeneous group of muscular dystrophies presenting in early adulthood with limb girdle weakness.
- *Oculopharyngeal muscular dystrophy* is an autosomal dominant trinucleotide repeat disorder presenting in the 4th to 6th decades of life with facial weakness, bilateral ptosis with normal eye movements, and dysphagia. The disease is slowly progressive leading to involvement of the axial and laryngeal muscles.
- *Emery-Dreifuss muscular dystrophy* is an X-linked recessive disorder presenting in the first decade of life with proximal upper limb and distal lower limb weakness. Patients develop severe contractures with extended neck, flexed elbows, and ankle deformities.

What are the inflammatory myopathies?

Polymyositis, dermatomyositis, and inclusion body myositis comprise the inflammatory myopathies.

- *Polymyositis* presents with slowly progressive symmetrical proximal muscle weakness affecting both the upper and lower limbs. Dysphagia and dysphonia may be associated with this condition due to the involvement of the oesophageal and laryngeal muscles. Disease may progress to involve the respiratory muscles.
- *Dermatomyositis* includes the features of polymyositis with characteristic skin involvement. Patients have a purple coloured rash (*heliotrope*) of the eyelids, an erythematous macular rash over the shoulders and back (*shawl's sign*), erythematous maculopapular rash over the extensor surfaces of the MCP and PIP joints (*Gottron's papules*), and painful cracked skin of the fingertips (*mechanic's* hands).

Both conditions have associated features that include fever, arthralgia, interstitial pulmonary fibrosis, myocarditis, and Raynaud's phenomenon. Anti-mi2 and anti-Jo antibody titres are typically raised.

- *Inclusion body myositis* begins in the 5th to 6th decades of life and typically presents with slowly progressive skeletal muscle weakness of a variable pattern. In 20% of patients there may be associated facial weakness, dysphagia and cardiac involvement. The ESR and CK are normal or mildly elevated in comparison to polymyositis and dermatomyositis. Muscle biopsy showing muscle fibre necrosis, vacuolar degeneration, and an inflammatory infiltrate is diagnositic.

What malignancies are associated with dermatomyositis?

- Ovarian
- Lung
- Breast
- Gastrointestinal
- Non-Hodgkin's Lymphoma

Patients diagnosed with dermatomyositis should undergo annual screening for malignancy that includes a clinical examination and radiological investigations (plain chest radiograph, abdominal and pelvic ultrasound scan or CT scan if high risk, mammography, and colonoscopy).

Tell me about Guillan-Barré Syndrome

Guillan-Barré syndrome, or acute inflammatory demyelinating polyradiculoneuropathy (AIDP) is an autoimmune disorder that causes progressive areflexic weakness and mild sensory changes. The classical presentation is with progressive, symmetrical weakness which ascends over 2–6 weeks. Back pain and hip pain is also common and may precede weakness. Oropharyngeal or respiratory weakness is a presenting symptom in 40%, and about 1/3 of patients require mechanical ventilation due to respiratory failure. Autonomic dysfunction causing postural hypotension and arrythmias is also common, and all patients should have cardiac monitoring.

Several variants have been described, including the Miller-Fisher syndrome with opthalmoplegia, areflexia, and ataxia. This is seen in 5% of patients with AIDP, and is characterized by anti-ganglioside GQ1b antibodies.

Imaging is usually required to rule out spinal cord and nerve root disease, and nerve conduction studies and EMG are required to confirm demyelinating nerve injury. Treatment is typically supportive, including nutrition, skin care, and ventilation and cardiac monitoring if required. Additionally, immunomodulation with IVIg and plasma exchange has been shown to hasten recovery and decrease disability.

Further reading

1. Dalakas M and Hohlfeld R, Polymyositis and Dermatomyositis, Lancet. 2003; 362.

Case 36 ◆ Haematuria

INFORMATION FOR THE CANDIDATE

Dear Doctor,

This 34-year old gentleman has recently registered with our General Practice and was found to have a positive urine dipstick for blood and a blood pressure reading of 160/98 mmHg on his initial visit. He admits to recent 'flu-like' symptoms and episodes of frank haematuria.

Many thanks for your opinion.

Acquiring the history

A. History of presenting complaint:

The history should aim to determine whether the haematuria is a result of a local or systemic cause. It should also be structured to exclude a urological cause.

Diagnoses in <45 years	Diagnoses in >45 years	Diagnoses to consider in all age groups
Pulmonary-renal syndromes:[*] Goodpasture's syndrome, Wegener's granulomatosis, Microscopic polyangiitis	**Malignancy:** Renal cell carcinoma Transitional cell carcinoma of ureter/bladder Prostate Carcinoma	Renal calculi **Infection:** Pyelonephritis Infective Endocarditis Cystitis
Glomerulonephritis:[*] IgA nephropathy, post-infectious glomerulonephritis, Alport syndrome (hereditary nephritis), sickle cell nephropathy	**Benign:** Benign Prostatic Hypertrophy **Infection:** Prostatitis	TB **Drugs:** Anticoagulants Cyclophosphamide
Vasculitis:[*] Polyarteritis nodosa, Henoch-Schonlein purpura		**Other:** Bleeding disorders Trauma: catheterisation
Connective Tissue Disease:[*] Lupus nephritis, Systemic sclerosis		Radiotherapy/chemotherapy

[*] Pulmonary-renal syndromes, vasculitis, and connective tissue diseases can cause microscopic haematuria but don't usually cause frank haematuria.

Age of onset.
Characteristics
- Onset and number of episodes of haematuria
- Colour of urine—bright red, pink, or brown?
- Has the patient passed any clots? Size and shape? Rounded clots arise from the bladder and elongated clots from the upper urinary tract.
- *'When during the stream do you notice the blood; at the beginning, throughout or at the end of the stream?'.* Blood at the beginning of the urinary stream suggests bleeding from the lower urinary tract (urethra and prostate). Blood seen throughout micturition indicates bleeding from above the bladder (bladder, ureter, and kidneys), whereas terminal bleeding suggests the bladder base and prostate as the source.

Associated symptoms
- **Urinary**
  - Urgency, dysuria, and frequency suggesting a urinary tract infection
  - Obstructive symptoms in men: poor stream, hesitancy, dribbling, incontinence, and nocturia suggesting prostatic disease
  - Loin or suprapubic pain. Colicky pain is characteristic of a ureteric calculus and clot retention, whereas constant pain suggests inflammation or infection.
  - Passage of stones
  - 'Frothy' urine appearance of proteinuria
- **Respiratory**
  - Recent upper respiratory tract infection followed by haematuria suggests IgA Nephropathy.
  - Haemoptysis occurs in the pulmonary-renal syndromes
  - Cough, rhinorrhoea, wheeze, and epistaxis are clinical features of Wegener's Granulomatosis
  - Pleuritic chest pain and pleural effusions may occur in SLE
  - Dyspneoa

- **Rheumatological**
  - ◆ Rash. Non-blanching purpuric rashes are characteristic of Henoch-Schonlein Purpura or Wegener's Granulomatosis; a malar rash of SLE may be present.
  - ◆ Arthralgia and myalgia are features of SLE and vasculitis.
  - ◆ Tight skin, painful and cold fingers (Raynaud's phenonomenon) as part of systemic sclerosis
  - ◆ Easy bruising and mucosal bleeding from other sites (e.g. bleeding gums).
- **Systemic symptoms**
  - ◆ Fever and rigors can occur in pyelonephritis, infective endocarditis, and vasculitis
  - ◆ Weight loss and anorexia suggest malignancy or vasculitis
- Recent trauma causing renal injury or rhabdomyolysis. The latter causes myoglobinuria giving dark urine resembling haematuria. Other causes of rhabdomyolysis are burns, exercise, falls, seizures, and statins.

Precipitating factors
Recent trauma or vigorous exercise (long-distance running, marching, drumming) may cause exercise-induced haematuria

B. Relevant medical and family history:
Past medical history
ASK specifically about:
- Previous UTIs and calculi
- Diabetes, hypertension, and their complications
- Rheumatoid arthritis and SLE as causes of renal disease
- Radiotherapy and chemotherapy (cyclophosphamide) for malignant disease causing haemorrhagic cystitis
- Bleeding disorders
- Gout may cause uric acid calculi

Family history
- Ask specifically about any family history of bleeding disorders
- Enquire about a family history of renal disease. A general question may be *'Does anyone in your family suffer with problems with passing urine?'* If necessary, expand the question by explicitly asking about problems with kidneys, bladder, or prostate. Consider Polycystic Kidney Disease, and Alport's Syndrome (in Alport's syndrome there may be a history of sensorineural hearing loss).
- Urinary tract malignancy
- Renal calculi.

C. Medications and interactions:
Drugs causing haematuria
- Anticoagulants
- Cyclophosphamide

Drugs and foodstuffs causing dark urine
- Rifampicin
- Beetroot

Recreational drugs
Illicit drug use can cause infective endocarditis, and drugs such as ecstasy and heroin can cause rhabdomyolysis and hence dark urine.

D. Social issues:

- Occupational history: Enquire specifically about work in the dye, rubber, and dry-cleaning industry. Exposure to hydrocarbons solvents such as benzenes and ethylenes are associated with an increased risk of transitional cell carcinoma of the urinary tract.
- Smoking is a risk factor for renal cell and transitional cell carcinoma.
- Travel history: enquire about fresh water swimming in areas with schistosomiasis (e.g. Lake Malawi). Infection causes bladder inflammation, obstructive symptom, and increases the risk of squamous cell carcinoma of the bladder.
- Sports: long-distance running, marching, boxing can cause exercise-induced haematuria.

Formulating a plan of action

- Explain to the patient that the cause for the haematuria will require investigation. Explain the possible causes suggested by the history.
- Tell the patient that initial tests are urinalysis and blood tests, and the results of these will determine further management.
- Investigations required in all patients presenting with haematuria are:
  - **Urinalysis** for blood, protein, nitrites, and leucocytes. A midstream urine sample should be sent for microscopy, cytology, and microbiology.
  - **Urine microscopy** is performed for red cell count and morphology to determine true haematuria. Red cell casts are pathognomonic of glomerulonephritis, leucocytes will be present in infection, and crystals will be seen in the presence of calculi.
  - **Blood tests:**
    - FBC for blood loss, thrombocytopenia and leucopenia in SLE and vasculitis, and a leucocytosis in infection.
    - ESR is raised in connective tissue disorders, vasculitis, and infection.
    - U&Es and estimated glomerular filtration rate (GFR) for assessment of renal function and staging of chronic renal disease.
    - Serum calcium and urate in patients with suspected calculi.
    - Clotting screen and LFTs for bleeding disorders
  - **Imaging:**
    - Plain abdominal X-ray of kidneys, ureter, and bladder may reveal radio-opaque calculi.
    - Ultrasound and CT KUB (CT—kidneys, ureter, bladder). These have superseded the intravenous urogram. Ultrasound of the renal tract is the initial choice of investigation in patients presenting with any urinary symptoms or renal failure to exclude obstruction and structural abnormalities. CT KUB is considered in patients with a strong history suggestive of calculi or malignancy
- Investigations to consider in accordance with history are:
  - Three early morning midstream urine samples for suspected renal TB
  - Urine albumin:creatinine ratio, or 24-hour urinary protein collection, to quantify proteinuria if glomerular disease is suspected.
  - CK will be raised in rhabdomyolysis
  - Random fasting glucose +/– oral glucose tolerance test for diabetes
- Autoantibody screen: ANA and ds-DNA are positive in SLE, anti-sm is specific for SLE, ANCA is positive in Wegener's Granulomatosis (cANCA) and Microscopic Polyangitis (pANCA) and usually negative in Polyarteritis Nodosa, Anti-GBM is positive in Goodpasture's Syndrome.
  - Immunoglobulins IgG and IgM are raised in SLE
  - Complement C3 & C4 are low in active SLE.
  - Prostate Specific Antigen (PSA)

◆ CXR is indicated in patients with pulmonary symptoms for haemorrhage.

◆ Renal biopsy may be carried out when urological causes have been excluded. It is also indicated for patients presenting with nephrotic and nephritic syndromes, new onset of acute renal failure and when there is evidence of systemic disease.

◆ Transrectal ultrasound scan for prostatic symptoms, flexible cystoscopy for bladder disease, and renal angiogram/digital subtraction angiography for renal artery disease (renal artery disease may cause hypertension but does not cause frank haematuria).

Questions commonly asked by examiners
What are the indications for cystoscopy?
Cystoscopy has a low yield in men under the age of 40 and in low risk women. The predominant indications are risk factors for bladder cancer, or if the original work-up for haematuria (including imaging and urine cytology) is negative or equivocal. High risk groups for bladder cancer are men over the age of 50, and those with specific risks such as cigarette smoking, work in the dye industry or prior use of phenacetin or cyclophosphamide.

What are the pulmonary-renal syndromes?
The pulmonary-renal syndromes are clinical entities that are characterized by pulmonary alveolar haemorrhage and glomerulonephritis causing renal failure. Common causes are Wegener's Granulomatosis, Microscopic Polyangiitis, and Goodpasture's Syndrome.

What is Rapidly Progressive Glomerulonephritis and how is it managed?
Rapidly Progressive Glomerulonephritis (RPGN) is a syndrome consisting of haematuria, proteinuria, and rapidly deteriorating renal function leading to end-stage renal failure within two weeks of onset if left untreated. Histologically RPGN is characterized by glomerular necrosis, crescent formation with or without immune complex deposition. Causes include any type of glomerulonephritis but particularly ANCA associated vasculitis, SLE, and Goodpasture's Syndrome. Treatment entails immunosuppresion with high-dose corticosteroids, and cyclophosphamide or mycophenolate mofetil. Plasma exchange may be indicated in patients with high antibody titres (ANCA and/or anti-GBM) or associated pulmonary haemorrhage. Maintenance therapy is with low-dose corticosteroids and immunosuppressants. Renal prognosis is poor in patients with creatinine greater than 600µmol/L at presentation.

Case 37 ◆ **Polyuria**

INFORMATION FOR THE CANDIDATE

Dear Doctor,

Thank you for seeing this 57-year old lady with a 4-week history of thirst, excess urine, and blurred vision. She also reports some blurring of the vision and frequent headaches. She has previously been treated for an invasive ductal carcinoma of the breast with surgery and chemotherapy. She is not on any regular medications.

Many thanks for your opinion.

Acquiring the history

True polyuria is the passage of greater than 3 litres of urine per day. Causes include:

- **Inability to concentrate urine**
  - Diabetes insipidus: cranial and nephrogenic
- **Osmotic diuresis**
  - Diabetes mellitus (osmotic diuresis)
  - Diuretics
  - Chronic renal disease
- **Primary polydipsia**
  - Psychogenic polydipsia
  - Habitual excessive drinking

A. History of presenting complaint:

Age of onset

Mode of onset, duration and progression of symptoms

- Sudden onset of polyuria, occurring over a number of days to weeks, is characteristic of cranial diabetes insipidus (DI) of any cause, but especially post-traumatic and surgical causes.
- Gradual onset of polyuria is seen with nephrogenic DI, osmotic diuresis, and primary polydipsia. Familial cranial DI may sometimes present in adulthood.

Characteristics

- Determine the frequency of micturition by asking *'How many times a day do you pass urine?'*
- Attempt to enquire about the volume of urine passed during a 24-hour period to differentiate true polyuria from frequent passage of small amounts of urine, although the patient is unlikely to be able to provide an accurate answer.
- Ask about nocturia *'How often do you have to get up to pass urine during the night?'*. Nocturia is an early sign of chronic renal disease, due to loss of tubular concentrating function, as well as of obstructive uropathy due to bladder or prostate disease.
  - Ask about polydipsia *'Do you feel more thirsty than usual? Do you have to get up in the night to drink water because you are woken up by thirst?'* Patients with DI have a preference for cold drinks. In primary polydipsia, it is rare for the patient to drink during the night.
  - Establish the amount of fluid intake per day including alcohol. Begin with an open question such as *'In a typical day from when you wake up in the morning, how much fluid do you drink?'* Specifically ask about intake of tea, coffee and alcoholic beverages, and also amount of intake just before bed.

Associated symptoms

- **Other urinary symptoms**
  - Dysuria, urgency, abdominal/loin pain as well as frequency of micturition suggest urinary tract infection. However, the volume of urine passed is normal.
  - Urgency, hesitancy, terminal dribbling, haematuria, and nocturia are features of prostatic disease. Again the volume of urine passed is normal.
- **Symptoms of diabetes mellitus.** Polyuria and polydipsia may be the first presentation of diabetes mellitus, including diabetic ketoacidosis, and results from the osmotic effects of hyperglycaemia. Ask about other symptoms:
  - Weight loss, lethargy
  - Abdominal pain, nausea, and vomiting secondary to ketosis.

- ◆ Blurred vision from the osmotic effect of hyperglycaemia on the lens
- ◆ Recurrent urinary tract infections and thrush
- **Features of anterior pituitary hypofunction.** Symptoms are slow in onset, and the order of onset reflects the sequence of failure of hormone secretion (see Vol 1, Case 103 Hypopituitarism).
    - ◆ In men, enquire about loss of body hair, reduced libido, and impotence reflecting deficiency of LH and FSH.
    - ◆ In women, ask about oligomenorrhoea and amenorrhoea due to LH and FSH deficiency, and menorrhagia in secondary hypothyroidism. Infertility, hot flushes, and loss of body hair also occur with low levels of LH and FSH.
    - ◆ Ask about features of hypothyroidism such as cold intolerance, weight gain, constipation, dry skin, proximal muscle weakness, hoarse voice, and low mood.
    - ◆ Nausea, vomiting, weight loss, and dizziness occur with adrenocorticotrophic hormone (ACTH) deficiency.
- **Features of hypothalamic hypofunction**
    - ◆ Ask about galactorrhoea, 'Have you noticed a discharge from the nipple?' due to disinhibition of prolactin secretion by the pituitary.
    - ◆ Weight gain secondary to impaired satiety.
- **Neurological**
    - ◆ Frontal headaches, blurring of vision, nausea, and vomiting are manifestations of hypothalamic and pituitary masses.
    - ◆ Sudden onset headache should alert one to the possibility of pituitary apoplexy.
    - ◆ Ask about fever, neck stiffness, photophobia, nausea, and vomiting suggesting meningitis.
    - ◆ Diplopia may result from involvement of adjacent cranial nerves from extension of a hypothalamic or pituitary mass.
    - ◆ Visual abnormalities, including visual field loss, may be caused by pituitary masses.
    - ◆ Ask about recent head injury.
- **Respiratory**
    - ◆ Some respiratory diseases may be associated with hypercalcaemia which can lead to nephrogenic DI, (eg. squamous cell carcinoma, aderocarinoma, small cell carcinoma, sarcoidosis, Langerhan's histiocytosis.) Enquire about dry cough and exertional dyspnoea. In addition, consider the extrapulmonary features of sarcoidosis such as neck swelling (lymphadenopathy), skin rash, arthralgia, and eye symptoms (redness, pain, visual loss).
    - ◆ Haemoptysis suggests tuberculosis or lung cancer.
- **Psychiatric**
    - ◆ If a psychiatric disorder is suspected, ask openly about changes in mood and obsessional behaviour.

B. Relevant medical and family history:

Past medical history

- Diabetes mellitus: ask about diabetic control (recent HbA1c level) and presence of complications.
- Previous head injury, neurosurgery, and cranial radiotherapy are the common causes of cranial DI.
- Malignancy, particularly breast and lung, may metastasize to the pituitary gland causing cranial DI. They may also be associated with hypercalcaemia which may lead to nephrogenic DI.
- Multiple myeloma leading to chronic renal disease and hypercalcaemia can cause nephrogenic DI.

- Chronic renal disease of any cause.
- Tuberculosis, sarcoidosis, and Langerhan's histiocytosis are infiltrative causes of hypopituitarism.
- Ask about psychiatric illness—psychogenic polydipsia occurs in some cases of schizophrenia. Patients with bipolar disorders may be on Lithium, which may cause nephrogenic DI.

Family history

Both cranial and nephrogenic DI have familial forms, therefore enquire about this in patients presenting in childhood.

C. Medications:

- Lithium associated nephrogenic DI is well recognized.
- Ask about medications that cause a dry mouth, such as diuretics and anticholinergics.

D. Social issues:

- Ask about alcohol consumption.
- Ask about travel abroad to areas where tuberculosis is endemic.
- Determine the impact of the patient's symptoms in daily activities and the patient's occupation.

Formulating a plan of action

- Explain to the patient that a full clinical examination is required, along with blood and urine tests.
- Consider the following investigations in all patients presenting with polyuria:
    - **Urinalysis** for glucose, protein, and ketones suggesting diabetes. The presence of leucocytes and nitrites points towards a urinary tract infection.
    - **24-hour urine collection** will differentiate true polyuria from urinary frequency.
    - **Blood count** may show a raised white cell count indicative of an infection. A normocytic normochromic anaemia may be due to chronic renal disease.
    - **ESR** will be raised in inflammatory conditions and malignancy.
    - **Serum glucose** is raised in diabetes mellitus.
    - **Urea, creatinine, and electrolytes.** Urea and creatinine will be raised in chronic renal disease. Sodium levels are usually within normal limits if the thirst axis is intact, to replace sodium loss. Hypernatraemia indicates uncompensated polyuria due to inadequate oral intake. Dilutional hyponatraemia occurs in primary polydipsia. Potassium levels may be low in nephrogenic DI, or normal to high in chronic renal disease.
    - **Estimated GFR** for the degree of chronic renal impairment.
    - **Serum corrected calcium.** Hypercalcaemia leads to nephrogenic DI.
    - **Serum ACE** may be elevated in sarcoidosis.
    - **Plasma osmolality** is low in primary polydipsia and high in DI.
    - **Urine osmolality** greater than 600mOsm/Kg excludes DI as a cause.
    - **Tests of pituitary function**
        - Thyroid function tests, a low TSH and free T4 indicate secondary hypothyroidism.
        - LH, FSH, and sex hormones may be low.
        - Short ACTH stimulation test is impaired and ACTH levels are low in secondary adrenal insufficiency.
        - Low IGF-1 level or impaired insulin tolerance test indicates GH deficiency.
- **Water deprivation test** to differentiate between primary polydipsia and DI.

- **DDAVP (desmopressin acetate (synthetic analogue of vasopressin)) test** to differentiate between cranial and nephrogenic DI if the water deprivation test is positive.
  - **Imaging**
    - Plain chest radiograph may reveal lung cancer, tuberculosis, or bilateral hilar lymphadenopathy suggesting sarcoidosis.
    - MRI scan of the head for hypothalamic and pituitary lesions.
    - CT scan of the thorax, abdomen, and pelvis may be indicated for identification and/or staging of primary malignancy.
  - **CSF analysis** if neurosarcoidosis, tuberculosis, or meningitis are suspected.

Questions commonly asked by examiners

What are the causes of diabetes insipidus?

Diabetes insipidus is the production of greater than 40ml/Kg of dilute urine in a 24 hour period. Two types are recognized:

Cranial DI due to antidiuretic hormone (ADH) deficiency.
Nephrogenic DI in which the collecting duct of the kidney is resistant to the action of ADH.

Cranial diabetes insipidus	Nephrogenic diabetes insipidus
Post-surgical (transfrontal and transphenoidal)*	**Drugs**
Head injury*	• Lithium (chronic use)
Radiotherapy*	• Ofloxacin
Neoplastic	• Amphotericin
• Craniopharyngioma	• Orlistat
• Meningioma, glioma	• Demeclocycline
• Pituitary metastases (breast, bronchus)	• Foscarnet
• Pituitary adenoma with extension	**Chronic renal disease**
Infection	**Electrolyte disturbance**
• Tuberculosis	• Hypokalaemia
• Meningitis	• Hypercalcaemia
• Cerebral abscess	**Familial**
Inflammatory	
• Sarcoidosis	
• Langerhan's Histiocytosis	
Vascular	
• Pituitary apoplexy	
• Aneurysm	
Idiopathic (autoimmune)	
Familial	

* Most common causes

How is diabetes insipidus diagnosed?

The water deprivation test is performed to

1. differentiate primary polydipsia from DI
2. differentiate cranial and nephrogenic DI

The patient is kept fluid restricted overnight. Baseline weight, plasma, and urine osmolalities are measured and every 2 hours thereafter for 8 hours. The test is discontinued if there is weight loss greater than 5% from baseline, to avoid excessive dehydration. Desmopressin is administered subcutaenously, if:

1. there is 3% reduction in body weight and a plasma osmolality greater than 300mOsm/Kg at any time during the test, or
2. urinary osmolality is <600mOsm/Kg at the end of the 8 hour period.

The normal response to the water deprivation test is a urine osmolality of >600mOsm/Kg, indicating normal renal concentration of urine following water deprivation. Plasma osmolality should remain within normal limits. Cranial DI is confirmed when the urine osmolality *increases to more than 600mOsm/Kg* after desmopressin administration, indicating a lack of endogenous ADH but normal renal responsiveness to synthetic ADH. Nephrogenic DI is diagnosed when the urine osmolality *remains less than 300mOsm/Kg* after desmospressin, reflecting the resistance of collecting ducts to ADH. In primary polydipsia, the kidney retains some concentrating capacity, therefore the urine osmolality rises after desmopressin administration but does not reach normal values.

How is diabetes insipidus managed?

The underlying cause of any type of DI should be treated. Intranasal desmopressin is the treatment for cranial DI. Hormone replacement is initiated in cases of hypopituitarism. Nephrogenic DI can be treated with thiazide diuretics and NSAIDs, which are thought to enhance the sensitivity of the collecting ducts to ADH, in addition to withdrawal of the offending drug if possible.

Case 38 ◆ **Acute Confusion**

INFORMATION FOR THE CANDIDATE

Dear Doctor,

Thank you for seeing this 82-year old lady who lives with her husband. He tells me that she has been confused for a few days and 'not quite herself'. She has a history of recurrent urinary tract infections, Parkinson's disease for which she takes levodopa and hypertension treated with bendroflumethiazide.

Many thanks for your opinion.

Acquiring the history

A collateral history must be obtained for any patient presenting in a confusional state. The focus should be to differentiate delirium from other causes of cognitive impairment such as hypothyroidism, vitamin B12 deficiency, mood disorders, and dementia.

- *Delirium* is the **sudden onset** and **fluctuating** impairment in cognitive function and consciousness. It is **reversible.**
- *Dementia* is the **progressive** and **irreversible** decline in global cognitive function from a premorbid level without any impairment in consciousness. The higher cortical domains usually affected are memory, along with one other from: speech, executive function, praxis,

and stereognosis. One should be aware that patients with known dementia can present with acute-on-chronic confusion secondary to a reversible cause.

A. History of presenting complaint

Age of onset

The aetiology differs between age groups. In younger patients, consider drug and alcohol use and withdrawal, meningitis, encephalitis, and as causes of acute confusion. The common causes of delirium in the older age group are polypharmacy, infection of any cause, electrolyte imbalance, and stroke.

Mode of onset and duration of symptoms

- Sudden onset of confusion of short duration (hours to days) is characteristic of delirium. The confusion may also fluctuate during the day. An insidious onset with gradual progression over a period of months to years favours dementia (see Case 39 Memory Loss).
- Ask about previous similar episodes of confusion

Assessment of confusion

Use open questioning to determine the nature of the confusion from the eyewitness. A general question may be *'In what way is her behaviour different from normal?'*. Ask for examples of episodes of confusion before asking the following specific questions for the diagnosis of delirium using the Confusion Assessment Method (CAM) tool:

1. Acute onset and fluctuating course: *'Is this a dramatic change in behaviour from baseline?'*; *'Does the abnormal behaviour come and go during the day?'*.
2. Inattention. *'Does he/she have difficulty focusing or is he/she easily distracted?'*
3. Disorganized thinking. *'Do you have difficulty following his/her conversation?'*.
4. Altered level of consciousness. *'Does he/she have episodes of drowsiness or agitation?'*

The diagnosis of delirium requires the presence of 1 and 2 plus *either* 3 or 4.

It is also important to establish the patient's premorbid baseline function and mental state to establish the degree of deterioration.

Associated symptoms

A thorough systems review is necessary in determining acute illnesses which may precipitate acute confusion in the elderly:

- **Neurological:** ask focused questions about
  - Meningitis: headache, fever, photophobia, neck stiffness, and rash
  - Head injury: Ask about recent head injury, trauma, or falls. In the elderly consider subdural haematoma as a cause for confusion.
  - Stroke: sudden onset of limb and/or facial weakness, sensory disturbance, dysphasia, visual impairment, vomiting, vertigo, and dysphagia.
  - Seizures of any type may cause periods of post-ictal confusion. Enquire about seizure activity (see Case 33 Seizures).
  - Encephalitis: fever, behavioural, and personality change.
- **Urinary:** dysuria, frequency, urgency, incontinence, and suprapubic pain suggest urinary tract infection. Anuria and suprapubic pain suggest acute urinary retention, a further cause of delirium in the elderly.
- **Respiratory:**
  - Chest infection: cough, productive sputum, dyspnoea, and pleuritic chest pain.
  - Pulmonary embolus: pleuritic chest pain, haemoptysis.

- **Cardiac:** chest pain, dyspnoea, orthopnoea, paroxysmal nocturnal dyspnoea, ankle swelling, palpitations, dizziness, and syncope suggest congestive heart failure, myocardial infarction, or arrhythmia.
- **Gastrointestinal:**
  - Acute abdominal pain with systemic features may indicate intra-abdominal pathology.
  - Hepatic encephalopathy is suggested by jaundice and abdominal distension due to ascites.
  - *Clostridium difficile* colitis is a cause of acute confusion and hallucinations in the elderly. Therefore, enquire about diarrhoea and recent antibiotic use.
- **Psychiatric:** Visual hallucinations and fleeting delusions occur frequently in acute confusional states and delirium tremens. Behavioural problems such as aggression and personality change suggest encephalitis.

B. Relevant medical history:

- Dementia: known dementia is a risk factor for delirium, and reversible causes for sudden deterioration in cognition should be sought.
- Diabetes: hyperglycaemia and hypoglycaemia can present with confusion.
- Decompensated liver disease may cause hepatic encephalopathy.
- Epilepsy causing post-ictal confusion.
- Parkinson's disease: confusion is a common side effect of dopaminergic medications used to treat Parkinson's disease.
- Malignancy. Consider cerebral metastases in patients with known or previous malignancy.
- HIV predisposes to opportunistic CNS infections. Consider cryptococcal meningitis, toxoplasmosis, and progressive multifocal leucoencephalopathy in such patients presenting with acute confusion. Consider AIDS-dementia complex or CNS lymphoma in patients presenting with cognitive impairment in the absence of fluctuating consciousness.

C. Medications:

A thorough drug history is essential.

- Ask about current drug regime and enquire specifically about:
  - addition of new medications
  - changes in doses of current medications
  - abrupt withdrawal from medications such benzodiazepines and opiates.
- Antihypertensive drugs, particularly thiazide, loop and potassium-sparing diuretics, may cause hyponatraemia leading to cerebral oedema and confusion.
- Ask about timing and frequency of medications. Overdose and toxicity of prescription drugs can be a precipitant for delirium. Drugs that have this potential are:
  - Insulin and oral hypoglycaemics
  - digoxin
  - lithium
  - opiates
  - sedatives such as benzodiazepines and barbiturates
- Some medications can cause confusion as a side effect. Examples include:
  - anticholinergics
    - benzatropine and procyclidine used in Parkinson's disease
    - tricyclic antidepressants such as amitryptilline and imipramine
    - SSRIs, especially citalopram and sertraline
    - oxybutynin used as a bladder stabilizer in urinary incontinence

- opiates: codeine and tramadol can cause marked confusion in the elderly
- dopamine agonist such as levodopa used in the treatment of Parkinson's disease
- corticosteroids cause a wide range of psychiatric symptoms such as psychosis, hallucinations, and euphoria.
- Recreational drug use and withdrawal should be considered in younger patients presenting with an acute confusional state.

D. Social issues:

- Enquire about the patient's premorbid functional status and determine the extent of deterioration in function. In the elderly, ask specifically about mobility and level of independence to perform activities of daily living.
- Ask about alcohol consumption and recent attempts at cessation. Alcohol dependence predisposes to:
  - Delirium tremens, presenting within 48–72 hours of alcohol withdrawal. It is characterized by acute confusion (disorientation, agitation, and inattention) vivid visual and auditory hallucinations and autonomic symptoms.
  - Wernicke's encephalopathy due to thiamine deficiency secondary to malnutrition. This is characterized by a triad of encephalopathy, ophthalmoplegia, and gait disturbance, although any one of these features may be present in isolation.

Formulating a plan of action

- Explain that a thorough clinical examination and investigations are required to determine the cause for the confusion.
- An abbreviated mental test score (AMTS) is necessary in all patients to establish the cognitive deficits present on admission and for a baseline score against which progress can be assessed.
- Consider the following investigations in all patients:
  - **Bedside tests**:
    - Capillary blood glucose for hypo or hyperglycaemia.
    - Urinalysis for blood, nitrites, and leucocytes indicative of a urinary tract infection. Send a mid-stream urine sample for microscopy, culture, and sensitivity if any of these are detected. Ketones and glucose in the urine suggests diabetic ketoacidosis.
    - Urine toxicology screen.
    - ECG for myocardial ischaemia, pulmonary embolus.
  - **Blood tests**
    - Blood cultures if patient has symptoms and signs of sepsis
    - Blood count. A raised white cell count may indicate an infection
    - CRP or ESR will be raised in an infection or malignancy
    - Urea, creatinine, and electrolytes for renal impairment and electrolyte imbalance
    - Corrected calcium. Hypercalcaemia is a cause of confusion
    - LFTs may be deranged in hepatic encephalopathy
    - Thyroid function tests
    - Digoxin and lithium drug levels if indicated
    - Arterial blood gases for hypoxia, hypercapnia, acidosis, and alkalosis
    - Cardiac enzymes if myocardial infarction is suspected
    - D-dimer if there is clinical suspicion of PE
    - ECG may show cardiac disease, PE or digitals toxicity

- **Imaging:** Imaging is directed by the history and clinical examination.
  - Chest X-ray for respiratory infection, congestive heart failure. An erect chest X-ray may be indicated in patients with an acute abdomen for a pneumoperitoneum.
  - Indications for a CT scan of the head:
    - (a) no cause of the confusion is found with above investigations
    - (b) history of head trauma
    - (c) history suggestive of a neurological cause, for example, limb weakness, sudden onset headache, and seizures
    - (d) focal neurological signs on examination
    - (e) to exclude mass lesion before lumbar puncture
    - (f) in patients with known malignancy when cerebral metastases are suspected
    - (g) in HIV/AIDS patients with confusion.
  - Lumbar puncture is warranted when meningitis or encephalitis is likely, or when there is a strong clinical suspicion of a subarachnoid haemorrhage in the presence of a normal CT scan.

Questions commonly asked by examiners

What are the causes of delirium?

Diagnoses to consider in young patients 65 years	Diagnoses to consider in elderly	Diagnoses to consider in all ages
Recreational drug use and withdrawal	Polypharmacy or recent changes in medications.	Electrolyte disturbance
Meningitis/encephalitis	Stroke/subdural haematoma	Infection of any cause
HIV/AIDS	Infections: urinary tract infection, respiratory are common.	Metabolic disturbance: hepatic encephalopathy, uraemia, hypo- or hyperthyroidism
	Acute urinary retention	Cerebral tumours and metastases
	Faecal impaction	Myocardial infarction
		Pulmonary embolus
		Alcohol intoxication and withdrawal syndromes: delirium tremens, and Wernicke's encephalopathy

What factors predispose to delirium?

- Age > 65 years
- Dementia
- Multiple co-morbidities
- Visual and hearing impairment
- Recent surgery
- Polypharmacy
- Drugs and alcohol dependence
- HIV/AIDS

How is delirium managed?

- **Supportive management** involves assessment of the patient in a quiet room with adequate lighting. Reassure and orientate the patient in time, place, and person.

- **Medical management:**
    - ◆ Identification and treatment of the underlying cause is the cornerstone of management of delirium.
    - ◆ Review the patient's medications and stop causative agents if possible.
    - ◆ Consider pharmacological treatment if the patient has not responded to supportive measures alone, is in a severe hyperactive state or is a danger to themselves and/or others. Intramuscular sedation may be used:
        - – **Antipsychotics.** Haloperidol is used in for rapid sedation. Atypical antipsychotics (olanzapine and risperidone) may be considered for longer sedation but are contraindicated in patients with cerebrovascular disease.
        - – **Benzodiazepines.** Short-acting lorazepam is particularly useful in alcohol and drug withdrawal states. It can also be used in conjunction with haloperidol. Chlordiazepoxide is a longer-acting alternative, but should be used with caution in liver disease due to the risk of precepitating encephalopathy.

Case 39 ◆ **Memory Loss**

INFORMATION FOR THE CANDIDATE

Dear Doctor,

Thank you for seeing this 74-year old gentleman, whose wife tells me he has been progressively confused over recent months. She reports that he has been getting forgetful, neglecting his personal care, and has failed to recognize her at times. He has a history of TIAs, hypertension, and hyperlipidaemia for which he takes aspirin, ramipril, and simvastatin. She is finding it increasingly difficult to cope at home, and is concerned that he may have Alzheimer's disease.

Many thanks for your opinion

Acquiring the history

Most patients with dementia do not complain of memory loss—self-reported memory loss does not correlate with the development of dementia. It is often a spouse or family member who brings the condition to medical attention, therefore this collateral history is essential in the assessment of a patient presenting with memory impairment.

Dementia is defined as a *progressive* and *irreversible* decline in global cognitive function from a higher premorbid level, resulting in significant functional impairment. The higher cortical domains usually affected are memory with one other from: speech, executive function, praxis and stereognosis. These symptoms must not be accounted for by delirium, psychiatric disease, or an alternative systemic or brain disorder.

In any patient presenting with cognitive impairment, an assessment for reversible causes of cognitive impairment must be made before diagnosing dementia.

A. History of presenting complaint

Age of onset

In younger patients (<65 years), consider CNS space-occupying lesions, familial Alzheimer's disease, Huntington's disease, cerebral vasculitis, AIDS dementia-complex, Korsakoff's syndrome and Creutzfeldt-Jakob disease (CJD) (including *new variant* CJD).

Characteristics of cognitive impairment

A collateral history is essential to establish the nature of cognitive impairment. Begin by asking an open question such as *'What changes have you noticed?'* Follow with specific questioning about daily activities, focusing on the type of task and the degree of disability:

*   **Memory.** Ask about examples of memory loss and whether short- or long-term memory is affected.
    *   *Anterograde episodic memory loss* (memory of new events) is seen in early Alzheimer's disease:
    *   *'Does Mr X easily forget recent events?'*
    *   *'Does he forget new information he has just been told?'*
    *   *'Does he forget where he puts things?'*
    *   *Long-term memory loss* is seen in the later stages of Alzheimer's disease:
    *   *'Does he forget the names of familiar people?'*
    *   *'Can he still recall events of the past?'*
*   **Attention and concentration.** Inattention and concentration are affected early in the course of dementia with Lewy bodies.
    *   *'Does Mr X find it difficult to concentrate on tasks, like counting money or paying a bill?'*
*   **Orientation**
    *   *'Does Mr X need to be frequently reminded of what time it is or where he is?'*
    *   *'Does Mr X get lost in familiar places?'*
*   **Language and comprehension**
    *   *'Does Mr X use the wrong words for familiar objects?'* suggesting word finding difficulty or expressive dysphasia.
    *   *'Does Mr X have difficulty understanding written information or writing?'*
    *   *'Does Mr X use the same word(s) to answer different questions?'*. Perseveration is a feature of frontotemporal dementia.
*   **Praxis**
    *   *'Does Mr X have difficulty dressing, washing or using household equipment?'* suggests dyspraxia.

Mode of onset, duration, and progression of memory impairment

*   Sudden onset cognitive impairment suggests delirium (see Case 38 Acute Confusion).
*   Gradual onset over a period of months to years favours a possible diagnosis of dementia.
*   Determine the progression of symptoms over a period of time by asking *'How quickly have the symptoms progressed over time?'*.
    *   Slow progression is characteristic of Alzheimer's disease and frontotemporal dementia.
    *   Rapid decline in cognitive function over a period of days to weeks is seen with subdural haemorrhage and CJD.
    *   Rapid decline in cognition over a period of months is a feature of CNS tumours, dementia with Lewy bodies, and dementia associated with the Parkinson Plus syndromes.
    *   A stepwise deterioration of symptoms (a rapid decline in function followed a plateau followed by a further decline) is seen with vascular dementia.

Associated symptoms

- **Neurological**
  - ◆ Focal signs such as limb weakness, sensory disturbance, or visual disturbance, may be due to cerebrovascular disease or CNS space occupying lesions.
  - ◆ Altered or fluctuating consciousness may suggest delirium of any cause or subdural haemorrhage. However, Lewy body dementia may be confused with delirium because fluctuations and visual hallucinations are common and prominent.
  - ◆ Ask about gait disturbance and balance (see Case 31 Gait Disturbance).
    - – Shuffling gait, hesitation, and freezing *with* loss of arm swing are features of Parkinson's disease and the Parkinson Plus syndromes
    - – Small steps and broad based gait *without* loss of arm swing is the characteristic gait of normal pressure hydrocephalus (characterized by gait disturbance, cognitive impairment, and urinary incontinence).
    - – Hemiplegic gait is typical of stroke or space occupying lesion.
    - – Unsteady, ataxic gait due to cerebellar dysfunction may be seen in alcohol-related dementia.
  - ◆ Postural instability and falls occur in Parkinson's disease, Parkinson Plus syndromes and normal pressure hydrocephalus.
  - ◆ Ask about the presence of a movement disorder in particular
    - – Tremor *'shaking of hands or other body parts'*. A resting tremor occurs in Parkinson's disease, dementia with Lewy bodies and Wilson's disease. An intention tremor may occur in Wilson's disease.
    - – Chorea *'writhing movements'* seen in Huntington's disease.
    - – Myoclonus *'sudden jerking of limbs'* is a feature of CJD.
    - – Dystonia *'stiffness or cramps of the limbs'* occurs with Wilson's disease.
  - ◆ Headaches, seizures, nausea, and vomiting exacerbated by postural changes are features of raised intracranial pressure caused by space-occupying lesions.
  - ◆ Ask about urinary incontinence *'Do you ever lose control of your urine?'* seen in normal pressure hydrocephalus and frontal lobe dysfunction such as frontotemporal dementia.
- **Psychiatric**
  - ◆ Ask about visual hallucinations which occur in dementia with Lewy bodies with a question such as *'Do you sometimes see things that other people don't see?'*. Ask the patient to describe the hallucinations.
  - ◆ Enquire about mood by asking the patient *'How do you feel within yourself?'* or the carer *'How would you describe Mr X's mood recently?'*. Depression in the elderly is commonly misdiagnosed as dementia. Elicit other depressive symptoms such as anhedonia *'Does Mr X still enjoy the activities and hobbies he used to?'*, low energy and sleep disturbance. Determine any triggers if depression is suspected.
  - ◆ Ask about recent behavioural and personality changes such as disinhibition and aggression, which are features of frontotemoporal lobe dementia and advanced Alzheimer's disease.
- **Other**
  - ◆ Screen for features of hypothyroidism such as weight gain, lethargy, hoarseness of voice, and cold intolerance. Remember that weight gain can be side-effect of antidepressants and antipsychotics (see Case 21 Weight Gain).
  - ◆ Cushing's syndrome can lead to cognitive impairment, particularly short-term memory, inattention and poor concentration as well as other neuropsychiatric symptoms. Screen for features of Cushing's syndrome such as weight gain, muscle weakness, diabetes, and hypertension.

B. Relevant medical and family history:

Past medical history

Enquire about the following:

- Cerebrovascular disease, ischaemic heart disease, and vascular risk factors (hypertension, diabetes, hyperlipidaemia). The presence of these would favour vascular dementia.
- Ask about Parkinson's disease and when the motor symptoms first started. The onset of cognitive impairment before or within one year of extrapyramidal features suggests dementia with Lewy bodies, whereas cognitive decline occurring more than one year after the onset of motor symptoms is suggestive of Parkinson's disease with dementia.
  - Ask about previous history of malignancy which may point towards cerebral metastases.
  - Enquire about HIV/AIDS by asking the patient 'Have you ever been tested for HIV?'. Consider AIDS dementia complex in patients with a known diagnosis of HIV presenting with cognitive decline.

Family history

Family history of neurodegenerative conditions with a genetic component such as Alzheimer's disease, Parkinson's disease, and Huntington's disease should be sought and considered in younger patients.

C. Medications:

- Take a thorough drug history to determine the use of medications which can cause cognitive impairment, such as anticholinergics, opiates, and anxiolytics. Antipsychotic drugs exacerbate the motor symptoms and cognitive impairment in dementia with Lewy bodies.
- Ask about compliance with regular medications, since cognitive impairment may impair compliance leading to inadequate treatment of co-morbidities which may in turn worsen cognitive impairment.
- Ask about the use of recreational drugs.
- Aluminium based phosphate binders in patients on dialysis.

D. Social issues:

- Ask about alcohol consumption. Chronic alcohol misuse can lead to Korsakoff's syndrome as a result of thiamine deficiency. Unlike dementia, which is a global decline in cognitive function, Korsakoff's syndrome is a selective disorder of anterograde and retrograde memory. Attention and social behaviour are usually preserved, such that patients may confabulate to cover their memory loss.
- Enquire about any exposure to heavy metals or organic solvents.
- Obtain a detailed account of the patient's social circumstances from a relative, friend or general practitioner. The following should be asked about for planning of social care:
  - Current living arrangements. Determine the type of accommodation the patient lives in, ownership, and other residents.
  - Find out if the patient is known to social services and if there is a package of care already in place.
  - Ability to carry out daily activities such as personal care and housework. Personal neglect is commonly encountered with cognitive impairment.
  - Risk assessment.
    - Determine whether the patient can go out of the house safely.
    - Establish if there have been episodes when the patient has put themselves or others in danger. For example, has the patient left the gas on, or the front door open?

- Determine if the patient still drives. Impairment in executive function and judgement makes this hazardous.
- Ask about episodes of violence or abuse towards others and self-harm. These are features of advanced dementia. Moreover, patients with dementia are vulnerable to physical, mental, and financial abuse by others, and this should be explored in detail if suspected.

♦ Ask about the management of financial and legal affairs and whether the patient has appointed a lasting power of attorney.

♦ Establish the impact of the patient's health status on the family and/or carers and determine whether they are able to cope with the current situation.

Formulating a plan of action

• Explain to the patient and the wife that a full cognitive assessment and clinical examination is required for a complete assessment.

• Explain that there are a number of possible diagnoses for the patient's symptoms and investigations will be required to determine the cause. Also explain that a diagnosis of Alzheimer's disease is a clinical process, following the exclusion of other causes of cognitive impairment.

• Address the wife's concerns elicited in the history, and reassure her that a full social assessment will be made for the provision of an appropriate package of care.

• Complete a bedside cognitive assessment using the Mini Mental State Examination (MMSE) to highlight areas of cognitive deficit. A score of less than 23 out of 30 is suggestive of cognitive impairment.

• Consider the following investigations to search for reversible causes of dementia:
  ♦ **Blood tests.** The following blood tests comprise the dementia 'screen', although the yield is low and there is no evidence to support routine testing.
    - Blood count for anaemia and red cell indices.
    - Haematinics: red cell folate, vitamin B_{12}, ferritin. Consider intrinsic factor and antibody for pernicious anaemia.
    - ESR
    - Serum glucose
    - U&Es
    - LFTs
    - Corrected calcium, magnesium and phosphate
    - Thyroid function tests for hypo- and hyperthyroidism
    - Copper studies (if <40 years of age): serum copper, caeruloplasmin, and urinary copper
    - Syphilis serology: EIA, TPHA, and VDRL.
    - HIV test if appropriate

• **Imaging**
  ♦ CT head (or MRI) is indicated in young patients (<65 years) and patients with:
    - History of recent head trauma/fall to exclude haemorrhage, subdural haematoma
    - Sudden onset and rapid cognitive impairment
    - History suggestive of a stroke, space occupying lesion, or normal pressure hydrocephalus
    - History of malignancy raising suspicion of cerebral metastases

- **Specialist investigations**
  - Cardiac investigations for embolic source: echocardiogram and carotid dopplers.
  - Autoantibody screen for vasculitis (ANA, anti-dsDNA, anti Ro, La, anticardiolipin, lupus anticoagulant, anti-glycoprotein)
  - MRI or cerebral angiography if primary cerebral angiitis is suspected.
  - Toxicology screen if appropriate
  - CSF analysis
  - Electroencephalogram in suspected CJD (very rare)
  - SPECT HMPAO scan (perfusion scan)—specific patterns of abnormalities are seen with dementia with lewy bodies, frontotemporal dementia, and Alzheimer's disease.

Questions commonly asked by examiners

What are the causes of dementia?

Dementia can result from primary CNS abnormality or secondary disease. Some secondary conditions leading to cognitive impairment are potentially reversible (15% of all cases) and therefore must be excluded.

Primary causes of dementia	Secondary causes of dementia
Neurodegenerative conditions	**Metabolic**
• Alzheimer's disease	• Vitamin B$_{12}$,* folate,* and thiamine deficiency
• Parkinson Plus syndromes	• Hypothyroidism*
◆ Dementia with lewy bodies	• Cushing's syndrome*
◆ Corticobasal degeneration	• Wilson's disease*
◆ Progressive supranuclear palsy	**Vascular**
◆ Parkinson's disease with dementia	• Cerebrovascular disease
• Frontotemporal dementia	• Subdural haematoma*
• Creutzfeldt-Jakob disease	• Primary angiitis of CNS
Other	• Antiphospholipid antibody syndrome
• Vascular dementia types	**Neoplastic**
• Normal pressure hydrocephalus*	• Primary CNS tumours
	• Metastases
	Inflammatory
	• SLE
	Drugs and toxins
	• Anticholinergics*
	• Chronic alcohol misuse (Korsakoff's encephalopathy)
	• Heavy metal exposure
	Infection
	• Syphilis*
	• AIDS dementia-complex

* Reversible causes of dementia

What is subcortical dementia and what types do you know about?

Subcortical dementia results from lesions in the basal ganglia, thalamus, deep cerebral white matter, and brainstem. The classical clinical features are executive dysfunction causing bradyphrenia (psychomotor 'slowness'), impairment in planning and judgement, change in mood, low affect, speech disturbance, and extrapyramidal motor features. These cognitive deficits predominate over memory impairment which if present is mild. Causes include:

- Vascular dementia
  - Large vessel disease: multi-infarct dementia, strategic infarct dementia
  - Small vessel disease: Binswanger disease, lacunar state, cerebral autosomal dominant arteriopathy with subcortical infarcts and leucoencephalopathy (CADASIL)
- AIDS dementia-complex
- Neurodegenerative disease
  - Parkinson's disease and progressive supranuclear palsy
  - Huntington's disease
- Wilson's disease

In contrast, cortical dementia involves the cerebral cortex and examples include Alzheimer's disease and CJD. Dementia with Lewy bodies, corticobasal degeneration, and frontotemporal dementia are mixed cortical-subcortical types of dementia.

What is the current medical management of Alzheimer's disease?

Acetylcholinesterase inhibitors such as donepezil, rivastigmine, and galantamine may be considered in patients with mild to moderate Alzheimer's disease with an MMSE score of between 10 and 20. Treatment should be initiated by a specialist in dementia and patients should be reviewed every six months with a repeat MMSE, behavioural, and functional assessment. Treatment is continued if there is no deterioration in function and the MMSE remains above 10. Treatment may also be initiated in people with severe functional impairment in comparison to premorbid status with a MMSE score above 20.

The use of these drugs is also recommended for the management of severe and challenging non-cognitive features of Alzheimer's disease of any severity, when non-pharmacological treatment has failed and antipsychotic drugs are contraindicated.

Memantine, an NMDA (N-methyl-D-aspartic acid) receptor antagonist, is licensed for use in severe (MMSE score 3–14) Alzheimer's disease in the setting of clinical trials.

These drugs are not recommended in dementia with Lewy bodies or vascular dementia.

Recent work has implicated chronic Herpes Simplex 1 infection with the development of amyloid plaques in Alzheimer's, and trials are currently evaluating the efficacy of antiviral therapy for Alzheimer's disease.

What is the role of antipsychotics in the management of non-cognitive features of dementia?

Antipsychotic drugs are recommended for the treatment of severe non-cognitive features of Alzheimer's disease such as psychosis, and severe challenging behaviour which is z risk to the patient and others only. Antipsychotics should be used with caution due to the increased risk of cerebrovascular events. They are contraindicated in dementia with Lewy bodies due to sensitivity and exacerbation of extrapyramidal features of the disease.

Further reading:

1. National Institute for Health and Clinical Excellence, Dementia: Supporting people with dementia and their carers in health and social care, NICE, London; November 2006.

2. Cummings JL, Alzheimer's Disease, New Engl J Med., 2004; 351,1:56–67

3. Scarpini E et al, Treatment of Alzheimer's disease: current status and new perspectives, The Lancet Neurology. 2003; 2:539–47

4. Mckeith I et al, Dementia with Lewy Bodies, The Lancet Neurology., 2004; 3:19–28.

5. Roman GC et al., Subcortical ischaemic vascular dementia, The Lancet Neurology. 2002; 1: 426–36.

Case 40 ◆ **Deliberate Self Harm**

INFORMATION FOR THE CANDIDATE

Dear Doctor,

This 29-year old lady presents after having taken an overdose of paracetamol, ibuprofen, and diazepam of unknown quantities. There is no past medical history of note. She is divorced and has recently lost her job.

Many thanks for your opinion.

Acquiring the history

Patients who have deliberately harmed themselves frequently present to the emergency department. The history requires detailed evaluation of:

- the immediate consequences of the act of self harm
- the nature of self harm
- current medical and mental status
- risk assessment for suicide
- recent life events and social issues
- previous medical and psychiatric history

Candidates should be able to demonstrate the ability to establish a rapport with the patient to assess the risk of suicide. The particular skills of empathic questioning and use of silence will be employed by the skilled candidate. Open questioning about the patient's situation and motivation to self harm, followed by direct enquiry about intentions is a useful approach. A collateral history from witnesses is also useful.

Approximately 90% of cases of deliberate self harm involve self poisoning commonly with non-opiate analgesics. Other acts of deliberate self harm include self-cutting and burning. More violent methods such as drowning, falling from height, hanging, and shooting are clear indications of intent to die.

A. History of presenting complaint:

Begin with an open question such as *'Can you tell me what happened today?'* to allow the patient to volunteer information about the deliberate self harm. With patience, appropriate use of silence, empathic responses and appropriate body language, the majority of the history can be gathered from open questioning. The skilled interviewer will allow the patient to volunteer the history of presenting complaint along with their psychiatric symptoms. The following questions should be used for clarification following this initial dialogue.

Features of self harm

1. Method of self harm

- Overdose

    - **What has been taken?** Ask directly about over the counter medications, prescribed drugs, drugs prescribed for other individuals in the household. Follow up the question by asking *'Did you take anything else with the tablets, for example alcohol?'* Household products such as bleaches, detergents, and antifreeze are examples of other agents deliberately ingested.

    - **Route of administration?** Most often oral preparations are taken in overdose, however it is equally important to ask the patient if they have taken anything via another route; inhalation, injection, or intradermal.

    - **Quantity?** Determine the amount ingested by asking *'How many tablets or packets did you take? What was the strength of the tablets?'* This is often difficult to determine as patients use indiscriminate and unquantifiable terms but can be estimated by examining empty packets or containers that may be found with the patient, although the initial quantities of these may be unknown.

    - **Time of ingestion?** Establish the timing of the overdose, or if a staggered overdose is taken, by asking *'What time did you take the tablets? Did you take all the tablets together or at intervals?'* This will determine the time at which drugs levels should be obtained (>4 hours after initial ingestion) and if methods for drug elimination such as activated charcoal and gastric lavage can be employed (within the first hour of overdose). Drug levels must be taken 4 hours from the last overdose if initial levels are within the non-toxic range in the context of a staggered overdose. Furthermore, delayed effects of the drugs may be expected in such cases or if long-acting preparations have been ingested.

    - **Symptoms?** Enquire about any symptoms related to the overdose. Symptoms are often non-specific but should be sought as they may give a clue to the substance(s) taken. Symptoms of commonly encountered drug overdoses are:

Drug	Symptoms
Paracetamol	Initially asymptomatic. After 24–48 hours: nausea, vomiting, anorexia, jaundice, and right upper quadrant pain.
Salicylates	Nausea, vomiting, tinnitus, deafness, abdominal pain, hyperventilation, sweating, fever, confusion, drowsiness, coma, convulsions.
Opiates	Nausea, vomiting, drowsiness, respiratory depression.
Benzodiazepines	Drowsiness, slurred speech, lethargy, respiratory depression.
Tricyclic antidepressants	Dry mouth, blurred vision, drowsiness, convulsions
SSRI	Nausea, vomiting, agitation, tremor, 'serotonin syndrome'
Hypoglycaemic agents	Sweating, irritability, slurred speech, drowsiness, seizures. Metformin specifically causes abdominal pain, diarrhoea, vomiting, and confusion
Corrosives	Drooling, odynophagia, dysphagia, stridor, hoarseness, abdominal pain, haematemesis.
Methanol	Nausea, vomiting, abdominal pain, blurred vision, blindness.
Ethylene glycol	Apparent intoxication, nausea, vomiting, haematemesis, diplopia, blurred vision, tetany, seizures.
Lithium	Nausea, vomiting, tremor, muscle weakness, seizures

- *Self injury*

Ask the patient direct questions to establish the nature and extent of injuries sustained by self harm. Some patients who repeatedly inflict superficial, non-fatal self injuries do so without intent to die. Ask the following questions to determine the reasons for self injurious behaviour. Obviously, more dangerous methods such as drowning, hanging, or falling from a height indicate clear intent to die.

  - *'How did you harm yourself?'*
  - *'What made you harm yourself in this way?'*
  - *'How did you feel at the time? How do you feel about it now?'*
  - *'Has this happened before? What makes you harm yourself in this way?'*

2. **Planning, precautions, and final acts.** Active planning and taking precautions to avoid being discovered indicate high risk for a fatal repeated attempt. Factors suggesting high risk for further suicide attempts must be elicited in the history.

- **Factors indicating high risk attempts**
  - Planned act (carried out in isolation, taking precautions to avoid interventions and discovery, and purchasing or saving tablets)
  - Final acts such as writing a will or organizing finances in the anticipation of death
  - Suicide note
  - Communicating suicidal intentions to others
  - Not seeking help after the act is carried out
  - Previous attempts

- *'Did you plan to harm yourself? How long have you been thinking about harming yourself?'* This will differentiate impulsive acts from a carefully planned attempt that the patient believes will be fatal.
- *'What did you do to make sure you weren't found?'* Taking precautions such as making sure the patient was alone at the time, locking the door, etc. are associated with a higher risk of further suicide attempts.
- *'Did you tell anyone that you might harm yourself?'*
- *'Did you write a suicide note?'*
- *'Did you write a will, organize your affairs, or take out insurance?'*

3. **Actions after the act of self harm**
- *'What did you do after taking the tablets and/or harming yourself?'*
- *'Did you contact anyone afterwards for help?'*
- *'How were you found? How do you feel about being found?'*

4. **Expected outcome and fatality of deliberate self harm**
- *'What did you think the outcome would be?'*
- *'Did you think you would die?'; 'How certain were you that this would lead to death?'*
- *'Did you want to die at the time?'; 'Do you still feel the same?'*

5. **Previous attempts**
- *'Have you harmed yourself like this before?'; 'How many times has this happened before?'*
- *'What was different this time?'*

6. **Precipitants**
- *'What made you think about taking an overdose or harming yourself?'*

7. **Current mental state.** In particular ask about mood, anhedonia, and biological symptoms of depression.
- *'How has your mood been lately?'; 'Do you feel low within yourself on most days?'*
- *'Do you feel hopeful about the future?'*

- 'Do you still enjoy doing things you used to?'
- 'Are you having trouble sleeping?'; 'Do you have difficulty falling asleep?'; 'Do you wake up early in the morning?'; 'What keeps you awake at night?'
- 'How is your appetite at the moment?'; 'Has your weight changed recently?'

8. Risk of suicide. Establish any further intent to self harm or others.
- 'How do you feel about what has happened now?'
- 'Do you still feel that you want to end your life?'
- 'What might stop you from harming yourself or ending your life?'
- 'Have you thought about harming anyone else?'

B. Relevant medical and family history:

Past medical history

Ask the patient about any current medical problems and previous episodes of psychiatric illness. Chronic medical illness or terminal illness is often a precipitating factor for depression and suicidal ideation.

Other specific conditions to screen for include:

- Malignancy—Ask about known malignancies. Ask about unintentional weight loss and night sweats.
- Hypothyroidism—Ask about weight gain, constipation, cold intolerance, neck swelling, and menorrhagia in women.
- Autoimmune disease—Ask about fevers, rash, joint pains, or mouth ulcers.
- Neurological disease—Neurodegenerative conditions in particular are associated with an increased risk of suicide. Ask about tremor, weakness, and memory loss.

Family history

Enquire about family history of psychiatric illness.

C. Medications:

- Take a detailed drug history of prescribed medications that the patient may have taken in overdose. For example, opiates, benzodiazepines, analgesics, anti-depressants, anti-arrhythmics, and hypoglycaemic agents are commonly ingested in overdose.
- Specific medications associated with psychiatric disease are: glucocorticoids, high-dose reserpine, and interferon.
- Ask about the use of over-the-counter medications.
- Make direct enquiries about the use of recreational drugs and routes of administration.
- Take a detailed history about alcohol consumption.
- Ask witnesses or household members if the patient is likely to have access to other prescribed medications in the house that may have been taken in overdose.

D. Social issues

Several aspects of the social history are important in establishing potential triggers for the act of self harm.

- Ask about living arrangements.
  - 'Where do you live? Is this your own home or rented?'
  - 'Who else lives with you?' Follow up this question about relationships with partner and family members, looking for any problems which may be a trigger for self harm. In particular ask about any problems that *others* are experiencing (financial, health, bereavement, etc.) that may be affecting the patient.

- *'How are things at home?'*
- Enquire about occupation and financial problems
  - *'What do you currently do for a living? Are there any problems at work such as difficulty keeping up with the workload and problems with other staff?'*
  - *'Are you experiencing any difficulties keeping up with payments such as bills, mortgage, and debts?'*
- Ask the patient about concerns about their own health.
  - *'Do you have any concerns about your health?*
  - *'Do you worry that you may become ill?'; 'What makes you worried about your health?'* This is important to ask if the patient has experience recent bereavement especially if the event was unexpected.
- Ask about support networks
  - *'Is there anyone that you can share your problems and thoughts with?'*

Formulating a plan of action

- Explain the medical effects of the act of self harm to the patient and the need for observation, investigations, and treatment.
- Explain the need for a psychiatric assessment and offer appropriate help with any practical problems that the patient may be experiencing (e.g. social services for housing, drug and alcohol services, day centres, and counselling services to deal with social isolation).
- Investigations to consider:
  - Urine toxicology screen for unknown substances. Screening blood tests for paracetamol and salicylates.
  - Drug levels for known substances in overdose are essential for appropriate management. Drug levels can be estimated for ethanol, paracetamol, salicylates, lithium, theophylline, phenobarbitone, carbamazepine, sodium valproate, iron, digoxin, methanol, and ethylene glycol. Repeat measurements may be required for staggered overdoses.
  - Urea, electrolytes, and creatinine. Electrolyte disturbances can occur with the ingestion of substances in overdose. For example, hypokalaemia in theophylline and insulin overdose, hyperkalaemia with digoxin, and hypocalcaemia in ethylene glycol poisoning. Haemodialysis or haemoperfusion may be necessary.
  - LFTs. Raised transaminases in paracetamol overdose suggest hepatocellular damage and occurs 18 hours post-ingestion. Maximal liver damage as assessed by transaminases and prothrombin time occurs 72–96 hours post ingestion.
  - Clotting. Coagulopathy as determined by prothrombin time indicates liver damage and prognosis in paracetamol overdose (see below).
  - Glucose levels. Hypoglycaemia and hyperglycaemia occur with salicylate overdose and hypoglycaemia may suggest insulin or oral hypoglycaemic poisoning.
  - Arterial blood gas for acid-base disturbance.
  - ECG changes may be seen with poisoning with specific substances. For example prolonged PR and QRS intervals occur with tricyclic antidepressants, prolonged QT interval with quinine,
  - A trial of antidotes may be required in unconscious patients in whom the toxic agent is *known* (for example iatrogenic opioid (trial of naloxone) or benzodiazepine (trial of flumazenil) poisoning. However, these drugs should be *avoided* in mixed overdoses or if chronic opiate or benzodiazepine use is suspected, since they may precipitate seizures.

Questions commonly asked by examiners

What is the difference between haemodialysis and haemoperfusion in the context of poisoning?

Haemodialysis is the elimination of toxins in the blood by diffusion of substances across a semipermeable membrane down its concentration gradient in an extracorporeal circuit. Haemoperfusion elimination techniques involve the diffusion and adsorption of poisons by adsorbents such as activated charcoal present in the extracorporeal circuit. Both haemodialysis and haemoperfusion are more effective that peritoneal dialysis.

What are the indications for haemodialysis or haemoperfusion in poisoning?

Haemodialysis is indicated in poisoning if there is evidence of severe acute renal failure, severe metabolic acidosis, and, rarely, for the elimination of poisons in patients with clinical deterioration and high levels of toxins in the blood. Toxins which have a low volume of distribution that can be eliminated using these techniques include:

- Ethanol (levels >7500mg/L)
- Ethylene glycol (levels >615 mg/L)
- Methanol
- Lithium
- Salicylates (levels >700mg/L)

When should single- and multiple-dose activated charcoal be used in poisoning?

Activated charcoal is a porous adsorbent. It is useful in reducing the absorption of substances ingested in toxic amounts and includes:

- Salicylates
- Paracetamol
- Barbiturates
- Carbamazepine and phenytoin
- Theophylline
- Digoxin
- Quinine
- Dapsone

The use of single-dose activated charcoal (50g) is limited to patient's presenting *within 1 hour* of ingestion of a potentially toxic amount of drug that is known to be absorbable.

Multiple-dose activated charcoal is effective in the elimination of absorbable toxins by providing a greater quantity of absorbent to reduce enteric absorption and by enhancing diffusion of toxins down their concentration gradient from the mucosa into the lumen. However, it has not been shown to reduce mortality and morbidity associated with poisoning. The dosing regimen commonly employed in practice involves an initial dose of 50–100g followed by 50g every 4 hours until the passage of charcoal in stool, drug levels fall to a non-toxic range, or clinical recovery of the patient.

It is *ineffective* in absorbing metals, ethylene glycol, and ethanol.

The administration of activated charcoal is contraindicated in patients with a low Glasgow Coma Score, compromised airway, or bowel obstruction/perforation.

What factors are associated with poor prognosis in paracetamol overdose?

Factors associated with a poor prognosis, and therefore discussion with liver transplant unit, are:

- Prothrombin time greater than the number of hours since ingestion (or if the INR is >2 at 24 hours, >4 at 48 hours, and >6 at 72 hours) indicates significant hepatocellular damage.
- creatinine >200µmol/l
- pH <7.30
- systolic BP < 80mmHg after adequate fluid resuscitation
- Encephalopathy or signs of raised intracranial pressure

The King's College criteria for liver transplantation in paracetamol induced acute liver failure

- pH <7.30 or lactate > 3.0 mmol/L after adequate fluid resuscitation
- **or all 3 of the following within 24 hours**
    1. Creatinine >300µmol/L
    2. PT >100s (INR >6.5)
    3. Grade 3 or 4 encephalopathy

Transplantation is strongly considered if lactate is >3.5 mmol/L after adequate fluid resuscitation.

Station 4 ◆ **Communication Skills and Ethics**

Core Concepts and Overview

Capacity

Consent-seeking and Refusal

Confidentiality and Information Sharing

Professionalism, Probity, and Accountability

Core concepts and overview

Capacity

Core concept	Case discussed
Capacity presumed in adults and a capacitous decision cannot be overridden	Case 41
	Case 42
Capacity is at the ethical heart of clinical practice because from it flows meaningful autonomy and self-determination, i.e. the freedom to choose or refuse care	Case 41
	Case 44
Capacity is a general clinical skill but a legal concept	Case 41
Relevant law relating to adults is found in the Mental Capacity Act 2005	Case 41
	Case 42
Incapacity can only be assumed where a patient is unconscious. Capacity is a dynamic and decision-specific concept that can fluctuate, rendering some patients capable of making some decisions but not others	Case 41
	Case 43
	Case 42
The Mental Capacity Act 2005 sets out the criteria to be met for a patient to have capacity, i.e. the ability, to (i) understand; (ii) retain; and (iii) weigh up information; then (iv) communicate a decision	Case 41
Capacity is a fluid concept and doctors can do much to enhance (or impair capacity)	Case 46
Assumptions about capacity based on diagnostic labels should not be made	Case 41
	Case 46
Advance decisions can be made under the Mental Capacity Act 2005 for a time when a patient no longer has capacity	Case 44
The ethical rationale for recognizing advance decisions is the principle of autonomy, i.e. they foster 'future' autonomous decisions provided they are informed	Case 44
Where patients lack capacity and have no advance statement or legal proxy, they can be treated in their best interests (which are broader than merely best medical interests) being as minimally restrictive of rights and freedoms as possible	Case 46
The Code of Practice that supplements the Mental Capacity Act 2005 sets out in greater detail the ways in which clinicians can evaluate a patient's best interests	Case 41
	Case 46
Patients may nominate a proxy under the Mental Capacity Act 2005	Case 45
	Case 46
Capacity in minors under 16 is assessed using the *Gillick* criteria	Case 42
The Independent Mental Capacity Advocacy Service exists to serve the interests of those patients who lack both capacity and a third party to represent them	Case 46

Consent

Core ethico-legal concept	Scenario
Valid consent is the legal translation of the importance of autonomy and self-determination	Case 47
	Case 50
	Case 54
	Case 57
	Case 58
	Case 59
There are four criteria for consent to be valid: (i) capacity; (ii) voluntariness; (iii) sufficiency of information; and (iv) continuing consent	Case 47
	Case 52
	Case 53
Seeking consent may, in itself, have therapeutic value and is an opportunity to build a relationship with the patient	Case 47
	Case 50
	Case 53
	Case 57
	Case 58
Consent need not be written but documentation may provide evidence of the consent process	Case 47
	Case 50
	Case 51
	Case 52
	Case 54
	Case 59
If a patient lacks capacity, it is a legal nonsense to seek consent	Case 53
A capacitous patient is entitled to refuse treatment and express a preference between options, but cannot demand treatment	Case 48
	Case 49
	Case 50
	Case 51
To proceed in the face of a capacitous patient's refusal or without valid consent is to commit an assault and or the tort of battery	Case 47
	Case 43
	Case 54
	Case 57
	Case 58
	Case 59
It is important to be honest both about what is known and what is uncertain when providing patients with information to seek consent. Furthermore, information should cover both the risks/benefits of treatment and non-treatment	Case 47
	Case 48
	Case 50
Consent for screening should be carefully managed taking into account the reliability of the information that may be obtained and its potential consequences	Case 48
After death, the consent process is legally regulated by the Human Tissue Act 2004 and particular provisions apply for (i) organ and tissue donation; (ii) hospital and coroner post-mortems	Case 55
	Case 56
There are particular considerations when seeking consent from a patient to participate in biomedical research (Research on human subjects and animals take place in two distinct legal and governance frameworks)	Case 54
Seeking consent from patients to participate in teaching or training is an essential part of clinical education and subject to the same principles as seeking consent for treatment	Case 53

Core ethico-legal concept	Scenario
The old distinction between living and cadaveric organ donation no longer exists, and the Human Tissue Act 2004 regulates both forms of organ donation	Case 55
The consent for a hospital post-mortem requires clarity about purpose, e.g. investigation of cause of death, teaching or research	Case 56
Refusal of treatment, i.e. refusal to give consent may appear unwise or even bizarre, but if the criteria for seeking valid consent are met, such refusal cannot be overridden	Case 57 Case 58 Case 59

Confidentiality and Healthcare Information

Core ethico-legal concept	Scenario
Confidentiality is integral to the development and maintenance of trust between doctor and patient	Case 60 Case 61 Case 62
Confidentiality is not an unfettered duty and there are three common law justifications for sharing confidential information, namely: (i) consent; (ii) in the patient's best interests but unable to obtain consent; and (iii) in the public interest	Case 60 Case 61
The public interest was legally defined in a case called *W v Egdell* as the risk of serious physical harm to an identifiable individual or individuals	Case 60 Case 61
The public interest qualification amounts to a justification for breaching confidentiality, but not a duty or obligation to do so	Case 60
Even where there is a public interest justification for breaching confidentiality, it is preferable to seek and, if possible obtain, patient consent prior to sharing information	Case 60 Case 61
Relatives, partners, and next of kin have no greater right to confidential information than any other third party unless acting as a legal proxy	Case 62 Case 63
There are several statutory requirements to share confidential information, e.g. notifiable diseases, gunshot injuries, and knife wounds.	Case 67 Case 68
It is easy to breach confidentiality inadvertently and the telephone can present particular risks to the unwary	Case 63 Case 64
Access to healthcare records and medical notes is governed by the Data Protection Act 1998, and it is good practice to write notes as if each patient were to seek access to their records.	Case 64
Requests for information from the police are common. In general, such requests are legally governed by the common law qualifications to confidentiality and the requirements of the Police and Criminal Evidence Act 1984. However, there are also specific statutory exceptions requiring information to be provided, e.g. terrorism and certain road traffic offences	Case 61 Case 66 Case 67
Notifiable diseases must be reported in accordance with the Public Health legislation and failure to do so is a criminal offence	Case 68

Professionalism Probity and Accountability

Core ethico-legal concept	Scenario
Professionalism encompasses 'pure' bioethics and working within the law but extends to other elements of practice such as effective communication, self-awareness, commitment to learning, team-working, and maintaining safe boundaries.	Case 69 Case 71 Case 73 Case 75
The way in which individuals respond to conflict and complaints is very powerful and can prevent further dispute and even legal action	Case 70
Most, if not all, doctors will make mistakes—response to mistakes is a crucial component of professionalism	Case 70 Case 71 Case 72
Proper processes should be followed when a critical incident or adverse event occurs with the emphasis on meaningful learning	Case 70 Case 71 Case 72
Competence can be a slippery concept and the majority of clinicians will work below their best at some stage in a long career. However, patient safety is the priority and individual competence must be reviewed and maintained throughout medical practice	Case 72 Case 73 Case 75
There is a distinction between negligence and competence with negligence being a legally determined lapse in the standard of care that is usually concerned with a single episode	Case 70 Case 72
The collegiate culture of medicine can make it very difficult to give colleagues honest feedback and express concerns about their performance	Case 74 Case 75
Doctors are required to act if they believe that a colleague is putting patients at risk and are afforded the protection of the Public Interest Disclosure Act 1998 provided concerns are raised in good faith	Case 74 Case 75

Capacity

Patients with Capacity: Clinical Cases

Case 41 ◆ **Assessing capacity to consent to a joint injection in a confused older patient**

You are working as an F2 doctor in rheumatology out-patients. Bill Marshall has come in today for a steroid injection into his frozen shoulder, to increase mobility and decrease pain. He is 72 years old, a widower living in warden-managed accommodation and somewhat forgetful. The consultant is aware of Mr Marshall's tendency to become confused and has asked you to assess Mr Marshall's capacity to consent to the injection.

Core concepts

- Capacity is at the heart of ethical decision making. Capacity to make choices about healthcare will rarely, if ever, be assessed without the benefit of input from a clinician. Often it is assumed that a psychiatrist should be involved where there are doubts about capacity, but the criteria for assessing capacity are relatively straightforward and it is a core skill in which all doctors should be competent, calling psychiatrists only in situations of doubt or complexity. Capacity is a legal rather than a medical concept, i.e. its definition is drawn from the law. As such, no doctor should engage in an assessment of a patient's capacity without understanding the relevant legal processes. As capacity is a legal concept, the standard of proof that is used in assessing capacity is that which is applicable to civil law in general, i.e. on the balance of probabilities rather than beyond reasonable doubt.

- The legal test used in assessing capacity to make decisions and choices about healthcare was first established in the case of *Re: C (Adult: Refusal of Treatment)*. Since October 2007, the Mental Capacity Act 2005 and its accompanying Code of Practice is the source for guidance on capacity. The principles in Box 3 underpin the legislation and are particularly important to note:

Box 3 Underlying principles of the Mental Capacity Act 2005

- Every adult has the right to make his/her own decisions and to be assumed to have capacity unless proved otherwise.
- Everyone should be encouraged and enabled to make his/her own decisions, or to participate as fully as possible in decision-making, i.e. given help and support to make and express a choice.
- Individuals have the right to make apparently eccentric or unwise decisions.
- Proxy decisions should consider best interests, prioritizing what the patient would have wanted.
- Proxy decisions should be 'least restrictive of basic rights and freedoms'.

The specific legal criteria for capacity are shown in Box 4.

Box 4 Criteria for adult capacity under the Mental Capacity Act 2005

The patient should be able to:

(a) understand the information relevant to the decision;

(b) retain that information;

(c) use or weigh that information as part of the process of making the decision, and

(d) communicate his decision (whether by talking, using sign language or any other means).

Application of core concepts to Case 41

- The task in this scenario is to assess capacity, but clearly to do so effectively a candidate will need to employ appropriate communication skills to explore whether the patient is able to meet the criteria of capacity (see section "Key concepts"), namely:
  - the patient's comprehension of information
  - the patient's ability to retain that information
  - whether the patient can weigh information in the balance to reach a considered decision; and
  - communicate the decision.
- Candidates should begin with an appropriate introduction telling the patient their full name and role and checking the patient's identity and preferred form of address.
- The patient should be invited to tell the doctor why he is attending and what he expects to happen at the consultation.
- Allowing the patient time to share his expectations and understanding of the procedure will enable candidates to offer appropriately relevant information at the right level of detail.
- Assessing comprehension: candidates should offer the patient information in simple terms explaining that the injection is intended to alleviate pain and increase mobility. As well as describing the purpose of the procedure, candidates should offer some guidance on possible disadvantages, e.g. but that sometimes the pain may worsen before it improves and it is not always successful in managing pain/mobility problems.
- Checking retention: candidates should explicitly demonstrate that they are checking the patient's understanding and retention by asking, for example, *'I realize I've given you a lot of information, what do you understand so far?'*, and *'Is there anything you would like explained further'*.
- Exploring whether information is being 'weighed in the balance': all this rather arcane legal expression means is that capacitous patients draw on information about common pros and

cons when making healthcare decisions. A simple way to explore this aspect of capacity assessment is to ask *'How do you feel about the injection now we've discussed it a bit?'* or *'Now you've heard more about the injection, what are your thoughts about the procedure?'*

- Communication of decision: this is a step that is often overlooked in capacity assessments. Having explored whether a patient is capacitous to make a decision, don't forget to give the patient the opportunity to communicate whether he has actually reached a decision! It is also good practice to summarize the consultation, invite further questions from the patient, and explain that you will share your discussion with the patient with your consultant.
- Throughout the consultation, candidates should verify understanding, check pace, be alert to non-verbal communication, and invite the patient to ask questions.
- A systematic and organized approach should be the aim throughout.

Further information

- Assessment of capacity is not a single, irrevocable and static judgement. Capacity is often a fluctuating concept and, in practice, patients may be somewhere along a continuum of capacity. As such, a patient might be capacitous to consent to one type of treatment and not another. Doctors must be wary of relying too much on previous assessments. Assessments of capacity should be regularly reviewed. Furthermore, the assessment of capacity is a matter of judgement and there are more areas of grey in assessing capacity than areas of clear black and white. The way in which a doctor asks questions or gives information can enhance or diminish a patient's capacity as can factors such as timing, pain, fatigue, and environment. Practical considerations in assessing a patient's capacity are summarized in Box 5.

Box 5 Practical issues in assessing capacity

- **Starting point**—Adults are presumed to be capacitous. If there is doubt about a patient's capacity, an assessment should be carried out. The assessment must be carried out with reference to the particular decision to be made, i.e. with reference to the specific intervention or treatment recommended. If you are the person carrying out the assessment, you should establish what it is you are being asked to assess. If you are the person asking for the assessment, you should explain exactly what it is you want assessed.

- **Pre-existing diagnoses**—the test of capacity is completed unrelated to any pre-existing diagnoses that might apply to patients *including diagnoses of mental illness or disorder*. The fact that a patient has a particular disorder does not mean that a formal test of capacity should not be performed. The test of capacity is concerned with function and not with diagnostic labels.

- **Non-cooperation with assessment**—simply because a patient refuses to cooperate with an assessment of capacity, it does not mean that the patient can be assumed to be incapacitous. Therefore doctors may need to be imaginative and patient in attempts to engage patients in capacity assessments.

- **Influencing factors on capacity assessment**—the way in which explanations are given, a doctor's manner, and demeanour and the surrounding environment can all enhance or diminish a patient's potential for capacity. It is expected that doctors will seek to enhance a patient's ability to understand information by explaining it in clear and simple language and being as reassuring as possible. Options that can be explored to maximize a patient's understanding include treating an underlying condition that is inhibiting decision-making, writing down information, drawing diagrams, using educational models, videos and audiotapes, using translators, letting the patient choose a friend or relative to be present, finding a private place for the consultation etc.

(Continue)

- **Confidentiality**—a doctor may need to seek the perspectives of other parties when assessing the capacity of a patient whom he or she does not know at all or well. Such information must, of course, be sought if it is clinically relevant. However, a doctor must have due regard to the principles of confidentiality and should seek to preserve the privacy and confidentiality of the patient so far as it is practicable.

- **Documentation**—it is essential that all assessments of an individual patient's capacity are fully and accurately recorded in the patient's medical notes.

Case 42 ◆ Relative's objection to capacitous patient's decision regarding active treatment

You are working on a general medical firm at a large hospital. You have been looking after Melvyn Oakham, aged 76 who has had congestive heart failure for three years. Mr Oakham was originally admitted with acute pulmonary oedema to the Intensive Care Unit (ICU) where he was intubated and ventilated. On the third day of his stay in the ICU, Mr. Oakham had ventricular fibrillation from which he was successfully resuscitated. Mr Oakham is now on a ward, and he is awake, alert, and aware. Jenny Parkes, the patient's daughter, regularly visits her father on the ward. Jenny has asked if she can 'have a private word with you'. Mrs Parkes tells you that she has been watching her father become 'progressively sicker' and 'less able to cope to the point where he really has no life at all'. She tells you that when her father was in ICU, she witnessed him having ventricular fibrillation and heard the resuscitation as she was led by a nurse outside the cubicle. Mrs Parkes feels that the resuscitation was 'brutal, a bit shocking and demeaning'. Mrs Parkes asks whether 'it would be possible to make one of those orders where everyone decides a patient shouldn't be resuscitated in case it happens again'. Mrs Parkes stresses that she is 'really grateful for everything you're doing for Dad, but it can't be right to stick needles and tubes in him just to bring him back to a life barely worth living' adding 'he's had a good life, and I don't want to prolong his suffering'.

Please discuss Mrs Parkes request.

Core concepts

- The significant piece of ethico-legal content relates to decision-making and DNAR (do not attempt resuscitation) orders. This is an area of clinical practice that is confusing and varies enormously, but what follows is a description of optimal practice regarding resuscitation decision-making.

- If no DNAR discussion or decision has taken place and the patient arrests, the initial presumption should be to resuscitate.

- If the clinical team (led by consultant level expertise) believes that CPR (caridopulmonary resuscitation) would not be successful and the patient does not raise the issue of resuscitation, it may not be necessary to discuss DNAR status. However, information should not be withheld because it is not easy to discuss or feels uncomfortable. Direct questions must be answered honestly and there should be careful thought as to why a patient who is alert should not be told if a DNAR order is made in the notes. And, of course, patients are entitled to see their medical records which could mean that they learn of their DNAR order in a way that is more upsetting than having an open discussion and could significantly compromise their trust in the clinical team.

- Where a patient lacks capacity, he may have a valid advance directive to inform resuscitation decision-making; see Case 50 Patient Preferences and Requests 3: DNAR and Older Patient for further discussion of advance directives.

- DNAR is, of course, specific to resuscitation. The relationship of CPR to other interventions and treatments, e.g. ventilation, hydration, nutrition, analgesia, etc., should be considered and discussed. It is important to be clear that even if a patient is 'not for resuscitation', the clinical team will do all that can be done to ensure he or she remains comfortable. DNAR does not equate to no care at all.

- DNAR orders occur in the realms of uncertainty about prognosis, recovery, and quality of life. The perceptions of patients, clinicians and families about the value of resuscitation can differ widely leading to misunderstanding. A crucial part of ethical practice in the context of resuscitation therefore is to explore existing understanding and be honest about both what is known *and* unknown with regard to the patient and the disease process.

- DNAR orders are overseen by the consultant in charge of a patient's care but should involve the multidisciplinary team and, if the patient has capacity, the patient himself and anyone whom the patient nominates. Indeed the UK Resuscitation Council recommends that the agreement of every member of the clinical team should be verified if possible and advises that, in the event of doubt, further senior clinical advice should be sought.

- DNAR orders should be recorded in the way set out by the local NHS Trust or hospital. Inadequate communication can lead to poor outcomes. Processes differ,[1] but each NHS Trust is required to have a publicly available policy regarding resuscitation status and decisions based on the current guidance from the UK Resuscitation Council.[2] Clinical practice should reflect the published policy.

- DNAR decisions should be clearly communicated to those who have clinical contact with the patient, being alert to the roles played by the wider clinical team, e.g. physiotherapy, occupational therapy, etc.

- It is important to discuss DNAR decision-making openly, factually, and honestly being clear about what is factually true, what is uncertain and without assumption. Remember what clinicians know about resuscitation (or indeed any other aspect of practice) is not necessarily known by patients and their families.

Application of Core Concepts to Case 42

- Mrs Parkes is likely to be frightened, tired, and upset at what has happened to her father. However, she is not the patient—her father is—and it is essential to remember that throughout this challenging discussion.

- You are going to have to tell Mrs Parkes that you are unable to discuss her father's care without his express permission, i.e. this is a scenario where you will have to demonstrate empathy for her whilst remaining firm about the boundaries of clinical confidentiality.

- You are likely to have to respond calmly in the face of emotion. Mrs Parkes will probably express frustration and even anger. However, although you cannot discuss her capacitous father's care with her in detail, you are able to both listen to, and acknowledge the legitimacy of, her distress, concerns, and anxieties.

- Mr Oakham is, we can assume, from the scenario, capacitous. Despite being seriously ill a few days previously, he is alert and aware of everything that is happening to him. As such, Mr Oakham is entitled to make his own choices about his healthcare and decide who, if anyone, he wishes to involve.

- The first task therefore is to explain clearly and sensitively to Mrs Parkes that you are unable to discuss her father without his express permission. Note there is a difference between simply telling someone that you cannot give them any information and actually *explaining* kindly and courteously why you are not able to talk to them about their family member.

- One task is to explain to Mrs Parkes how and why healthcare decisions about capacitous adults are made, both generically and specifically in the case of resuscitation decisions. Although you are unable to fulfil her immediate request, you can enhance her understanding of resuscitation decision-making.

- Where a patient, such as Mr Oakham, has capacity, resuscitation decisions should be discussed with him sensitively and clearly, *avoiding* euphemisms (such as' *'we wondered if you wanted any heroics?'*, *'do you want us to pull out the stops?'* etc.).[3]

- A DNAR order cannot be made simply because Mrs Parkes has asked for it. Mrs Parkes may ask whether you would be willing to make such a decision and 'not tell' her father—the answer to this question is, of course, that DNAR orders cannot be made without a patient's knowledge on the basis of a familial request.

- In this case, if Mr Oakham is capacitous, it is for him to reflect on whether and when he believes that resuscitation would be too burdensome or deleterious to his dignity. He may or may not wish to involve his daughter in those deliberations.

- Not being able to accede to Mrs Parkes's wishes and respecting Mr Oakham's confidentiality does not mean that candidates can offer her nothing by way of information and support. For example, it is possible to have a general discussion with Mrs Parkes about her concerns whilst remaining alert to verbal and non-verbal cues without breaching her father's confidentiality or promising a DNAR order will be made.

- It may be possible to facilitate a discussion with her father, but proceed with caution as it is Mr Oakham's decision whether or not to share information with his daughter because he is the capacitous patient.

- Avoid making judgemental comments about either the patient's quality of life or his daughter's perception of her father's quality of life.

- Seek to maintain an organized, calm, and empathic approach throughout this challenging scenario.

Further information

- Although you are unable to make a DNAR order because his daughter has asked, her request does highlight the ethico-legal tension in resuscitation decisions. People have, by virtue of the Human Rights Act 1998, a right to life and a right not to undergo degrading treatment. The weighting given to those two rights is at the heart of much DNAR discussion. DNAR orders must not be made on the basis of age, although age may be a clinically relevant variable to consider along with co-morbidity, function, etc. It has been suggested that patients such as Mr Oakham who are over the age of 75 will be given DNAR status sooner than younger patients, irrespective of prognosis.[4] To make age determinative however is to be discriminatory.[5] All resuscitation decision-making should be predicated on an individual assessment of each patient with opportunities for discussion and review.

- 'Futility' is commonly cited as a rationale for DNAR decisions without necessarily involving the patient. Indeed, so commonly is the concept of futility invoked to inform ethico-legal decision-making in resuscitation practice, that it has led to a quasi-bioethical movement named the 'Futilitarians'.[6] It is an approach that, of course, looks to outcome, or rather predicted outcome, to determine the moral worth or otherwise of an intervention. Perhaps predictably, the challenge about who should define 'futility', and how, complicates such an approach. After all, every medical treatment is ultimately futile because all human beings ultimately die.

Case 43 ◆ Assessing an adolescent's capacity in A&E

Jessica is a 14-year old girl who has come unaccompanied to the Accident and Emergency Department (A&E). You are working in your capacity as an F2 doctor. You ask Jessica why she has come to A&E. Jessica explains that she **'got carried away'** *with her boyfriend last night and didn't* **'use anything'**. *You establish that Jessica has had sexual intercourse within the last 48 hours and did not use any contraception. Jessica asks you for* **'the tablet you can take afterwards to stop pregnancy'**.

Core concepts

- The issues of consent and confidentiality in respect of minors have prompted much academic debate and some of the most significant legal decisions in the history of medical law. The trend (perhaps in common with a more general trend towards respect for patient autonomy) has been towards the recognition of children's rights, a trend borne out both by statutory and common law developments.
- The key case from which the law regarding the capacity of minors to consent to medical treatment is drawn is that of *Gillick v West Norfolk and Wisbech Area Health Authority* [1985]. Mrs Victoria Gillick challenged a Department of Health circular concerning the prescription of contraception to girls under the age of 16. The case eventually was heard in the House of Lords, where, by the narrowest of majorities, the court found in favour of the Health Authority. The principles that emerged from the *Gillick* case are clear and gave rise to the term '*Gillick* competent'. In recent years, that has been some debate about the use of the term '*Gillick* competence'. As a result, the term '*Fraser* competence' is also sometimes used (after Lord Fraser who was one of the judges in the House of Lords hearing the case). Aside from the fact that 'capacity' is now the preferred term, rather than 'competence', the apparently interchangeable use of the terms '*Gillick*' and '*Fraser*' competence is technically incorrect and has even created an ethico-legal urban myth. The term '*Gillick* competence' delineates how minors will be assessed when making decisions about healthcare, including but not limited to the provision of contraception and sexual health advice. The 'Fraser guidelines' describe the practical application of '*Gillick* competence' when an adolescent seeks contraception.
- This situation is a very good example of an area where the law is actually limited in its practical usefulness (indeed when examined alongside the legal age of consent for sexual intercourse, the law appears to be totally contradictory), and a great deal of discretion has

been left to the individual doctor. Indeed, it has been suggested that whilst *Gillick* was frequently described as marking the demise of paternalism, the paternalism to which reference was being made was not *medical* paternalism but *parental* paternalism.

- Whether a minor is sufficiently mature to consent to treatment and procedures must be approached on a case-by-case basis, considering the individual child and with regard to the child's level of understanding in respect of a particular treatment. Moreover, it is perfectly possible (and perhaps likely) that a child may be considered capacitous to consent to one treatment but not another. Indeed, some research suggests that it is experience of a particular type of treatment or procedure that is most relevant in determining capacity and not the age or intelligence of the child.

Application of core concepts to Case 43

- The principal aim of this scenario is to evaluate the candidate's ability to assess the capacity of a teenage patient to make her own decisions about her health. Although you will be discussing contraception and sexual health, this is *not* the primary aim of this assessment.
- Candidates should begin with an appropriate introduction telling the patient their full name and role and checking the patient's identity and preferred title.
- The patient should be invited to explain why she has come to A&E in her own words.
- Candidates should confirm the patient's age in a way that is non-judgemental.
- Allowing the patient time to share her expectations and understanding of sexual health will enable candidates to offer appropriately relevant information at the right level of detail.
- When approaching this scenario, candidates must establish whether the five criteria in Box 6 are met.

Box 6 The criteria for assessing capacity in a minor seeking contraception or sexual health advice

- Although the patient is under 16, she can understand the doctor's advice;
- The doctor cannot persuade the patient to inform her parents or to allow him to inform her parents that she is seeking contraceptive advice;
- The patient is very likely to have sexual intercourse with or without adequate contraception;
- Unless the patient receives contraceptive advice or treatment her mental or physical health (or both) are likely to suffer; and
- The patient's best interests require the doctor to give her contraceptive advice, treatment, or both without parental consent.

- It is important that candidates can show that they are able to use their discretion sensitively, appropriately, and professionally. In practice, this requires candidates to recognize the influence their own communication skills and approach have on a young person's capacity to understand sexual health advice.
- In relation to this scenario, candidates have to assess how much the patient understands about sexual health and contraception, including post-coital contraception. The patient in this scenario appears to have reasonable base line knowledge of sexual health and contraception. Candidates should take their lead from the words used by the patient, i.e. explore what she means by 'getting carried away' and 'not using anything' before discussing the possible prescription of emergency contraception.
- Candidates need to consider how to translate the criteria shown in Box 6 into clinical practice. Ways of establishing the patient's understanding of sexual health and contraception

have already been discussed. In addition, candidates should decide how to ask about the possible involvement of parents and the consequences of not prescribing contraception. For example, phrases such as *'Have you thought about telling your mum or dad?'*, *'Is there an adult family member to whom you could talk?'*, and *'If I weren't able to help you today, what do you think might happen?'* may be useful in exploring whether parents can be involved and the minor's best interests. These questions should be asked in a neutral way.

• Candidates should be alert to verbal and non-verbal cues from the patient.

• Throughout the consultation, candidates should verify understanding, check pace, be alert to the patient's emotions, respond empathically where appropriate, and invite the patient to ask questions.

• When candidates have finished discussing the patient's request, they should make a decision that can be mapped against the criteria in Box 6. If candidates believe that the patient is *Gillick* competent, they should include a discussion of future contraceptive options and advise of places where confidential sexual health advice and treatment can be obtained.

• A systematic and organized approach should be the aim throughout.

Further information

• This scenario is neither an emergency nor involves life-saving treatment, but candidates should know that the courts have distinguished between cases according to the seriousness of the condition and the urgency of the treatment required. For example, two minors who were practising Jehovah's Witnesses and refused treatment with blood products for terminal conditions (one was suffering from leukaemia and the other from thalassaemia), were deemed not to understand the consequences of their refusal and therefore could not be considered *Gillick* competent. Significantly in one of these cases, the boy continued his opposition to the treatment and on becoming an adult (and therefore able to exercise the right to refuse treatment previously denied him as a minor) he died.

• Although this scenario involves a minor seeking rather than refusing treatment, candidates should know that a distinction has been drawn at common law between consent to, and refusal of, treatment whereby the application of the *Gillick* test has been limited to the former situation. It has been suggested (per Lord Donaldson in *Re R*) that in cases of *'fluctuating understanding and mental capacity'* the *Gillick* test of capacity may be inappropriate and that understanding must be demonstrated not only of the proposed treatment but also of the consequences both of treating and, this is stressed, of failure to treat in such circumstances. More significantly, the decision of *Re W* decided that whilst a *Gillick* compe-tent child could not have their right to choose treatment usurped by their parents, the same child could have their right to *refuse* treatment so usurped. This sits extremely uneasily with the ethos of the *Gillick* decision. Indeed in the *Gillick* case, Lord Scarman explicitly noted that a legally mature minor was able to take over parental power both to approve *and to decline* treatment).

• The case of *Re W* actually concerned a girl over the age of 16. The law relating to minors between the ages of 16 and 18 years old is contained in the Family Law Reform Act 1969, s 8. By virtue of that section consent given by a young person between 16 and 18 is said to be *'as effective as it would be if he were of full age'*. However, in *Re: W* it was suggested that as s 8 does not explicitly refer to refusal of medical treatment the principles of full capacity embodied by the provision did not apply in such circumstances. It should be noted, though, that these cases in which the courts distinguished between consent and refusal pre-date both the Human Rights Act 1998 and the Mental Capacity Act 2005. The Mental Capacity Act 2005 appears to follow the Family Law Reform Act 1969 and require that patients aged 16 and 17 should be treated as adults save for the purposes of advance decision-making and appointing a lasting power of attorney. If faced with a patient of 16 or 17 who appears capacitous but is refusing treatment (but not in advance), the current advice is to proceed with 'extreme caution' and to consider the young person's preferences.

Case 44 ◆ Advance decision-making under the Mental Capacity Act 2005

Mr Peter Jacobsen is a 57-year old man who has motor neurone disease. He is under the care of the neurology team which you have recently joined. Today Mr Jacobsen has come in to the clinic because he **'wants to discuss his future care with people who know me well'***. Establish specifically why he has come to clinic and offer Mr Jacobsen appropriate advice.*

Core concepts

- Advance directives (sometimes also described as 'living wills') are statements expressing wishes about future treatment or interventions. The statements are made by capacitous patients in anticipation of a time when they cease to have capacity. Advance directives have historically been poorly understood by the medical profession. In 1998, despite the publication of the original BMA guidance on advance decision-making in 1995, a paper reported that in a survey of 214 doctors only 49% were aware that advance directives, properly drafted, have legal force.[7] Policies on advance directives are increasingly common in NHS Trusts particularly since the Mental Capacity Act 2005 came into force thereby affording statutory recognition to advance statements. However, awareness of the existence of policies has been startlingly low in some areas.[8] Furthermore, simply being aware of a policy on advance directives is insufficient to achieve ethical and lawful medical practice. Doctors need training and practice in the specific ethico-legal issues surrounding the status of directives. The implications of patients seeking advice from doctors when drafting advance directives are significant. Doctors need help in applying statute, Codes of Practice, and professional guidelines.
- The statutory recognition given to advance statements or directives is one of the most significant provisions of the Mental Capacity Act 2005 which came fully into force in October 2007. Given that advance statements do now have statutory force and some high profile cases involving patients who seek to make decisions in advance of deterioration, it is likely that more people will consider making an advance directive.
- There are four criteria that must be met for a patient to make a legally valid advanced statement or living will. Those criteria are show in Box 7.

Box 7 Criteria for legal validity of advance directives, advance statements, or 'Living Wills'
• Capacity (is the patient capable of making a decision?).
• Voluntariness (is the patient doing this freely and of his or her own volition?).
• Information (does the patient understand the implications of the choices and preferences he or she has?).
• Specificity (is the advance statement specific enough about possible future situations as to make clear what the patient wants in a given situation?).

- The ethical rationale for the acceptance of advance directives is respect for patient autonomy. If, as is well-established in law, competent patients are entitled to make a free and informed choice about healthcare, it has been suggested that it is difficult to distinguish morally between the right to make free choices in the present and the extension of that right to future decision-making. Thus, advance directives are frequently described as an effective way to extend a patient's autonomy when they lose capacity. However, it could also be argued that none of us is ever competent to make decisions about our future care because the person we become when ill is qualitatively different from the person we are when we are healthy. Furthermore, doctors have an ethical responsibility to be aware of their own discomfort when faced with the patient who appears to favour death over life whilst not letting this personal discomfort or anxiety compromise the fundamental requirement of respecting the patient's autonomy. Finally, patients who have had the opportunity to express their concerns, preferences and reservations about the management of their health are likely to trust their doctors more and to enjoy a more honest and effective relationship with healthcare professionals.

- Perhaps the most important training, however, is in communication skills that will allow doctors to facilitate informed and calm reflection by patients thinking about an advanced directive. Conversations about future ill health, suffering, and death are not easy and many doctors are insufficiently trained to feel confident about engaging in such communication. Patients cannot properly consider their options without the honest, disinterested (note not uninterested), and impartial advice of their doctors. This is perhaps the greatest challenge of all in relation to advance decisions.

- A further point to note is that advance decisions should be periodically reviewed. Any amendments, revocations, or additions can be made in the same way as a codicil is made to a will assuming, of course, that the person is still capacitous. Any changes must, of course, be communicated to all parties who have access to the advance directive, e.g. GP, any hospital departments, solicitors, relatives, carers, etc. There is a common misapprehension with regard to advance directives that refusal of treatment applies to all intervention including even basic care. Ethical practice demands that even where there is an advance directive, basic care must continue to be provided and the dignity of the patient preserved. Advance directives are further limited in content such that there is a distinction between expressing preferences and demanding treatment. An advance directive is generally assumed to be a statement of refusal with respect to specific treatments or interventions. What is the position with regard to requests for specific treatment on intervention? In general, no patient has the right to demand or request treatment that is not clinically indicated. Therefore it would be odd and inconsistent to allow patients to include in their advance directives requests for specific treatments, procedures or interventions that they would like to receive in the future in the event of them ceasing to have capacity: a point that was confirmed in the case of Lesley Burke.[9] For example, if Mr Jacobsen were to include in his advance statement a request that he be treated with an experimental drug against the advice of the clinical team, that request could legitimately be disregarded.

Application of core concepts to Case 44

- The principal aim of this scenario is to assess the candidate's ability to provide accurate information about making an advance statement or directive (also commonly called a 'living will') in an empathic and professional manner.

- Although to do so candidates are likely to be discussing neurological disease, this is *not* the primary aim of this assessment.

- Candidates should begin with an appropriate introduction telling the patient their full name and role and checking the patient's identity and preferred title.

- This is a sensitive area to discuss—the patient is facing the possibility, even probability of deterioration and eventually death. The patient has come to seek specific advice on the issue of advance directives and it is essential first to explore sensitively Mr Jacobsen's understanding of advance directives, and his apparent desire to make an advanced statement now. Patients will have a range of triggers for seeking advice and will have different appreciation of what an advance statement is and how it might apply to their situation. Some may have seen 'living will' packs in WH Smith; others may have read an article or spoken to a friend. The important point is that the starting point for the consultation is to discover what Mr Jacobsen both knows and wants to know.

- Candidates should make it clear to Mr Jacobsen that it is possible to make a valid advance directive in English law. The Mental Capacity Act 2005 sets out the legal framework in which advance statements should be applied and candidates should explain that there are four criteria (shown in Box 7) for a valid advance statement.

- Candidates should take time to explain each of the criteria shown in Box 7, and explore Mr Jacobsen's wishes in the context of these criteria. A valid advanced directive must be made by a capacitous person. Mr Jacobsen appears to have capacity and, as adults are presumed to be competent, candidates should not spend time assessing capacity. However, it would be sensible to explain that for an advance directive to be implemented there has to be certainty that it was made by a capacitous person and voluntarily. Candidates should therefore discuss ways in which Mr Jacobsen can demonstrate that, e.g. by having the advance directive in written form and witnessed by someone who can attest to the patient's capacity (using the criteria for assessing capacity described above).

- Candidates should spend time exploring Mr Jacobsen's specific concerns, e.g. feeding, resuscitation, treatment of infections, etc. and discussing his preferences. It is not necessary, nor probably possible, to cover every eventuality. It is sufficient for candidates to demonstrate awareness that to be valid an advance statement must be informed and specific to situations likely to occur in the future.

- Candidates can assure Mr Jacobsen that he can take his time in drafting a statement and can change his mind about the content of his advance directive should he so choose.

- The information that a doctor provides in this consultation is likely to be complex and has potent emotional resonance for the patient. It is essential therefore to pace the discussion. Information should be offered in discrete chunks, checking for understanding, and leaving time for the patient to take in what is being said and ask questions.

- No matter how accurate or valuable the information provided, the patient may feel a bit overwhelmed and rather emotional. To hear about the exacting criteria that must be met to make a valid living will may remind the patient of the seriousness both of this decision and his condition. It is important to remain alert to verbal and non-verbal cues from the patient and adapt the consultation accordingly.

- Allow space for the patient to ask questions and demonstrate empathy where appropriate.

- You may ask whether the patient has discussed, or will discuss the issue of making an advance directive with his family. Listen carefully to the patient's response and explore the options for sharing information without judging or passing comment on what a partner should or shouldn't be told, when and by whom—that is not your role.

- It is unlikely that a patient would be able to decide whether and how to make an advance statement during a single meeting in an outpatient clinic. Therefore, candidates should acknowledge the difficulty and significance of the choices Mr Jacobsen may make and offer appropriate follow up as he makes his decision, e.g. subsequent appointments, involvement of GP, discussion with family, patient-led organizations, written literature, etc.

- Summarizing, offering time to think, and reminding the patient that he is welcome to discuss this further at future appointments is a good way to close the consultation. This is not likely to be something that is resolved in an initial meeting and giving the patient time is as important as giving him accurate information about making an advance directive.

• A systematic, empathic and organised approach should be the aim throughout.

Further information

• The more informal and non-specific the advance directive is, the more likely it is to be challenged or disregarded as being invalid. Whilst advance decisions can be verbal, in cases involving life-saving or sustaining treatment, the Mental Capacity Act 2005 requires that the statement be in writing, signed, and witnessed.

• In practice, it is the requirement of specificity that is most difficult for patients to fulfil because of the inevitable uncertainty surrounding future illness and the amount of knowledge an average patient is likely to have about potential treatments or interventions. These principles have been extrapolated from the case of Re: T.[10] This was a case in which a woman due to undergo a caesarean section refused blood products in advance. Hospital staff had misled the patient as to the implications of her refusal and had been unduly reassuring. The court ordered that the transfusion proceed because the patient had been insufficiently informed about the consequences of her refusal.

• A further practical point in relation to advance decision-making is how to make the advance statement available to clinical teams who may be meeting a patient for the first time with minimal or no information and in an emergency situation. The law requires only that clinicians make reasonable attempts to establish whether there is a valid advance statement and the presumption is to save life where there is ambiguity about either the existence or content of an advance statement.

• At present, advance directives and statements remain relatively rare but are likely to become increasingly common as the legislation becomes better known. Indeed, there have been several high profile campaigns led by national organizations such as 'Help the Aged' and The Alzheimer's Society to encourage people to plan ahead and make advance statements or directives, making it an area of increasing ethico-legal importance in routine clinical practice.

Incapacitated Patients: Clinical Cases

Case 45 ♦ **Proxy decision making under the Mental Capacity Act 2005—Lasting Power of Attorney**

Mrs Rotini is 77. She has not been in good health for the last decade. She has osteo-arthritis, COPD, diabetes mellitus, mild dementia, and was recently diagnosed with lung cancer. Mrs Rotini has been living in a nursing home for 6 months when it became clear she could no longer cope alone at home. On receiving her diagnosis of lung cancer, Mrs Rotini asked her solicitor to come to the nursing home to advise her on how her son, Mr Joe Rotini, could take over the **'difficult decisions'**. *A Lasting Power of*

Attorney was duly granted. Mrs Rotini was admitted three days ago with pneumonia. She is intubated and unconscious on the intensive care unit. Mrs Rotini is not responding to initial treatment and is in fact becoming increasingly unwell. The clinical team needs to decide how to proceed and arrange a time to talk to Mr Joe Rotini.

Core concepts

- The Mental Capacity Act 2005 is one of the most significant changes in the law applicable to healthcare for a century. It is relevant to all specialties and it is incumbent upon all clinicians to be familiar with its principles and application to daily practice.
- Significantly, and for the first time in England and Wales, the Mental Capacity Act 2005 also provides statutory recognition of advance directives, proxy or substituted decision-makers, and advocacy services for those patients without friends or family via the Independent Mental Capacity Advocacy Service.
- Proxy or substituted judgement for people lacking capacity can be given by a person who has been granted a Lasting Power of Attorney.[11] Once a person's lack of capacity has been registered with the Public Guardian[12] and the lasting power of attorney granted, the person holding the power of attorney is charged with representing a patient's best interests. Therefore, for clinicians, it is important to (a) establish whether there is a valid lasting power of attorney in respect of an incapacitous patient and (b) to adhere to the wishes of the person acting as attorney.
- The only circumstances in which clinicians need not follow the wishes of the attorney is if it is believed that the attorney is not acting in the patient's best interests in which case the matter should be referred to the Court of Protection.[13]

Application of core concepts to Case 45

- Mrs Rotini is very unwell and may previously have led clinicians to reflect on the concept of 'futility'. Indeed, so dominant was the notion of 'futility' in the ethical analyses of end of life decision-making that the genus 'futilitarians' emerged in some quarters of the ethico-legal literature.[14] However, this is exactly the sort of situation where the Lasting Power of Attorney that Mrs Rotini arranged for her son applies.
- Mr Joe Rotini is, by virtue of the Mental Capacity Act 2005, empowered to act as Mrs Rotini's proxy. As such, his representation of his mother's best interests has the legal force equivalent to any capacitous patient.
- It is to be hoped that, as part of the process of establishing the Lasting Power of Attorney, Mr Rotini and his mother discussed the possibilities of deterioration in her health. Candidates should remember though that this is still likely to be a difficult conversation. Mr Rotini may feel the burden of *'doing the right thing for his mother'* and is being asked to make some significant decisions at a time when he is probably distressed and tired.
- Just as with a capacitous patient, the task is to explain clearly and compassionately what is happening to Mrs Rotini, outlining the treatment she has received (and to which she has not responded) and the remaining options. Remember that what clinicians may take for granted because it is so familiar, may not be known or understood by Mr Rotini. For example, clinicians may readily understand the withdrawal of active treatment to mean that analgesia will continue and the patient made 'comfortable'. Whilst Mr Rotini may assume or worry that 'withdrawing active treatment' will cause his mother a painful and distressing death.

- It is increasingly rare for people to see the dying process and, understandably, many relatives are afraid of what is unknown. Gentle explanation of how Mrs Rotini is likely to respond if treatment is withdrawn and what constitutes 'a good death' may be useful for Mr Rotini.

- Remember that merely because the legal issue is 'solved' by Mr Rotini being a nominated proxy, ethical practice requires much of the clinical team in the form of patience, honesty about both what is known and unknown, empathy, and skilful communication. Mr Rotini may seek time and space to reflect before making a decision. He may wish to ask questions either immediately or later. He may want to involve other family members. The point is that the meeting with Mr Rotini should be paced according to his wishes and needs. Candidates need to be flexible and adapt to Mr Rotini according to his priorities. Establishing and maintaining an effective relationship is as essential as the Mental Capacity Act in enabling Mr Rotini to fulfil his role as his mother's proxy and represent her best interests.

Further information

- The legal recognition of proxies via the lasting power of attorney provisions in the Mental Capacity Act 2005 is a significant change for clinical practice. Previously, third parties had been limited to taking over financial and legal affairs and had no remit in healthcare. In common with publicity raising awareness of advance decision-making, there have been a number of campaigns aimed at encouraging the population at large to consider nominating a legal proxy for future healthcare decision-making. The ethical rationale being that 'prospective autonomy' is desirable and provides a preferable moral basis for care of the incapacitated patient than clinical determination of 'best interests'.

- Clinicians may consider whether it is part of their duty of care to raise the subject of future decision-making when treating patients in whom capacity is likely to diminish. Understanding that advance decision-making and the nomination of proxies is possible under the law potentially enables clinicians to work proactively to ensure that future healthcare is informed and chosen rather than well-intentioned but inferred.

- Finally, where a patient has neither made an advance statement/decision nor nominated a proxy, clinicians will have to weigh what is in the patient's best interests. Ways in which a clinician may obtain insight into a patient's wishes, preferences, and best interests include talking to family members, friends, carers, and professionals with whom the patient may have had a longer term relationship. It should be stressed that third parties in such a situation are not making determinative judgements but rather are being asked to give an informed sense of the patient and his or her likely preferences.

Case 46 ♦ **Proxy decision making under the Mental Capacity Act 2005—adult with learning disabilities**

Mr Holloway is 53. He has severe learning disabilities and cerebral palsy. He has been a resident in a nursing home for patients with physical and learning disabilities since he was 21 years old. Both his parents are dead and he has no siblings. There appear to be no other relatives and in over thirty years, he has never had a visitor other than volunteers. He has always been fed by one of three members of staff at the nursing home with whom he has a good relationship. Although feeding hasn't ever been easy, it was possible with a lot of patience on the part of his carers. Indeed, his carers believe that the prolonged contact Mr Holloway has whilst being fed is probably the most significant human interaction he has. Ten days ago, Mr Holloway developed a respiratory infection and he has since refused all food and had only small amounts of water. Mr Holloway has become increasingly unwell and was admitted last night. He is very distressed, appears frightened, and will let no one, except for the one of his carers, Mr Jahpur (who regularly comes to the hospital), touch him. Mr Jahpur says that he can see Mr Holloway is becoming increasingly malnourished and asks the clinical team for advice. The clinical team agrees that Mr Holloway needs feeding and suggest Percutaneous Gastronomy (PEG) tube feeding. Mr Jahpur is concerned about tube feeding Mr Holloway believing it will make him **'even more terrified of being in hospital and utterly miserable'.** *The clinical team is unsure how to proceed. You are asked to talk to Mr Jahpur about what should happen next.*

Core concepts

- Mr Holloway is an adult and therefore presumed to be capacitous. Many people with learning disabilities can be capacitous or facilitated to become capacitous with imaginative communication and patience and often the skills of a specialist learning disabilities team will assist in maximizing a patient's capacity. However, this discussion will proceed on the basis that Mr Holloway does not have capacity for the purposes of illustrating what happens in such cases.

- Assuming that there is no nominated proxy empowered to act for Mr Holloway via a Lasting Power of Attorney (and this is unlikely if he lacked capacity ever to appoint such a person), then the Mental Capacity Act 2005 requires that the clinical team contact the local Independent Mental Capacity Advocacy service.

- At present, the advocacy service can be used when a review of care is required, but more significantly, the Independent Mental Capacity Advocacy service must be involved in cases where significant medical decisions are being considered or in relation to accommodation decisions where a patient has been in hospital for more than 28 days. It is good practice to be aware of how and when to contact the local Independent Mental Capacity Service.

- The local Independent Mental Capacity Advocacy services exists to provide Independent Mental Capacity Advocates (IMCAs) in situations where a person does not have family or friends to represent their interests in relation to significant decisions about health or social care.

- The IMCAs are not proxy decision-makers but act as independent facilitators to ensure that an inclusive and thorough review informs the determination of a patient's best interests.

Application of core concepts to Case 46

- Candidates may be concerned about confidentiality and wonder whether they can speak to Mr Jahpur about Mr Holloway's care and, if so, on what basis. Confidentiality is not unlimited and there are, as described in Section 4 of this volume, several circumstances in which disclosure can be justified. One of the situations in which information can be shared is where it is in the patient's best interests to disclose but consent cannot be obtained. Mr Holloway lacks the capacity to consent to the clinical team sharing information about him with Mr Jahpur, but most would accept that it is in Mr Holloway's interests for decisions to be discussed with his carer who knows him best and appears to be one of the people with whom he has an established relationship.

- Candidates have to explain to Mr Jahpur that whilst his perspective and presence is invaluable to providing clinical care for Mr Holloway, he is not able to make decisions on his behalf because he is not a legally recognized proxy. It is important to be sensitive to the obvious attachment and mutual affection that exists between Mr Jahpur and Mr Holloway. To assume that a paid or professional carer is not distressed by Mr Holloway's condition and to forget that Mr Jahpur may be surprised to learn that he is unable to make decisions on Mr Holloway's behalf would be a mistake.

- Although Mr Jahpur is not the legally recognized decision-maker, his contribution is essential to Mr Holloway's well-being. This must be explicitly acknowledged. Candidates should convey understanding of the importance of Mr Jahpur to Mr Holloway and explore his response to the suggested PEG.

- It may be that Mr Jahpur has simple suggestions born of his long-standing relationship with Mr Holloway that will improve the patient's nutritional state without the use of the PEG, e.g. he may be able to suggest favourite foods, preferred bowls, plates, or cutlery and times of the day when Mr Holloway is more likely to be hungry. Indeed, one very basic but poten-tially effective option to consider is whether Mr Jahpur would be able to feed Mr Holloway himself.

- If, however, Mr Holloway remains malnourished and/or deteriorates such that a decision about PEG feeding has to be made. It has to be explained to Mr Jahpur that it is a require-ment under the Mental Capacity Act 2005 that, if Mr Holloway lacks the capacity to make his own decisions and there is no one to represent him as a legally appointed proxy, the clinical team has to contact the local IMCA service.[15]

- Care should be taken to explain the role of the IMCA, i.e. that he or she will be appointed, via a local service, to support Mr Holloway and represent his interests. Explaining to Mr Jahpur that it is likely that the insertion of a PEG tube falls within the broad category of 'serious medical treatment' which is specifically covered within the legislation and the urgency with which Mr Holloway's deterioration must be addressed is important.

- The lead clinician should make a prompt referral to the local IMCA service so that Mr Holloway can be seen as a priority. The notes should record that such a referral has been made and, where possible, the appointed IMCA should be involved in decision-making once he or she has made contact with Mr Holloway and had an opportunity to review his care.

- Whilst a key aim is to work effectively and inclusively with the IMCA to ensure that, as a vulnerable adult, Mr Holloway is supported and his interests represented throughout, the relationship with Mr Jahpur is also a priority—at all stages, he should be kept informed, valued, and respected for his expertise. It is likely that not only does Mr Jahpur bring much that is helpful to the clinical team, but his perspective is also likely to be invaluable to the appointed IMCA.

- Avoid making judgemental comments about either the patient's quality of life or Mr Jahpur's perception of Mr Holloway's quality of life.

- Seek to maintain an organized, calm, and empathic approach throughout.

Further information

- The IMCA service is a relatively recent addition and many working in the NHS will have limited experience of its role and value in decision-making. Indeed in a review of the pilot IMCA service, a team at Cambridge University found that healthcare professionals' uncertainty about the IMCA service was a significant bar to effective decision-making involving vulnerable patients.[16] It may therefore be wise for prospective candidates to spend some time reviewing the work of the IMCA service and considering how to access an IMCA in their own practice.

Consent-seeking and Refusal

Consent: The Basics

Case 47 ◆ Seeking consent for investigation (endoscopy)

Mr Hughes is 48 years old. He has been referred for an endoscopy by his GP following a history of dyspepsia which has not responded to treatment with antacids and H2 antagonists. Helicobacter Pylori has been excluded. Mr Hughes attends the endoscopy unit and you are asked to obtain consent.

Core concepts

- Consent is integral to ethical and legal practice. Obtaining informed consent is the legal *sine qua non* of patients making free choices and gives meaning to autonomy. Indeed, some authors argue that not only is the process of facilitating and obtaining valid consent of ethico-legal importance, but it is also therapeutically valuable.[17]
- Autonomous decisions are made by those capacitous so to do who are adequately informed and acting voluntarily. Incidentally, the term 'informed consent' is tautologous because consent has to be informed, otherwise it is not consent and therefore any actions would be unlawful and constitute assault and/or battery.
- Consent is integrated into clinical practice via written materials such as information leaflets, consent forms, and, less commonly, advance directives. The integrated nature of seeking consent can, perversely, diminish the quality of the consent that is obtained and has, notoriously, perpetuated legal nonsense such as clinicians signing consent forms on the part of incapacitous patients. In short, it may sometimes be that familiarity does not breed consent. Meaningful, valid consent depends on the ways in which individual clinicians work with particular patients to ensure that informed choices can be made and the criteria shown in Box 8 are met.

Box 8 Criteria for valid consent
For consent to be legally valid it must be:
• Capacitous (and the patient's capacity should be assessed using the process described above).
• Voluntary, i.e. free from undue pressure, coercion, or persuasion for any third parties.
• Informed.
• Continuing, i.e. patients should know that they can change their mind at any time.

- Whilst it is common and good practice for written information to be provided to patients attending for investigations such as endoscopy, the existence of written material and a consent form does not remove the responsibility to discuss the endoscopy with the patient to ensure valid consent is obtained.

- The four essential elements of consent—capacity, information, voluntariness, and its continuing nature—are described in Box 8.
- Consent in general, and consent forms in particular, can often seem obsessed with risks. Disclosure of risk is, of course, an integral part of obtaining informed consent. However, there are many medico-legal myths that persist about the extent to which risk should be disclosed with complicated equations calculating percentages in relation to severity often being cited. The essence is that risk disclosure is assessed in accordance with the standard of care test that applies to any other area of clinical practice, i.e. did the doctor disclose the risks in a way that accords with the practice of a reasonable body of his professional peers and does the degree of risk disclosure withstand logical analysis? Despite legal challenge, the law works to a standard of disclosure that is professionally-determined. The general position is that 'significant risks' should be disclosed—and significance may be assessed with reference to the frequency of occurrence, severity, or both.

Application of core concepts to Case 47

- Capacity can be assumed. Mr Hughes is an adult; there is no mention of possible incapacity in the GP referral and nothing in the scenario to indicate that he may lack capacity to make his own decisions about endoscopy.
- The next and probably most significant element of obtaining consent from Mr Hughes is the provision and exchange of information. Note that the exchange of information is as important as the dispensation of information from clinician to patient.
- The first task is to establish what Mr Hughes understands about why he has been referred, what he has been referred for and how the referral will inform his care. It is easy to assume that Mr Hughes's GP has explained the indications for an endoscopy given the ongoing history of dyspepsia and apparently textbook management excluding H. Pylori and prescribing antacid/H2 antagonists. However, it is essential to find out from Mr Hughes himself how he perceives his situation: a simple, open question asking Mr Hughes to share what has been happening would be sufficient and is likely to yield invaluable information rendering the process of obtaining meaningful consent both more genuine and effective.
- Having asked for Mr Hughes's account, it is, of course, essential to be responsive and to develop a proper dialogue. Mr Hughes may reveal points of confusion, uncertainty, or anxiety and information should be given that is responsive to the specific preoccupations of the patient attending to both verbal and non-verbal cues during the discussion. The worries of patients can be surprising and may be unanticipated by busy clinicians for whom endoscopy is a 'routine' investigation. It is only by encouraging Mr Hughes to talk that these concerns will ever be known, still less ameliorated.
- Risks, of course, must be located in the appropriate clinical context and discussed with reference to benefit. As such, when giving Mr Hughes information about the risk of endoscopy, e.g. bleeding, perforation, etc., the discussion should also encompass the likely benefits of performing the investigation and the value of the results derived from endoscopy for managing his poorly-controlled and chronic dyspepsia.
- In addition to information about the endoscopy itself, Mr Hughes should be informed as to possible ancillary activities such as sedation, biopsy, and/or the retention of tissue.
- Clinicians and units vary in their use of sedation. Is Mr Hughes entitled to insist upon sedation even if it is not the preferred practice of a clinician? Patients are entitled to refuse treatment and to express preferences, but not to demand that which is not clinically

indicated. However, 'clinically indicated' in relation to sedation is an elastic concept which can be variously interpreted by doctors.

- It is wise to avoid a situation where clinician and patient assume adversarial positions in respect of sedation and, instead explore why Mr Hughes wishes to have sedation and explain the reasons why the unit prefers not to use it, or vice versa. A few moments spent in open and non-defensive discussion is likely to be time well spent leading to trust, an effective therapeutic alliance, and ultimately improving care and outcomes for Mr Hughes *and* the endoscopy unit itself.

- Moving on to the remaining two elements of valid consent, voluntariness and its dynamic nature, Mr Hughes should understand that he has a choice. Merely being referred by a GP and entering the monolithic system of the NHS does not preclude patients from choosing care at each stage.

- Candidates should also note the continuing nature of consent. Mr Hughes will, if the task of seeking consent has been well done so far, have received considerably more information about endoscopy and the way in which it is likely to inform future care. Asking Mr Hughes if he has any further questions and reminding him that he can change his mind should he wish is a simple but necessary way to capture the essential concepts of voluntariness and ongoing consent.

- Only when the consultation has reached the point at which Mr Hughes has no further questions, should the consent form be introduced.

- It is good practice to talk Mr Hughes through the form locating the bare words in earlier discussion, and to be prepared to answer any further questions as you proceed. Assuming Mr Hughes is willing to sign the form, a signed copy should be placed in the notes before the procedure begins.

- Seek to maintain an organized, calm, and responsive approach throughout the consultation.

Further information

- Frequently actions based on invalid consent processes are predicated on claims of either inadequate or misleading disclosure of risk. However, it is extremely common for such legal action to fail because of the legal requirements of demonstrating causation, i.e. that the inadequate consent process directly contributed to the alleged foreseeable damage or loss.

- Even if risk is not disclosed or it is insufficiently well disclosed, the patient has to demonstrate that had risk been disclosed, his or her decision to proceed with the investigation, procedure, or treatment would have been different. To use the language of civil law, the patient must show that 'but for' the doctor's sub-optimal consent process, the investigation, procedure, or treatment would not have taken place. And it is extremely difficult for most claimants to show that they would not have proceeded with treatment had risks been otherwise disclosed.

- Following a case called *Chester* v *Afshar*,[18] a further layer has been added to the complications of causation in relation to disclosure of risk. In that case, the House of Lords held that a patient did not need to demonstrate that he or she would never have had the investigation, procedure, or treatment at all, but merely that he or she would have delayed having the investigation, procedure, or treatment to another time and with another clinician. The judgment therefore implicitly acknowledges that there are multiple variables that influence clinical risk and that changing the scenario may or even does alter risk. More importantly, the judgment acknowledges that patient choice, be it about the clinician, whether to seek a second or even third opinion, and determining the time of treatment, is an inherent part of informed consent.

Consent: Patient Preferences and Requests

Case 48 ◆ **Patient preferences and requests 1: Screening for bowel cancer**

*Mr Sorensen, age 42, attends the outpatient clinic for investigation of lower abdominal discomfort and continuing bowel symptoms. He discloses early in the consultation that his mother died from bowel cancer and he is '**very worried**' about the possibility that he has bowel cancer. Mr Sorensen has done some research on the internet, and knows that the NHS bowel cancer screening programme is routinely available to those aged 60–69. People aged over 70, can also ask to participate in the programme. Mr Sorensen wishes to discuss whether he should be screened for bowel cancer even though he is considerably younger than the age at which the national programme applies.*

Core concepts

- For consent to screening procedures to be meaningful, counselling must consist of more than simply quoting statistics on risk, sensitivity, and specificity. But how much more is required? Doctors are bound by the GMC to disclose information that they believe any reasonable person in the patient's position would require for an informed choice.

- Mason and Laurie[19] suggest that doctors need to establish whether patients are seeking information or advice. This is an ethical question that is frequently overlooked when discussing screening options. Indeed, on the subject of options, the national screening programme for bowel cancer screening has only recently become available to all eligible patients.[20]

- It is essential to be clear about the scope of screening for abnormality. As such, candidates need to know themselves how screening works, its effectiveness at detecting disease, the rates of identifying bowel cancer amongst those who have been screened and the range of results/treatment pathways.

- The question of choice following screening can be ethico-legally complex. Once a patient agrees to undergo most 'routine' screening, there is a potential chain of further investigations. If Mr Sorensen is recommended to have an invasive test as a result of screening, in what sense is his choice to undergo the invasive test 'free'? The way in which this issue is usually conceptualized is as what might be called 'contingent autonomy', i.e. if Mr Sorensen is properly counselled when deciding whether or not to have screening, he will be encouraged to consider what choices he would prefer to make if further investigations and/or treatment are indicated. This so-called 'contingent autonomy' emphasizes the importance of effective pre-screening consultations whilst not, of course, removing the need for Mr Sorensen to give valid consent to any future treatment.

Application of core concepts to Case 48

- After introductions, candidates should allow Mr Sorensen to explain, in his own words and time, his concerns about his symptoms in general, and bowel cancer, in particular. Careful and active listening will allow Mr Sorensen to convey most accurately what he both understands about bowel cancer screening and his priorities for the consultation.

- Even if Mr Sorensen decides he does not wish to pursue screening, he should be able to make that decision following a dialogue with clinicians that enable him to leave feeling more informed about his options.

- Mr Sorensen is considerably younger than the people targeted by the NHS screening programme. He seems to perceive an increased risk because of his mother's medical history and it may be helpful to explain that understanding of the genetic component of bowel cancer is increasing (see Case 5 'Family History of Cancer').[21] However, candidates must not, of course, substitute an empathic response to Mr Sorensen's concerns with a lecture on genetics.

- For consent to screening to be valid and in accordance with good practice guidance on consent, candidates need to explain to Mr Sorensen that screening:

    ◆ has been shown to reduce the mortality rate in patients with bowel cancer[22] because it offers the possibility of earlier, and therefore more effective, intervention and treatment when the disease is not symptomatic.

    ◆ does not necessarily provide certainty. Indeed it may exacerbate anxiety by revealing to the patient what can best be described as 'partial knowledge'. In the specific case of screening for bowel cancer, polyps may be detected which are not cancer, but do have the potential to develop into cancer later in Mr Sorensen's life. It is essential that the consultation both raises the possibility of partial knowledge and explains to Mr Sorensen that he may subsequently have to decide whether he wishes to have any polyps identified removed.

    ◆ may lead to further investigations and interventions however 'routine', e.g. a colonoscopy and/or the removal of polyps.

- Honesty about uncertainty in medical screening is essential and candidates need a sound grasp of probabilities. For example, as well as the normal/abnormal result from bowel screening, approximately 4 patients in 100[23] will have ambiguous test results. The way in which these probabilities are communicated, and accurately reflect what is known, is crucial.

- Mr Sorensen is too young to receive a routine invitation to bowel cancer screening. However, it may be indicated because of the family history and his presenting symptoms. The decision whether to screen therefore falls within the remit of the usual 'standard of care' test, i.e. would a reasonable body of doctors offer screening to Mr Sorensen and does the decision whether to offer screening withstand logical analysis?

- There is a lot of complex information for candidates to discuss with Mr Sorensen (who is already anxious). It is essential therefore to pace the discussion as is remaining alert to Mr Sorensen's verbal and non-verbal cues. Information should be offered in discrete chunks, checking for understanding, and leaving time for the patient to take in what is being said and ask questions.

- This is a complex scenario and it may be that candidates are unable to answer all of Mr Sorensen's questions immediately, in which case an honest expression of uncertainty and an offer to find out more is the best option.

- Screening for bowel cancer is only one part of investigating Mr Sorensen's symptoms although it is the aspect he has highlighted as his priority, but the screening decision should be contextualized by summarizing the next steps available to him. This is unlikely to be a decision that Mr Sorensen makes immediately and candidates should explicitly invite him to think about the possibilities and perhaps point him to further resources in advance of a follow up consultation.

Further information

- It is worth noting that just as patients are not obliged to undergo screening, there is no 'right' to screening that is not indicated any more than there is a 'right' to any other form of medical investigation or treatment. However, if a doctor refuses to perform a test he or she must consider whether it would unreasonable or illogical in the eyes of others so to refuse the patient the test requested. If so, the doctor could be vulnerable to a claim of negligence.
- If a screening test gives a false negative result, an action for damages may only be brought if it can be shown that the test was performed negligently.[24]

Case 49 ◆ Patient preferences and requests 2: Access to resources for patient seeking Avastin

Mr Hari is 46 years old. He has metastatic colorectal cancer. He has become aware that Bevacizumab ('Avastin') has improved survival time in patients with metastatic colorectal disease. He attends the Oncology outpatient department and asks you why he is 'not receiving Avastin if it has proven benefits. It might help me live long enough to see my daughter's 18th birthday. Surely that's got to make it worth a try?'

Core concepts

- Questions of resource allocation are common and increasingly vexed as newer, more expensive drugs are licensed and the population served by the NHS increases. Although Mr Hari is a cancer patient, few, if any, areas of medicine are exempt from decisions which could be seen to have been taken on fiscal rather than clinical grounds.
- The law and accompanying regulations thus far have been explicit in declaring that clinical need must not be compromised by financial considerations. To date there have been a few key judicial decisions concerning the provision (or lack of provision) of medical treatment. One of the most notable was the refusal by Cambridgeshire Area Health Authority to fund further remedial (as opposed to palliative) treatment for a child, Jaimee Bowen:[25] the court was clear that whilst there was no duty to prescribe or give expensive treatment, such refusal to offer treatment must not be motivated *'solely or exclusively by financial consider- ations'.*[26] However, this case is distinguishable in that there was a clinical consensus that the treatment sought by Jaimee Bowen's parents was experimental, had a very small chance of success,[27] and was likely to have significant and debilitating side-effects which could not be in the patient's best interests given the prognosis.
- The distinction between needs and wants in the NHS has been affirmed by cases involving patients seeking treatments that are refused. What is a need? What is a want? The distinction

may sound seductively neat, but is a judgement made by human beings, albeit those with 'authority' to make these decisions and human beings are partial, value driven creatures with biases and preferences. For example, is screening a want or a need? Is pain relief in labour a want or a need? Is the prescription of 'Zyban' to a dependent smoker a want or a need? These are the judgements that have to be made and are not made uniformly.

- If it is accepted that there are few absolute 'needs', then how can a limited budget in a socially funded health system best be managed to achieve maximum advantage to the maximum number of patients when faced with myriad conflicting demands? It has been suggested that if a healthcare provider can demonstrate that any restriction on a particular drug has taken place in a logical, reasonable, and consistent way, then sanctions are not likely to be imposed.

- As doctors and, of course, drug companies became increasingly resistant to the perceived arbitrary rationing dictats of the Department of Health, the National Institute for Clinical Excellence (now called the National Institute for Health and Clinical Excellence) was established to offer a transparent process in which diverse interests could be considered and best evidence would inform the availability of treatment. The establishment of the National Institute for Health and Clinical Excellence (NICE) was intended to establish a formal, centralized, and independent process for reviewing the clinical and cost effectiveness of particular medicines. Therefore, local healthcare providers may sometimes want to wait until a particular medicine has been reviewed by NICE before approving it for general use on patients, even though the drug has a licence.

- Resources are inevitably constrained in the NHS. However, absolute bans on treatments or procedures on the grounds of cost are legally indefensible. Hence the declared approach of NICE to use evidence and efficacy to inform decisions about equitable access. Cost effectiveness is the most difficult to measure: Quality Adjusted Life Years (QALYS) have been used as a tool for attributing quantitative value to particular groups of patients, but are controversial.

- QALYS weigh a patient's life and the effect of an intervention, e.g. a year of healthy life expectancy is worth +1, a year of life compromised by ill health is worth −1. Healthcare interventions are measured according to the likely extension of years of life and improvement in quality of life. If all interventions are given an agreed QALY value, they can then be ranked against each other.

- However, QALYS assume that quality of life can and should be measured objectively. They could be said to be ageist in that quantity of life expectancy is important in making the calculation and may therefore infringe Human Rights and equality laws. Many interventions do not have an agreed QALY value. QALYS work at a population rather than individual level and therefore generalize about patients, diseases, and interventions. Pre-existing disabilities will influence the assessment of QALY, what has been described as 'double jeopardy'. Finally, QALYS focus on outcome rather than need—those who are likely best to benefit are treated not those who most need treatment.

- The existence of NICE notwithstanding, from the perspective of the clinician, there is often considerable discretionary power to shape, if not determine, resource decisions. The opinion of clinical staff is likely to be sought when difficult decisions about healthcare resources are being made.

- The difficulties surrounding the ethically and legally defensible allocation of resources are further exacerbated by the potential impact of the Human Rights Act, in particular article 14. If a particular group of patients can show that decisions about available treatments are based on criteria that could be considered discriminatory, e.g. age, gender, sexuality, marital status, etc., such decisions may contravene article 14 which provides for the right not to be subject to discrimination. In the case of Mr Hari, it does not appear that there is any question of discrimination but it is always a variable that should be considered in the context of resource allocation to ensure that particular groups are not discriminated against, either directly or indirectly.

- Mr Hari is a cancer patient and it is in the field of oncology that there has been discussion of mixing public and private provision. What would the position be if Mr Hari asked to combine standard NHS and publicly-funded treatment, such as chemotherapy and radio-therapy, with private treatment such as the prescription of Avastin? Although much of the recent debate about combining public and private healthcare provision has suggested that it is a new issue in healthcare, there are already examples of mixed provision, e.g. an NHS consultation may result in a private prescription. However, the general principle of the NHS is one of universal equality. As originally conceived, the NHS was intended to provide that all patients receive the same treatment irrespective of their social or economic status. This is a familiar ethical precept and is based on the Rawlsian[28] notion that equality and fairness require us to protect the weakest as a society. On that basis all the patients on a ward with the same diagnosis should be receiving the same treatment. If that treatment is sub-optimal, that doesn't justify giving preferential treatment to one patient over another. Indeed some would argue that to do so is to 'collude' and allow the NHS to provide for those who 'shout the loudest' rather than protecting the most vulnerable whose voices are not being heard. This is an ethical position that depends on notions of justice.

- As well as the advocacy role, there are interesting issues raised by cases like Mr Hari's for the doctor–patient relationship. First, if the patient is able to request and fund treatment, is the doctor relegated to the role of technician and does this matter?

- A further and important question in relation to this scenario is how doctors can ensure informed consent in the context of 'wonder drugs'? There may be a paucity of data with limited follow up and unclear information about side-effects which may be significant, e.g. cardiac toxicity in relation to Herceptin. The information available can be difficult to assess critically, even for the medical community; see for example Richard Horton's critique of the Herceptin trials in The Lancet[29] when the same trials were praised as 'revolutionary' by oncologists writing in the New England Journal of Medicine three weeks earlier.[30] And medicine is sadly familiar with drugs that are initially hailed as a revolution and yet later revealed as having adverse effects, e.g. consider the stories of Thalidomide and, in more recent times, Vioxx.

- An alternative perspective on mixing public and private provision is what might be called a 'libertarian' position in which individuals are free to supplement their care in a system that provides basic provision. This view would argue that for the hospital management to refuse any request from Mr Hari to combine NHS treatment with the private prescription of Avastin would be to infringe his autonomy. In one account of mixing NHS and private healthcare for patients on an NHS ward, nursing staff reported significant difficulties in providing differential care.[31] Whether the more familiar examples of mixed private and public provision can be considered 'more ethically justifiable' or not seems doubtful. The stakes are generally lower, therefore it might be argued that the ensuing inequality is less serious. However, such a conclusion assumes that it is the consequences of inequality that are the moral crux of the matter, whilst it may be that it is the fundamental notion of inequality and the ethical precept of justice that are the moral 'heart of the matter'.

- A fundamental question in the resource allocation debate is to whom these difficult decisions should be entrusted—patients, clinical staff, ethicists, hospital managers, politicians, all of us?

- There is ethical value in processes, particularly in resource allocation decision making, and the creation of a transparent and clear process—even if it has imperfect results—could be argued to be as important as the decisions eventually reached. There is greater moral legitimacy in decisions taken by public, acceptable, and well-understood processes rather than in secrecy or opacity.

- Individual doctors have to make individual choices about the extent to which they are cognizant of the less familiar and perhaps less appealing role of allocating resources. Centralization and committees notwithstanding, there remains local discretion, although many would argue it is diminishing. Furthermore, in the unlikely event that doctors have all their discretion removed in relation to treatment decisions, this does not equate to removing responsibility to consider these vexed questions and contribute to the debate. Ideally, this 'representation' is as inclusive as possible and has an eye on the silent patient who has healthcare needs but perhaps has a diagnosis that is not well-known or 'appealing', e.g. care of the elderly, mental health, a patient who is less able to engage the powerful (media, politicians, and even doctors themselves) in his or her cause.

Application of core concepts to Case 49

- Patients, such as Mr Hari, may not have 'long' to live nor enjoy good health by objective standards, but nonetheless will value extra time albeit in pain or discomfort because they want to see a grandchild born, celebrate a graduation, attend an assembly, etc.

- At the moment there are different decision-makers depending on the particular request: individual doctors have discretion on a micro level as to how they construct patient requests as either wants or needs, NHS Trusts and prescribing sub-groups will make locally applicable decisions about treatments and, nationally, NICE too will issue guidance about whether a treatment is sufficiently effective to warrant prescribing thereby implicitly making a judgement about whether a drug is a want or a need. One question to be considered in the context of this scenario is whether 'core' cancer services should be the priority given the prevalence of cancer in the UK or whether individual patients should be entitled to receive so-called 'last chance' drugs such as Avastin.

- Is Mr Hari's desire to receive Avastin and potentially prolong his life a need or a wish? Is it essential that Mr Hari lives as long as possible? Or even simply long enough to see his children grow up? Or is the extension of Mr Hari's life and his presence at his daughter's 18th birthday merely a 'desirable outcome'?

- If Mr Hari were to pursue his wish to receive Avastin, the local prescribing committee in its deliberation of national guidance would also probably ask whether his clinical team believe that he should receive the drug. The influence of medical opinion and the ability to 'make a case' to an authority therefore creates potential for the campaigning, 'active', or articulate empowered patient, who achieves access to healthcare via legal action. Doctors, therefore, may have to consider the extent to which they can advocate patients and the implications of so doing both for the individual and other patients.

- Exceptional circumstances can also be used as a reason for providing care and has been cited where controversial resource allocation decisions to refuse treatment have been reversed following high profile media campaigns by particular patients.

- What of the duty a doctor owes to a patient such as Mr Hari? Doctors have traditionally been the advocate of the individual patient. The relationship has been constructed as a dyadic one with little attention to broader notions of resource management even though the NHS is a fundamentally utilitarian system. Thus, the ethical preference has been to represent both the area in which one works and particular patients in extremis, i.e. in this situation, oncology and Mr Hari. Representing Mr Hari and other cancer patients to committees and the NHS managers who make funding decisions could be seen as part of the role of a doctor. However, increasingly there is a responsibility on everyone in the NHS, including doctors, to make resource decisions. The GMC requires doctors to make the patient their first concern but also to be aware of scarce resources–these may be difficult duties to reconcile, e.g. how are sick patients to have therapeutic relationships with those who are apparently 'denying' them treatment?

• For some patients, including Mr Hari perhaps, the drug that appears to offer benefit may harm. In any event, there remains considerable uncertainty surrounding the effect(s) of Avastin making meaningful consent a challenge. Information about risks and the inherent uncertainty of such new drugs must be part of the consent process and yet cautionary notes, negative effects, and clinical ambiguity are likely to be far harder for Mr Hari to hear than the 'miracle drug' stories, especially when he is vulnerable and desperate.

• There is no 'right' or easy answer to how clinicians balance these competing ethical claims, but candidates should be aware of the main arguments and be able to construct a logical argument to support their decision with regards to Mr Hari's request.

Further information

• The importance of the rationale for allocating resources was confirmed in the case of a patient seeking the prescription of Herceptin for breast cancer: Ann-Marie Rogers. Mrs Rogers took her local Primary Care Trust (Swindon) to court because they refused to fund the prescription of Herceptin for her even though clinical opinion was that she would benefit from the drug. Herceptin was not available on the NHS in the Swindon region save for 'exceptional cases'. Mrs Rogers challenged the policy. The court affirmed that clinical and cost effectiveness and social factors can be considered by local NHS bodies when deciding who should receive treatment.

• The effect of the persuasive patient who is receiving extensive publicity was evident in a series of cases that predated the Ann-Marie Rogers claim. In those cases, several women who were claiming that they should receive Herceptin led PCTs to capitulate rather than face ongoing publicity and judicial review.

• The implications of the Rogers case are not quite as they were represented by the media (although the case was also somewhat misrepresented by some NHS Trusts). The court held that Swindon PCT had been irrational and arbitrary in refusing to prescribe on the basis that their policy was flawed. The flaw was that the PCT specifically excluded cost as a consideration, therefore it appeared to be an inexplicable decision based on the available evidence and clinical need. By saying that cost was not a factor in their decision, the PCT could not, with the apparently ample funds the PCT cited, justify denying treatment on any rational grounds. The appeal therefore succeeded on a very narrow legal basis, rather than the broad 'treatment as of right' account that has been represented in much of the reporting of the case. Therefore the case actually confirms that costs could legitimately be *part* of an exercise in weighing access to treatments. The court also noted that different PCTs might adopt contrasting approaches to resource allocation. In other words, discretion was confirmed and cost may be part of the determination of resource allocation decisions which, taken with other factors such as efficacy and clinical evidence, combine to provide the rationale for choices made about healthcare on a case by case basis.

Case 50 ◆ **Patient preferences and requests 3: Resuscitation decision-making with a COPD patient**

Mrs Edith Miles is 78 years old. She has chronic heart failure, osteoarthritis which causes her considerable pain, and COPD. An exacerbation of COPD led to Mrs Miles being admitted to the ward. The consultant asks you to discuss resuscitation with Mrs Miles.

Core concepts

- The ethico-legal issues in treating the older patient are of increasing concern to healthcare professionals. As the numbers of patients over the age of 65 continue to rise, the NHS is faced with a growing body of patients who raise particular ethico-legal concerns.
- The decline in the extended family and the increasing ability of medical technology to prolong life (although not necessarily to prolong mental health) means that increasingly the care of older patients is falling to the social and healthcare systems.
- The autonomy of the older patient may be compromised by organic disease, e.g. dementia and/or socio-economic factors such as inadequate housing or lack of money.
- It is easy to make value judgements about the 'quality of life' of older patients. There are significant ethical questions to be asked however before such judgements should be made. How, for example, can it be known that an older patient with cognitive impairment does not enjoy a good quality of life? Is this simply a subjective judgement on the part of a doctor who may be a great deal younger than his patient and may have no idea about their patient's experiences and personality? It is clear that decisions about quality of life and non-treatment in the older patient must be based on the needs and desires of the individual and not on either the patient's age or diagnosis.
- If, as some believe, older patients are a particularly vulnerable group in the healthcare system, it is perhaps too easy to conclude that such a group should be treated paternalistically. However, unless the capacity of the patient is clearly compromised, patients should be involved in medical decisions as much as possible.
- The impetus for a paternalistic approach to healthcare for older patients may come not from the medical profession but from the patient's family or regular carers. There is no legal duty for children to care for their elderly parents and it has been suggested that 'elder abuse' is a significantly under-acknowledged crime.[32]
- The balance between the needs and wants of the patient, and the needs and wants of the patient's relatives can be particularly delicate when caring for the elderly. Good communication, a clear understanding of the principles of capacity and consent and multi-disciplinary support will aid the doctor in this fine balancing act.
- This scenario should be read in conjunction with Scenario 2.2.2 (Case 42 Relative's Objection to Capacitous Decision) which also concerns resuscitation decision-making, albeit with reference to third party objections to a capacitous patient's choices.

Application of core concepts to Case 50

- There are multiple sources for guidance on resuscitation decision-making including the United Kingdom Resuscitation Council, professional and specialty specific bodies, and the European Resuscitation Council.

- It is important that wherever possible resuscitation decisions are discussed honestly with patients and in advance of the patient deteriorating and emergencies. In general, if no DNAR discussion or decision has taken place and the patient arrests, the initial presumption should be to resuscitate.

- The emphasis of ethics guidance on resuscitation is that patients, and where appropriate, their families, should be involved in discussions. However, this is clearly a complex and sensitive conversation to have with Mrs Miles.

- Candidates have been specifically asked to raise the issue of resuscitation, and, as such, a truthful exchange is required. Information should not be withheld because it is not easy to discuss or feels uncomfortable. One of the challenges is to convey in a careful way to Mrs Miles the realities of resuscitation particularly in patients who are unwell and have several problems as she does. A crucial part of ethical practice in the context of resuscitation is to explore Mrs Miles's existing understanding of both her disease and resuscitation. Remember what clinicians know about resuscitation (or indeed any other aspect of practice) is not necessarily known by patients and their families. It is important to explore Mrs Miles's wishes and not to make assumptions that she either will or will not inevitably want to be resuscitated. Retaining an awareness of the significance of the decision in hand and appreciating that there is much more to Mrs Miles than her complex medical needs and co-morbidity is essential.

- DNAR is, of course, specific to resuscitation. The relationship of CPR to other interventions and treatments, e.g. ventilation, hydration, nutrition, analgesia, etc., should be considered and discussed with Mrs Miles. It is important to be clear with Mrs Miles that even if a patient is 'not for resuscitation', the clinical team will do all that can be done to ensure that she is well cared for and remains comfortable. DNAR does not equate to no care at all but Mrs Miles cannot be expected to know this and may well be very frightened at the prospect of being 'abandoned' by healthcare staff.

- Mrs Miles must be given the space to consider both what she is being told and asked. An explicit invitation to ask questions is important in allowing her the opportunity to clarify what she has understood and revealing her concerns and priorities. Direct questions must be answered honestly. Mrs Miles may misunderstand the basis of any resuscitation decision and perhaps fear it is based on her age or scarce resources rather than her clinical interests.

- Candidates should explain to Mrs Miles that DNAR orders are reviewable and will be recorded in her notes. Inadequate communication can lead to poor outcomes. Processes differ,[33] but each NHS Trust is required to have a publicly available policy regarding resuscitation status and decisions based on the current guidance from the UK Resuscitation Council.[34] Clinical practice should reflect the published policy.

- DNAR decisions should be clearly communicated to those who have clinical contact with the patient, being alert to the roles played by the wider clinical team, e.g. physiotherapy, occupational therapy, etc.

- It is important to discuss DNAR decision-making openly, factually, and honestly being clear about what is factually true, what is uncertain and without assumption.

Further information

- Sometimes the imperative to discuss resuscitation decisions with the patient if at all possible is confused with a requirement that patients should give explicit consent for a DNAR order. In fact, due to the legal principle that a patient can refuse treatment and express a preference but not demand a particular intervention, patients are not able to demand resuscitation in any eventuality.

- However, the aim should be to involve patients and explain why resuscitation is not considered to be beneficial. The provision of a second opinion may be valuable too. The ethical obligation to be compassionate, open, and considerate remains irrespective of legal principle.

- Finally, there has been considerable discussion in the ethical literature about whether family members and/or close friends should be present when resuscitation attempts are made. For a long time the conventional view was that witnessing resuscitation efforts would be distressing and potentially harmful. However, the evidence shows that of those people who did observe resuscitation, over 90% would wish to be present if the situation were to arise again in the future.[35] It has been suggested that when loved ones are able to be present during CPR attempts, they are better placed to accept the realities of bereavement and feel that it was important that they were there to witness the moment of death.[36] However, the positive effects of families being present at resuscitation attempts is not universal and many clinicians continue to express reservations about loved ones being in the room when CPR is undertaken.[37] What is clear is that if relatives are to be present during resuscitation efforts, attention to their needs is important and it is common for a member of staff to be responsible for briefing and supporting the family if they choose to stay during resuscitation efforts.

Case 51 ◆ Patient preferences and requests 4—Analgesia and the end of life

Mrs Robson has bone cancer and has been a patient on the ward for three days. She is in tremendous pain and has begged staff to 'put her out of her misery'. The clinical team agrees that she is very sick indeed and not likely to live long. After discussion with the consultant, you prescribe opiate analgesia in increasing doses. Mrs Robson's husband asks if 'so much pain relief will see her on her way to peace sooner rather than later?'

Core concepts

- At the outset, it is important to distinguish between patients with chronic illnesses who may be suffering great pain and patients who are terminally ill (who may also be in great pain) such as Mrs Robson in this scenario. Although patients with chronic conditions may share the levels of pain that are experienced by the terminally ill, their lives are not generally foreshortened in the same way as patients with terminal medical conditions; a fact that may have significant implications for the ways in which doctors define their duties to such patients in general, and Mrs Robson in this specific scenario.

• Most ethical duties are framed in terms of giving a 'benefit' to the patient. For example, the short-term discomfort caused by putting a line into a dehydrated patient is outweighed by the benefit of rehydrating the patient and restoring them to health. However, difficulties can arise about the way in which benefit is defined, particularly in the context of caring for patients with pain. Benefit may be seen as the symptomatic alleviation (temporary) of pain. Yet, there will frequently be side-effects of such pain relief that may become increasingly severe and debilitating. At some point in an illness in which pain is an overwhelming factor, the permanent alleviation of pain may be the expressed wish of the patient as seems to be the case for Mrs Robson who, we are told, has asked staff to 'put her out of her misery'.

• It is important to be clear about terminology when discussing end of life decision-making. Candidates should be familiar with the following terms and the concomitant legal position:

  ♦ Active euthanasia: describes an act that contributes to death. It is illegal.

  ♦ Physician Assisted suicide: a sub-set of active euthanasia. It is illegal.

  ♦ Passive euthanasia: an omission that contributes to death. May be lawful subject to the distinction between acts and omissions and proportionality.

  ♦ Suicide: causing one's own death. Since the Suicide Act 1961, suicide has not been illegal.

  ♦ Assisted suicide: contributing to another's death by act. Suicide pacts and assisted suicide are currently illegal in UK.

• The Human Rights Act 1998 has also been invoked in high profile end of life cases. The case law to date suggests that the right to life contained within Article 2 is being interpreted conservatively. For example, in the first instance hearing of the case of Dianne Pretty, the court stated that this article was aimed only at the protection and preservation of life, not at protecting a patient's right to his or her own death. The Pretty case further confirmed that the illegality of assisted suicide in the UK does not represent an infringement of human rights.

• Although assisted suicide remains a crime in the UK, there have been a number of high profile cases in which families and partners have accompanied relatives to jurisdictions where euthanasia is lawful.[38] No one has, to date, been prosecuted for travelling with loved ones who have been assisted to die abroad. Furthermore, following the House of Lords decision[39] in the case brought by Debbie Purdy, the Director of Public Prosecutions was asked to review and clarify the 1961 law relating to assisted suicide and its prosecution.

• Given that the law in the UK precludes active euthanasia or physician assisted suicide,[40] what role does the doctor have in caring for Mrs Robson? The situation is further complicated when the harms of opiate pain relief increase to such a point that the shortening of the patient's life and concomitant hastening of the patient's death are known to be possible or even likely consequences of treatment. It is an established principle in healthcare ethics and law that treatments which have foreseen (but not intended) harms must be justified by reference to the relative benefit.

• Is there a moral difference between an omission (i.e. to withhold active treatment or medical intervention) and an action (to intervene pharmacologically or otherwise) where the consequences of both are identical? For example, is there a moral distinction between deciding not to give an antibiotic to treat pneumonia in a terminally ill patient, and giving a lethal injection to the same terminally ill patient? Both actions have in common the relief of suffering for the terminally ill patient and both actions have accelerated the natural process of dying. However, it is a general principle of both medical ethics and law that it is harder to justify holding people responsible for what they do not do, rather than for their actions.

- A further important consideration in this example is causation. Thus, not to give an antibiotic is not causing the patient's death; pneumonia is the cause of death. Whereas if a doctor were to give a lethal injection of, for example, potassium chloride, that would directly cause the patient's death.

- The current law in the UK prohibits the intentional act of killing another human being. Thus even if the patient really believes that death would be the greatest available 'benefit' a clinician could provide, the healthcare professional is legally prevented from intending to take the life of the patient. The ways in which 'intention' is defined in UK law is complex. Suffice to say for the purposes of this text that foresight is an integral part of the process of defining intention for the purposes of the criminal law. This complex relationship between intention and foresight creates particular tensions and problems in the medical context.

- Whilst healthcare professionals are precluded, like anyone else, from intending to cause the death of a patient, it is, of course, perfectly permissible (indeed some would say ethical) for healthcare professionals to want to alleviate their patient's suffering by prescribing appropriate medication. As informed professionals, clinicians will know that such medication may have the foreseen effect of shortening the patient's life. Therefore the law applies the doctrine of double effect as a means of resolving this tension. The doctrine of double effect is the mechanism by which the law distinguishes between intention and foresight.[41] The name of the doctrine is a description of the dual consequences that may result from a particular type of treatment. For example, heavy sedation (e.g. Midazolam) in the palliative care of some patients with cerebral tumours may have two potential effects. First, it may result in the reduction of suffering on the part of the patient by alleviating distress. Secondly, it may shorten the life of the patient. The first effect is said to be intended. However the second effect is said to be foreseen but not intended.

Application of core concepts to Case 51

- It is lawful to prescribe opiates in increasing doses to Mrs Robson provided such prescription is clinically indicated and proportionate to the symptom burden she is experiencing. That the prescription of increasing doses of opiate analgesia may depress her respiratory function and even foreshorten her life does not make such treatment unlawful because of the doctrine of double effect which provides for the foreseen but unintended effects of opiate analgesia.

- To address Mr Robson's question honestly, a sound knowledge of the actual effects of opiates on both pain and respiratory function is required. It is common for the effects of opiates to be overstated and misunderstood. Clarification of the value of analgesia in his wife's care and openness about the unpredictability of disease progression and the difficulty of predicting the timing of death are key to answering Mr Robson's questions. His wife is close to death and Mr Robson should be supported without false reassurance or undue dissembling.

- The priority is to tell Mr Robson honestly that his wife is very unwell and not likely to live very long but that the team are doing all that can be done to ensure she is not in too much pain and remains as comfortable as possible. Whilst an awareness of the doctrine of double effect, the law relating to euthanasia and the distinction between acts and omissions is essential for doctors, discussing these provisions with a grieving man is not what is needed in this scenario. Openness, accessibility, and informed empathy are much more pertinent and valuable.

Further information

- Of the key cases that have involved doctors and the doctrine of double effect, that of Dr Cox is one of the most important to note. Dr Cox was a GP caring for his patient, Lillian Boyes. Boyes suffered from rheumatoid arthritis that was increasingly resistant to pain relief.

As her pain increased, Mrs Boyes (and her sons) asked Dr Cox repeatedly to end her life. Dr Cox administered an obviously lethal dose of potassium chloride and Mrs Boyes died within minutes. Dr Cox was charged with attempted murder rather than murder because it could not be shown that the injection had actually caused Mrs Boyes death as her body had been cremated. Dr Cox was convicted and sentenced to one year in prison. In sentencing the doctor, the judge in the case, Ognall J, expressed the view that the act of injecting Mrs Boyes with potassium chloride was a breach of an 'unequivocal duty' towards a patient. The judgment was approved in the later case of Bland,[42] although a number of the judges in the *Bland* case recognized the difficulty of distinguishing between withdrawing life sustaining treatment and taking steps to end the life of a patient. The decision to prosecute Dr Cox was much criticized,[43] and the lesson from the case for practising doctors and those in training appears to be that the inconsistent and legally constructed devices of the doctrine of double effect and the distinction between acts and omissions will continue to be of use so long as the drugs being given are powerful analgesics where a known consequence can be to accelerate death.

Consent and Particular Situations

Case 52 ◆ Consent for HIV and other serological testing following a needlestick injury from a patient

You are on a medical firm and working in A&E. Luke Hollins is a newly-qualified staff nurse who joined the team a few days ago. Luke asks if he can **'have a word in private'***. Luke says that he injured himself while taking blood from a patient a few minutes previously and asks* **'what shall I do?'**

Core concepts

- In order to conduct an HIV test, explicit consent is required. It used to be that consent was sought only following HIV-test specific counselling. This requirement was known as 'HIV exceptionalism' in the ethico-legal literature and dates from the time in the 1980s when HIV was both experienced and perceived as a hopeless, stigmatizing disease.

- Recently, and following increasing advances in the treatment of HIV which make early intervention desirable, there has been a call for wider testing and the cessation of any 'special' or 'particular' ethico-legal status for HIV testing.[44] Rather than there being a requirement that any special 'counselling' is undertaken, there should simply be the honest and sensitive provision of information as for any proposed test or treatment.

- As such, the principle is that there is a legal requirement, which finds statutory enactment in the Human Tissue Act 2004, that consent is sought in order to determine the patient's HIV status and, as such, the potential risk to the healthcare professional. Indeed, many laboratories will not proceed with serological testing unless the sample is accompanied by evidence of written consent.

- Consent should be sought from the patient by someone other than the person who sustained the needlestick injury. If the rationale for testing is explained carefully and sensitively, it is rare for patients to refuse consent. It has been suggested that a universal approach to seeking consent from all patients is more ethically appropriate because it militates against personal judgement, stereotyping, and labelling.[45]

- Where a patient lacks the capacity to be give consent to HIV testing, there is no point in seeking consent. In such situations, a distinction may be drawn between patients in whom capacity is temporarily impaired and those in whom incapacity is likely to be a longer or enduring state. In the case of patients were capacity is temporarily impaired, the advice is commonly to wait until capacity returns and then seek consent for serological testing in the usual way. In patients where capacity is likely to be impaired for a long time, testing is legally permitted only if, in accordance with the provisions of the Mental Capacity Act 2005, it is deemed to be in the patient's best interests to test for HIV and/or other blood borne viruses (assuming that there is no legal proxy to act on the patient's behalf; see the discussion of lasting power of attorney above (Case 45 Nominated Proxy and Pneumonia)).

- There are no exceptional requirements for counselling prior to testing for other blood borne viruses such as Hepatitis B and C save the standard expectation that reasonable information will be provided in order for the patient to give his or her valid consent.

- The information given to patients as part of seeking consent to serological testing for blood borne viruses should include an explanation both of the purpose of testing and the extent to which the information will be shared/be confidential, i.e. that the results of serology will be shared with the occupational health team and the professional who sustained the needlestick injury.

Application of core concepts to Case 52

- The scenario states that Luke is a new member of staff and so candidates should introduce themselves as if he were any other patient.

- In a situation such as this where time is important, candidates should be clear about what has happened and directive/informative as required. All NHS Trusts are required to have a policy regarding needlestick injuries and post-exposure prophylaxis.

- The key skills needed are (a) exploring and checking what actually happened to Luke and (b) giving him clear information about what should happen next in as honest and empathic a way as possible.

- Information is needed in order to respond to Luke appropriately. Candidates need to establish what happened so that the advice given is accurate and timely.

- points to verify are (a) when the incident occurred, (b) what Luke was using to take blood, (c) whether he was wearing gloves, (d) if he squeezed the blood out, (e) if he washed the wound and (f) whether Luke's immunizations are up-to-date.

- Whilst information about the patient and concomitant risk factors will be important, e.g. diagnosis, nationality, drug use, or blood borne viruses, the first priority is to advise Luke on the immediate management of the needlestick injury and refer him to occupational health for specialist advice.

- As the incident is very recent, the immediate advice to give Luke is to (a) squeeze or continue squeezing out the blood, (b) run the wound under cold running water, (c) attend occupational health as soon as possible to discuss post-exposure prophylaxis, and (d) complete an incident form.

- Be wary of offering information that would normally be the preserve of the occupational health team and may not be wholly informed or accurate such as evaluating specific risk and misleading Luke regarding the inevitability or otherwise of taking post-exposure prophylaxis.

Your task is to ensure good immediate management of the situation and ensure Luke is seen quickly by those with particular expertise in this area of occupational health.

- You should explain to Luke that in accordance with national guidance, another member of staff will seek consent from the patient to test for blood borne viruses.

- Luke should understand that consent must be sought and obtained if the patient has capacity. Where the patient lacks capacity, you need to explain that if the lack of capacity is temporary, consent will be sought at the time that the patient regains capacity. Where a patient is likely to lack capacity for a long, indeterminate, or enduring period of time, you must explain that by virtue of both the Human Tissue Act 2004 and the Mental Capacity Act 2005, testing can only be performed if either you have the consent of a legally appointed proxy or if it is considered to be in the patient's best interests to undergo serology.

- When Luke has responded to the immediate injury and received proper occupational health advice, completion of a critical incident or adverse event form is indicated and required at most NHS Trusts.

- Information should be chunked and understanding checked throughout.

- Luke is likely to be anxious and perhaps upset; remaining calm and being clear throughout is likely to be most effective.

Further information

- Where a patient is deceased and their HIV and other blood borne virus status is unknown, the provisions of the Human Tissue Act 2004 continue to apply, i.e. consent for testing should be sought from a legal proxy if one exists, or a 'qualifying relative' within the terms of the legislation. For discussion of the hierarchy of 'qualifying relatives' under the statute, see scenarios 3.4.4 and 3.4.5 below (Case 55 Organ Donation and Consent and Case 56 Post-mortems and Consent).

- Where a needlestick injury occurs and there is no know source, e.g. the injury is sustained from a discarded sharp, the evaluation of risk turns on the nature of the exposure and is properly conducted by a professional with appropriate expertise to determine whether post-exposure prophylaxis is indicated.

- Where clinicians know that they have a health condition or could have a condition that presents a risk to patient care, the GMC requires that advice and, if indicated, treatment is sought from a suitably qualified professional. If modifications to practice are recommended, these must be implemented and followed.[46]

Case 53 ◆ **Consent in medical education and clinical training—student working on the team**

Javick is a third-year medical student working on the medical firm on which you are a Senior House Officer (SHO). Your consultant met Javick after the ward round and asked him to clerk and examine Mrs Alessi, aged 86, who has been admitted with abdominal pain. The consultant had also told Javick that he would need 'to have a go' at performing a rectal examination. Javick had never performed a rectal examination before, although he had practised on models in the clinical skills cubicles. You observe Javick approaching Mrs Alessi who seems confused and appears distressed when Javick approaches her. Javick gives up and asks you what he should 'do next'. How would you respond to Javick?

Core concepts

- Much of medical education and training takes place in the clinical environment. Future doctors have to learn new skills and apply their knowledge to real patients. However, patients have a choice whether or not they wish to participate in educational activities even if they are being seen or treated in a 'teaching' hospital.

- As such, the concepts covered by this scenario are two core elements of ethical practice, namely assessing the capacity of a patient who is said to be confused and, depending on whether she is deemed to have capacity, either seeking her consent or determining what is in her best interests if she or a legally appointed proxy is unable to give consent.

- It is easy to overlook the precepts of ethical practice especially when students are keen to learn and their teachers are enthusiastic about sharing their expertise. However, demonstrating ethical practice is as integral to professional training as observing procedures and eliciting signs.

- The clinical environment can be ethically challenging for all and the phenomenon of ethical erosion is well-documented in the literature[47] and refers to the diminution of moral awareness and ethical behaviour as students and doctors progress through their training. The explanation for such moral decline being variously the pressures of real world practice, pressure from peers and seniors to 'fit in' and make 'pragmatic' decisions, compassion fatigue, de-sensitization, and emotional burnout. All clinicians have a responsibility to be alert to the possibility of ethical erosion within both themselves and those with whom they work.

Application of core concepts to Case 53

- This deceptively simple and brief vignette contains many points for rich ethico-legal discussion with Javick. Remember, you are the senior doctor here and sharing accurate ethico-legal knowledge with medical students is as important as sharing biomedical information and clinical skills. You are a powerful role model who is charged with educating Javick.

- The first issue to consider is whether Mrs Alessi has capacity to give or refuse consent for Javick to clerk her and take a history and/or perform an examination. To recap on points made elsewhere in this text, as an adult, Mrs Alessi is assumed to be capacitous unless there are reasons to doubt otherwise.

- The fact that Mrs Alessi is confused may raise some doubt about her capacity, in which case you might want to discuss with Javick how one goes about assessing a patient's capacity (and whether it is an appropriate task for a student to undertake).

- If Mrs Alessi is capacitous, Javick would have to ask her permission to take a history and perform an examination. This is, of course, obtaining informed consent. As discussed above, for consent to be legally valid, four criteria must be met:
  - the consent is given (or refused) by a capacitous person;
  - the person must be informed;
  - the consent should be given voluntarily;
  - the consent should be continuing.

- The issue of what constitutes sufficient 'information' for the purposes of consent in the case of Javick and Mrs Alessi warrants discussion.
- Questions candidates might ask Javick include:
  - what should he say to Mrs Alessi to ensure she is informed about who he is and his role in her care? For example, Javick has been asked to clerk Mrs Alessi which would presumably have to happen as part of her care and is not 'additional' to routine clinical care. There may be questions about the appropriateness of a very inexperienced medical student clerking a patient who is confused and distressed and candidates might think about how they would discuss this point.
  - Should he explain to Mrs Alessi that he has never performed a rectal examination on a real patient before if she is to be effectively informed?
  - How should he respond if Mrs Alessi asks him questions to which he doesn't know the answer?
  - Whether he should have a chaperone if Mrs Alessi gives consent for him to perform the rectal examination.
- If Mrs Alessi is not capacitous, then any healthcare interventions or treatment must proceed on the basis of her 'best interests'. You should encourage Javick to consider how the clinical team would go about assessing what is in Mrs Alessi's 'best interests'.
- The request for an examination, including a rectal examination is more problematic in the context of 'best interests'. Whilst the rectal examination is likely to be a routine part of Mrs Alessi's care, it is unlikely that the student's findings alone would be relied upon. As such, what is being proposed is over and above clinical care and is for educational rather than therapeutic purposes. If Mrs Alessi is unable to consent because she lacks capacity, it would be difficult to make the case for Javick carrying out the PR examination for the first time. Some would argue that if Javick is well-supervised and the procedure is one that is a necessary skill for a medical student to acquire to work as a Foundation year doctor, educational examinations can be carried out on incapacitated patients. However, there should be a strong case for conducting the procedure on a vulnerable patient rather than one who is able to determine for herself whether she wishes to participate in student education and learning. For eaxmple, it might be that one can only learn to take a history from a psychotic patient without consent, but a PR can be learned on a range of patients, the majority of whom are capacitous and from whom consent should be sought.
- Clear, professional role modelling and well-reasoned mentoring is the aim throughout this scenario. As the qualified doctor, this is an opportunity to model sound professional practice, impart and consolidate the student's ethico-legal knowledge, and demonstrate how to analyse a scenario ethically by highlighting the key issues, elucidating principles, challenging assumptions, and facilitating a practical solution to a real and common situation in clinical education.

Further information

- All healthcare staff should be aware of the phenomena of ethical erosion, compassion fatigue, and burnout and consider some of the possible reasons why they occur. Staff should be encouraged both to identify, and act as, positive role models. In so far as it is possible to expose what is hidden, the influence of the hidden culture should be named and challenged with reference to examples of sub-optimal professional behaviour.
- It should be explicitly acknowledged that medical professionalism is more than merely clinical knowledge and technical skills. There should be a recognition on the part of all staff that professionalism can be compromised irrevocably or instilled effectively by role

modelling—and all staff contribute to the process, both consciously and unwittingly. If teams can work to, and achieve, collective responsibility for creating organizations that produce and support competent, humane, reflective, and committed healthcare staff, the reward will benefit not only staff and their patients, but society at large.

Case 54 ◆ Consent to participate in research—clinical trial of anticonvulsant

Miss Collard is 20 years old. She has been diagnosed with grand mal epilepsy which is poorly controlled following numerous tonic-clonic seizures during the day and at night. The consultant neurologist is currently recruiting participants to a randomized controlled trial of a new anticonvulsant drug. You are asked to seek Miss Collard's consent to participate in the trial during her outpatient appointment.

Core concepts

- Since the Nuremberg trials and the promulgation of the Nuremberg Code, research on human subjects has been regulated. The key source of regulatory information on biomedical research on human subjects is found in the Declaration of Helsinki (which has been revised several times). In practice, the national and local regulation of research on human subjects falls within the remit of the appropriate Research Ethics Committee.[48]

- The National Research Ethics Service[49] is part of the National Patient Safety Agency and provides a national structure within which all local research ethics committees and governance processes operate.

- Ethical research practice requires that attention should be given to the core principles underlying any proposed research, namely: (a) scientific validity; (b) risk versus benefit; (c) informed consent; and (d) procedures for ensuring the ethical conduct of research.[50]

- Scientific validity is a fundamental ethical requirement of research. Any research will entail some degree of inconvenience and/or risk for the participants. As such, the potential benefits and scientific quality of the research must be scrutinized. Research must be designed so as to ask an important question with appropriate and adequate methodology so that an answer can be obtained within a reasonable period of time. However, the fact that a proposed study has scientific validity does not necessarily mean that the research is justifiable.

- Once a project has been determined to be scientifically valid, the relative risks and benefits must be considered. The Declaration of Helsinki distinguishes between therapeutic and non-therapeutic research for the purposes of evaluating risks and benefits and this distinction should be made clear.

- In therapeutic research the key principle is that, without the research, there can be no certainty as to which of the treatments or interventions being tested will be of benefit to the patient thereby justifying the random allocation of treatments to patients, i.e. the concept of equipoise. If it becomes clear during the course of a study that one particular treatment or intervention is more effective than another, then the research must cease.

Concomitant risks that arise during the research must be minimized wherever possible and safety of the participants is the primary concern.

- In non-therapeutic research, the rights of the participants are central. Many patients will agree to participate in such research (where there is no benefit to them) for altruistic reasons. Furthermore, participants who act as controls in therapeutic research are in the same position as participants in non-therapeutic research in that no benefit is likely to accrue to them.

- Particular ethical questions arise in respect of vulnerable participants, e.g. children, psychiatric patients, and cognitively impaired patients. For such patients, researchers may rely on assent from third parties where research is deemed to be in the incapacitous patient's best interests.

- Difficulties arise in relation to vulnerable patients and research where is unlikely to be any benefit to the patient. An absolutist perspective suggests that vulnerable patients should never be able to participate in non-therapeutic research. However, the repercussions of such a position for research, therapeutic development, and scientific progress would be huge. Therefore, it is more usual for ethics committees to adopt a risk assessment approach to vulnerable participants. Thus the greater the likely risk[51] to the patient the less justification there is likely to be for the proposed research.

- In all research, consent is essential not only because it demonstrates that a participant has evaluated the risks and benefits, but also because it demonstrates that participants are moral agents in their own right and not simply 'a means to an end' in deontological terms.

- Sometimes, it may be more appropriate for an independent third party to seek consent from possible participants. Payments are a vexed area in research. If a payment is too great, it may be perceived as an inducement and invalidates the essential voluntariness required for legal consent. However, it is usual for expenses to be reimbursed, and sometimes for inconvenience to be recompensed.

Application of core concepts to Case 54

- As with all situations where one is meeting a patient, a clear introduction is the first step in which candidates explain who they are and what they wish to discuss with Miss Collard.

- There are two elements to this appointment, namely (a) the routine clinical consultation; and (b) the potential recruitment of Miss Collard to a research trial. The former is expected by Miss Collard as part of her routine care, but the latter is distinct and particular ethical considerations apply. It is important therefore to ensure separation between discussion of clinical management and Miss Collard's possible recruitment to the trial. Candidates should be clear that they wish to ask Miss Collard about research and that is not part of her routine healthcare.

- In order for her to be recruited to the trial, she must give consent that is (a) capacitous; (b) informed; (c) voluntary; and (d) continuing. Miss Collard is, via the process of seeking consent, afforded moral status and respect.

- Miss Collard is presumed to have capacity as she is an adult and there is nothing to suggest that an assessment of her capacity is indicated.

- As regards information, whilst it is reasonable to assume that both a research ethics committee and the research and development governance process will have considered the scientific validity and relevance of the trial, it is important, in seeking Miss Collard's consent, to explain, in simple terms, why the trial is being conducted and the methodology of randomized controlled trials.

- Although there will be written participant information and the consent form for the trial is likely to be detailed, the essence of seeking consent is often in the discussion with a patient.

The consent form is only an acknowledgement that consent has been obtained, and it is not a substitute for a discussion in which the proposed research is fully explained (in non-technical language) and the patient's questions and concerns addressed. There is no substitute for talking to Miss Collard to explain why the research is being conducted and how she might experience being a participant particularly given the randomized methodology.

- In respect of the voluntariness of her consent, Miss Collard must be assured that a refusal to participate in research will not affect her medical care in any way. This is perhaps particularly important because, in this scenario, consent is being sought from an existing patient as part of a routine outpatient clinic.

- Clarity about the practicalities of the research, covering reimbursement, the attendance that would be required of Miss Collard, the duration of the trial, the treatment she may be required to take depending on the random allocation, the recording and use of data relating to her, communication of results and the relationship of the research to her ongoing clinical care, etc. should all be part of the process of giving Miss Collard the information she requires in order to choose whether she wishes to participate in the trial.

- Miss Collard should know how the research will be regulated, i.e. that the appropriate research committees and governance procedures are responsible for ensuring that research is conducted ethically. There should be a named point of contact for all participants in research and clear guidance on how adverse incidents or unexpected events will be managed should they arise during a trial.

- With regard to the continuing nature of her consent, Miss Collard should be told that she can withdraw her consent at any point and that should she choose to withdraw, her clinical care would continue as before.

- It is unlikely, perhaps even undesirable, that Miss Collard will make a decision about whether she wishes to participate in the trial at a single outpatient appointment. Following a thorough discussion in which the principles and practicalities of the research are explained, Miss Collard should be furnished with the relevant literature that describes the trial to potential participants and encouraged to discuss it with family or even her GP. It should be clear whom Miss Collard can contact should she have any further questions or concerns about the trial and reiterated that her decision about participating in research is entirely hers and will not affect her clinical care by the neurology team.

Further information

- The ethico-legal discussion relating to this scenario applies to research involving human subjects. For those conducting research that involves animals, there are distinct ethico-legal considerations. Research on animals has been regulated since the Cruelty to Animals Act 1876. The current law is found in the Animals (Scientific Procedures) Act 1986. The Declaration of Helsinki states that any health research involving human participants 'should be based on adequately performed laboratory and animal experimentation'.[52]

- Peter Singer[53] suggests that the key to understanding the debate about the use of animals is not equality of treatment but equality of consideration. He argues that after considering how animals should be treated, the conclusion may be that the logical thing is that they should be subject to different treatment and different 'rights'. However, Singer argues, we have not yet reached a position where we have afforded animals equal consideration, and therefore asks on what basis can differential treatment of animals be justified?

- 'Speciesism' is the term used by Singer to describe discrimination against non-humans. Singer argues that if society does not discriminate against human beings because they may be less intelligent or less able than the majority of people, there is no sustainable moral argument for treating animals differently simply because they are 'less intelligent' than us.

Interestingly, Jeremy Bentham expressed a similar idea well ahead of his time when he asked 'the question is not, Can they [animals] reason? Nor can they talk? But, Can they suffer?'[54]

- Thus suggests Singer, it is sentience not intelligence that is the criterion for the right to equal consideration (note not necessarily treatment). Indeed, Singer has suggested that mature cats, dogs, and mice are more aware of what is happening to them than human infants, and therefore the appropriate question for researchers is whether they would be prepared to conduct their research on a human infant. If the answer is 'no', Singer suggests that it is discrimination to perform the experiment on an animal. Thus, if sentience is the key point then there are two choices. First, does sentience entitle animals to the same consideration as non-animals? Or does the argument lead to rights to the same care and protection for animals. If it is the latter, the protection offered to animals should be the same as that given to humans who are incapable of giving consent. As such research could only be performed on animals where it is of direct therapeutic benefit to them or where there is a minimal risk of harm.

- If sentience is rejected as the principle by which we afford animals equal consideration, are there other ways in which human beings can be distinguished from non-humans? Can human beings be distinguished on the grounds of their unique capability for moral agency? Only humans have the capacity to make moral distinctions and to constrain their behaviour as appropriate. If this is the case, how can one protect humans in whom the capacity for moral agency is compromised or absent, e.g. babies or severely cognitively impaired adults? Campbell et al.[55] suggest these examples are distinguishable because of the capacity of babies to develop into moral agents as adults and because of the unique relationship mentally impaired adults have with their fellow humans. Our obligations to both children and impaired adults must exceed our obligations to animals, argue Campbell et al.

- Furthermore, what can be said in response to the point that benefit (which may be a benefit to humans or to other animals or to both) might arise, and indubitably has arisen, from animal experimentation? Research is a continuum and although one experiment may not of itself be obviously beneficial or significant, it may build on and develop the ideas and findings of earlier research and raise relevant questions to be asked in future experiments. Thus is it more appropriate to think of 'benefit' in terms of the micro effect of a single experiment, or the macro effect of a series of experiments within an institution, a country, or even globally? How far removed from the experimental process does the 'benefit' need to be before it can be considered significant?

- Indeed, the way in which the 'benefit' argument is addressed depends upon the way in which distinctions are drawn between human beings and animals. Thus, if we adopt Singer's test of sentience, it is not clear why experiments with obvious and proven benefits, which it is said could only be performed on animals,[56] could not be performed on humans for the same benefit. Thus benefit alone may not be enough to justify experimentation on animals unless we can distinguish and demarcate animals from humans in some intellectually convincing and morally significant way. As discussed above, Singer, of course, believes that intelligence is not the way to do this but sentience which results in there being parity and equality between the species. Moreover, if Singer's sentience criterion is used, the question has to be whether it is sentience of pain or simply an awareness of surroundings that should be significant since experiments may be painless.

- If sentience is not the means by which to attempt to distinguish humans from animals, what alternative arguments have been made? The basic principle to which philosophers most often return is that human life is intrinsically more valuable than animal life. What is it that makes so many commentators convinced of the increased value of human life? Some argue that it is the ability for spiritual or religious experience. Others cite the more complex constitution of the human as the rationale for the belief in the greater value of human life.

It is the fact that we enjoy a wider range of relationships, occupations, and purpose than animals. Our lives are more valuable because 'of the many more possibilities for enrichment they contain'.[57] However, such an argument does not help us with human beings whose quality of life may be undeniably poor (although we should be aware of the perils of making such moral judgements, e.g. how do we know whether the quality of life of someone with cognitive impairment is poor?). To adopt such a position one needs to be convinced that the quality of all human life is inherently richer and more valuable than that of any animal.

- Some of the main moral arguments for and against the use of animals in research are outlined above. There are many variations and subtleties in the debate, which are not discussed due to the constraints of space.

- As regards the law relating to research involving animals, the Animals (Scientific Procedures) Act 1986 requires that the Home Office, advised by the Animal Procedures Inspectorate, takes overall responsibility for the use of animals in experiments. The Home Office's policy on the regulation of animal experiments is often described as 'The Three Rs',[58] namely (a) replacement (non-animal methods should be used wherever possible, e.g. the use of computer simulators or tissue samples rather than animals); (b) reduction (the numbers of animals used experiments should be the minimum needed to give clear experimental results); and (c) refinement (the smallest degree of pain and distress should be inflicted and for a justifiable purpose).

- At a local level, all institutions carrying out research on animals must have an animal ethics committee and its remit is to establish ways in which the 3Rs can be practicably implemented. The committees are responsible (within the Home Office and statutory framework) for authorizing and monitoring all research proposed or taking place within an institution.

- Whilst the ethical dimensions of research are consistently captured in broad debates about the autonomy and rights of individuals and the social value or utility of research, the law and governance procedures are complex and change regularly. This scenario depends on a general awareness and application of the ethico-legal framework within which research takes place in the NHS. However, for those who are researchers, close attention to the large and growing literature and relevant national and international laws pertaining to research are an integral part of professional competence for the clinician involved in academic work.

Case 55 ◆ Organ donation–request to family following death of son in road traffic accident

Mr Hillier, age 27, is brought to A&E following a serious road traffic accident. He is transferred to intensive care but the prognosis appears poor following massive head injury. The team explains to his parents and girlfriend that Mr Hillier is brainstem dead. Mr Hillier was, prior to the accident, a fit and healthy man and would appear to be an excellent potential organ donor. There is no organ donor card in any of his personal belongings.

Core concepts

- The law relating to the donation of organs is found in the Human Tissue Act 2004 which, by repealing and replacing the Human Tissue Act 1961, the Anatomy Act 1984, and the Human Organ Transplants Act 1989, removed the distinction between living and cadaveric donors.

- Under the Human Tissue Act 2004, a new regulatory body was established, the Human Tissue Authority, replacing the Unrelated Live Transplant Regulatory Authority and the post of HM Inspector of Anatomy.

- The UK has one of the lowest organ donation rates in Europe. The BMA recently estimated that approximately 24% of the population is registered with the NHS Organ Donor Register.[59] Furthermore, of those who carry a donor card, a significant number of people are unaware that the NHS Donor Register exists as a confirmatory step in communicating their choice to become an organ donor.

- The Human Tissue Act 2004 makes provision for minimal steps to preserve a patient's organs whilst the wishes of the patient regarding organ donation are explored.

- The Human Tissue Act 2004 prioritized the wishes of the potential donor and therefore makes it lawful to proceed when a patient has expressed his wish to donate even if family members object. However, it is unclear how often clinicians override familial objection particularly given that such objections are expressed in a context of immense shock, emotion, and grief.

- Where there is no evidence of a patient's preferences about organ donation, the law requires that consent is sought from someone with whom the potential donor was in an established relationship. The Human Tissue Act 2004 uses the term 'qualifying relative'. The list of potential parties who can be approached is wide and includes parents, spouses, partners, siblings, grandparents, nieces, nephews, grandchildren, and long-standing friends. Step-parents and half-siblings can also be 'qualifying relatives'. Civil partners will be afforded the same status as heterosexual partners and spouses by virtue of legal order under the Civil Partnership Act 2004.

- 'Qualifying relatives' are ranked under the Human Tissue Act 2004 as follows:
  - spouse or partner
  - parent or child
  - sibling
  - grandparent or grandchild
  - niece or nephew
  - step-parent
  - half-sibling
  - friend of long standing

- Consent for organ donation should be sought from the highest ranking relative. Where there is more than one person who is an equally ranking relative, for example, parents or siblings, the consent of one person will suffice.

- The law provides that even if a relaive is of the highest rank to make a decision about donation on behalf of a deceased patient, that person is entitled to opt out of the decision-making process either because of preference or because he or she is unable to participate due to, for example, incapacity.

- The code of practice that accompanies the Human Tissue Act 2004 emphasizes that seeking consent in relation to organ donation is a process and requires that clinicians check that consent is continuing right up until the point at which donation is scheduled to begin.

- However, interim guidance from the Human Tissue Authority provides that once an incision has been made, consent for organ donation cannot be withdrawn and requires clinicians to explain the point beyond which consent cannot be rescinded to qualifying relatives.

- Local procedures may differ with some organizations involving, or devolving the task of seeking consent entirely to, a transplant coordinator and/or bereavement services staff. However, the leader of the clinical team is responsible for ensuring that delegation of the task is appropriate and consent is sought in accordance with the principles of the Human Tissue Act 2004.

- Where relatives disagree about organ donation, the law requires clinicians to consider whether the distress caused by proceeding with donation in the face of disagreement can justify going ahead with organ donation.

Application of core concepts to Case 55

- It is the Human Tissue Act 2004 which sets out how possible organ donation from Mr Hillier should be considered by the clinical team and his family.

- It appears from the scenario that Mr Hillier was not carrying a donor card. This is not unusual. The basic principle of the Human Tissue Act 2004 is that organ donation cannot proceed without establishing the wishes of Mr Hillier be it via a donor card, the NHS donor register, or a third party.

- In this scenario, there is no donor card and therefore the next step would be to ask Mr Hillier's family about donation. The law allows for a nominated representative or a third party to represent Mr Hillier's wishes about organ donation.

- The scenario refers to Mr Hiller's parents and his girlfriend. The question is who constitutes the 'qualifying relatives' for the purpose of the Human Tissue Act.

- In Mr Hillier's case, we are told that he has a girlfriend. The ranking of the patient's girlfriend as a qualifying relative depends on whether their relationship was an established partnership. In this acutely sensitive situation, exploration of the relationship will require considerable empathy and tact.

- If Mr Hillier's girlfriend is the highest ranking qualifying relative but she does not wish, or is unable, to be involved in decision-making about organ donation, this should be recorded in the notes with a brief, factual explanation.

- Whether it is Mr Hillier's girlfriend or parents who are the qualifying relative(s) for the purposes of lawful organ donation, the statute requires the clinical team to encourage qualifying relatives to involve other family members and persons where possible. As such, it may be that the ideal situation is to encourage Mr Hillier's parents and girlfriend to talk to each other about the possibility of organ donation.

- This is a situation where seeking consent is a difficult task. It is important to remember the basic rules of seeking and obtaining valid consent.

- Capacity should be maximized by attention to surroundings, patient explanation, and well-paced information.

- Voluntariness and the continuing nature of consent are supported by allowing time to opt out of discussions, to reflect on the process, and to have a named contact to whom to address questions.

- Sufficient information depends on honest accounts of the practicalities of organ donation that is responsive to cues and offers the preferred level of detail whilst remaining within the timescale required for successful donation.

- Candidates should remember that, as discussed above, the code of practice on the implementation of the Human Tissue Act 2004 stresses that seeking and obtaining consent for organ donation is a dynamic process. As such, clinicians ought to provide a named contact to whom the family can address concerns and questions and that person should be available until the point at which donation is scheduled to begin.

- Remember, it may be that Mr Hillier never discussed organ donation with either his parents or his girlfriend and, as such, there may be many questions and difficult discussions in which a clinical perspective may be (but should not be assumed to be) helpful whilst the options are explored.

- If Mr Hillier's girlfriend and parents were to disagree about organ donation, the law requires that clinicians consider whether the distress caused by proceeding in the face of disagreement justifies going ahead with organ donation. There is an ethical responsibility not to exacerbate distress, albeit that such exacerbation may be 'in a good cause' (organ donation) or inadvertent.

- Finally, if Mr Hillier's girlfriend and parents agreed to organ donation, they may ask about the intended recipient or recipients. It is common for information to be provided in broad terms about the benefits of organ donation but candidates must remember that the identity of recipient(s) is protected. Beware of making false promises or creating inappropriate expectations of ongoing relationships with the recipient(s) of Mr Hillier's organs.

Further information

- Unfortunately, where the wishes of the potential donor are unknown, evidence suggests that approximately 40% of qualifying relatives will not consent to organ donation.[60] The low levels of organ donation relative to other European countries and the limited numbers of people on the NHS Donor Register have lead to the current debate about presumed consent in which variations on an 'opt-out' system to replace the current 'opt-in' system have been proposed. However, the government-commissioned independent report from the Organ Donation Taskforce[61] rejected a system predicated on 'presumed consent' from which people would 'opt-out'.

- The recommendations from the Organ Donation Taskforce favoured a continued focus on engaging diverse groups and ensuring effective publicity for organ donation. Furthermore, the Organ Donation Taskforce's report concluded that moving to a system of presumed consent would potentially undermine progress that had been made in increasing the availability of cadaveric organs for donation and could have a significant negative effect on organ donation in general.

Case 56 ◆ Referral to the Coroner and discussion of post-mortem—death of patient following likely aortic aneurysm

Mrs Julliard, aged 58, was brought to A&E after her daughter discovered her collapsed at home. Mrs Julliard was unconscious, hypotensive, and appeared to be in haemorraghic shock on admission. Despite the efforts of the clinical team, Mrs Julliard died within ten minutes of arrival at A&E. Mrs Julliard was not known to be unwell and she had not been seen by her GP for over two years. Mrs Julliard's daughter, Ms Lukas, has been with her mother since she arrived at the hospital and knows she has died. You have been asked to talk to Ms Lukas about what happens next.

Core concepts

- Where a patient dies suddenly without being known to be unwell or having been seen by a doctor in the previous two weeks, the law requires that a report be made to the coroner who may require a post-mortem.
- The coroner's post-mortem is distinguished from what is commonly called the 'hospital' post-mortem, i.e. a post-mortem that is not required by the coroner but is requested so as to seek further information about the cause of death.
- Deaths should be referred to the coroner in the following circumstances:
    - if the death was sudden and unexpected;
    - if death occurred as a result of violence, unnatural, or suspicious circumstances;
    - accidents resulting in death;
    - deaths occurring during a stay in hospital, whilst medical and/or surgical treatment was being given; and
    - where the deceased had not been seen by a treating doctor within the previous fortnight.
- Approximately 50% of referrals to the coroner will lead to a post-mortem. Where a coroner requires that a post-mortem is conducted, the consent of the family or next of kin is legally irrelevant in that the post-mortem will proceed irrespective of their wishes. However, it is good practice to provide families with as much information about the process as possible.
- Bereavement services are likely to be very helpful to families and, if appropriate, faith group leaders can also provide active support particularly if there are specific cultural beliefs or religious concerns about death, post-mortems, and the timing of funerals or burial rites.

Application of core concepts to Case 56

- This death has to be reported to the coroner because Mrs Julliard died suddenly at home and was neither known to be unwell nor had she been seen by a doctor in the fortnight preceding her death.
- Although one key task is to inform Mrs Julliard's daughter, Ms Lukas, about the need to refer her mother's death to the coroner, remember that this is also an extremely sensitive situation in which communication with a distressed, bereaved relative is required. Do not be so 'task focused' that empathy, compassion, and the principles of good communication are forgotten.
- Remember that whilst death may be an integral part of medical practice, for Ms Lukas, this is a shocking and traumatic time. She may wish to be accompanied; she may need refreshment, a break, or a breath of fresh air before you talk.
- Candidates should explain first why it is that Mrs Julliard's death will be referred to the coroner. It may be alarming for Ms Lukas to hear that her mother's death is to be referred to a legal body and candidates must take care to explain why Mrs Julliard's death has to be referred, i.e. that it is because she died suddenly at home and having not seen a doctor for a fortnight prior to her death.
- It is important to be clear about why the death is being referred and what might occur next. Candidates should explain that the coroner may decide on a series of actions, one of which is a post-mortem.
- Ms Lukas should understand that the referral to the coroner and any subsequent action, including a post-mortem, are processes required by law. You are not seeking her consent either to refer the death to the coroner or for any subsequent post-mortem requested by the coroner, but rather you are explaining what is going to happen next and why.

- The level of detail about post-mortems should be dictated by Ms Lukas's preferences as the deceased's daughter. She may wish to know a great deal about the processes of coroners and the technical details of post-mortems, or she may prefer to know very little save for the most basic information about timescale, etc.
- Being alert to both verbal and non-verbal cues will enable candidates to respond appropriately to Ms Lukas and ensure that the discussion is personalized rather than a generic 'post-death' conversation.
- Informing Ms Lukas about bereavement services and telling her what pastoral care is available within the hospital may be helpful. Be guided by her response.
- Writing down details such as contact names, office hours, and direct telephone or extension numbers is likely to be valuable.
- Allow plenty of space for silence, processing of information, and invite questions.

Further information

- If Mrs Julliard had died in circumstances where referral to the coroner was not required, it may still be that a hospital post-mortem would be requested. In the case of a hospital post-mortem, the relevant law is the Human Tissue Act 2004. Just as with organ donation (see Case 55 Organ Donation and Consent), consent for a hospital post-mortem must be sought from a 'qualifying relative'.
- The hierarchy of 'qualifying' relationships for the purpose of seeking consent to a hospital post-mortem is:
    - spouse or partner
    - parent or child
    - sibling
    - grandparent or grandchild
    - niece or nephew
    - step-parent
    - half-sibling
    - friend of longstanding
- Like organ donation, consent to a hospital post-mortem can be sought and obtained from a patient in advance of his or her death. Some patients may nominate someone to act on their behalf following death in which case consent should be sought from the formal nominee. Most commonly, consent for a hospital post-mortem will be sought from the highest ranking qualifying relative as defined by the Human Tissue Act 2004.
- It should be made clear to families that a hospital post-mortem is not a statutory requirement but something voluntary, unlike the coroner's post-mortem. Whilst there is an exceptional power for the Secretary of State for Health to override the refusal of a qualifying relative, this is an extremely rarely used provision and is intended to apply only to exceptional situations, e.g. public health crises or epidemics.
- Consent for hospital post-mortems should be in writing, but the requirement that consent be written does not, of course, remove the obligation to discuss the post-mortem fully with families responding truthfully and accurately to any questions or concerns.
- There are different purposes for hospital post-mortems and it is important to be frank and clear about these with families. First, the hospital post-mortem may reveal more information about the cause of death and underlying disease or diagnosis. Secondly, the hospital post-mortem may provide tissue or data that are of value for educational or research purposes. The consent process attaches to the purpose rather than to the post-mortem itself. That is to say that doctors seeking consent for a hospital post-mortem must be

explicit about the different ways in which material may be used, i.e. diagnostically, education-ally, or for research. Consent must be obtained for each discrete purpose for which the post-mortem may be used.

- As part of the hospital post-mortem, tissue and organs may be removed. Part of the consent process requires that discussion with families explores whether they are willing for such removal to occur and, if they are so willing, whether they wish for the material to be returned or agree to it being retained for audit, research, teaching archives, etc.

- Be aware that the care of relatives and families does not cease when the post-mortem consent form has been signed. Good practice requires that families understand what will happen to the information gleaned from a hospital post-mortem.

- They should be advised when the post-mortem report is likely to be available and whom they should approach if they wish to discuss the report. Remember that families are likely to be in a shocked and distressed state, an experienced, responsive, and reliable point of contact, at the hospital and/or via a GP, will make the complexity of coping with death in the midst of grief a little easier to navigate.

Refusal of Treatment

Case 57 ◆ Negotiating a management plan—patient reluctant to take medication to control hypertension[62]

You are working as the new SHO in the outpatient hypertension clinic. Mr Warren has been referred by his GP who has been treating his hypertension for six months. Mr Warren's hypertension remains poorly controlled. The most recent 24-hour ambulatory pressure monitoring recorded an average BP measure-ment of 155/110. In his referral letter, Mr Warren's GP states that he is unsure whether Mr Warren is actually taking, regularly or at all, the medication that has been prescribed for him. Mr Warren is a 57-year old, obese man who has never smoked and drinks moderately. Mr Warren has few other risk factors for cardiovascular disease, other than a family history. You have explained to Mr Warren that it is important to treat hypertension and refer, in your explanation, to the evidence that untreated hypertension contributes to premature disease and even death. Mr Warren challenges you, saying, 'You doctors are always coming up with "evidence" for something you do or don't want us to do, and it changes every five minutes. I've read all about the so called evidence on the internet—no one can even agree what a blood pressure should be, let alone how to treat it.' Mr Warren then declines your advice regarding further treatment. Mr Warren goes on to say 'My father put all his trust in doctors and yet not long after he started taking blood pressure tablets, he was dead.'

Core concepts

- If a patient makes an autonomous, but seemingly bizarre, decision that satisfies the capacity criteria discussed above, that decision must be respected even if harm or death occurs. To act without, or in opposition to, a patient's expressed, valid consent is to commit an assault.

- The question of information, specifically what is sufficient information, is a recurring theme in discussions of consent. Essentially, the information given to a patient should be that which a 'reasonable person' would require whilst being alert to the particular priorities and concerns of individuals. The content of the information shared should cover risks and benefits, possible consequences of treatment and non-treatment, options and alternatives, and delineation of both what is known and not known about the patient's care.

- Disclosure of uncertainty should be as much part of the discussion as sharing what is well-understood. And it is a discussion: patients should be given the opportunity to ask questions and express their concerns, priorities, and preferences rather than being subjected to an uninterrupted clinical monologue.

- Clinical decision-making both for the novice and experienced professional is often difficult. Judgements have to be made in a complex environment, balancing the needs, wants, and knowledge of the patient with the best available evidence. Decisions are taken in the context of a professional relationship, which may differ in the degree of trust and respect between the two parties, as well as in their belief systems. In effect every clinical encounter is unique, and ethical and moral principles to guide these actions are both necessary and unavoidable. The inherent uncertainty renders the reconciliation of individual circumstance, complexity, evidence, and ethical decision-making particularly challenging. Clinical guidelines are now often developed (although not necessarily used)[63] to help this complex decision-making process, but because the interaction of the clinician, the patient, and the guideline is complex, and the outcome sometimes unpredictable, ethical principles are important in determining the outcome of this interaction.

- Before a decision is made, there are usually a number of alternatives (which may be understood quite differently by different individuals even if the situation is apparently identical). After the decision is made it becomes part of history and influences the subsequent options open to the individual. Thus the decisions made in one consultation will affect those made in the next. Each patient and each doctor contribute to, and are influenced by, their individual and collective histories in making even commonplace decisions. An apparently throwaway phrase by the doctor can have far-reaching effects on the patient, or vice versa (as in the case study), particularly where such innocuous remarks reveal the different belief systems sometimes held by doctor and patient.

- Currently, the GMC arguably continues to equate ethical behaviour predominantly with precepts and rules. In medicine, many clinicians assume that there is one right answer to a medical problem and also one correct way to act. This positivist backdrop frames biomedicine and therefore influences, albeit not exclusively, the belief system of those who have had a biomedical training. Training variably emphasizes the social, interactionist, and psychological dimensions of medicine, but universally building on a predominantly positivist base in which the world is presented as ultimately predictable, whereby if we understood all the laws of physics and had enough information, we could know everything. If this search for explanation, consistency, and replicable knowledge parallels, even subconsciously, the thinking of the clinician, it begins to become clear why one might struggle with potential ambiguity or even conflict in guidelines.

- Commonly, most physicians continue to work to eliminate uncertainty and primarily act as though there were a cause and effect for the illness of each patient. Although sociologists have explored the ways in which uncertainty pervades even the work of doctors working in specialties as diverse as haematology,[64] surgery,[65] cardiology,[66] genetics,[67] and paediatrics,[68] the aim is largely to recreate the clinical encounter to present, if not certainty, at least tolerable uncertainty by providing diagnosis (and treatment) for the patient. Consequently, many tests and investigations are performed to minimize clinical uncertainty. In many cases even more certainty could be sought by performing more investigations and this lies at the heart of the mismatch between demand and resources in the NHS.

- What appears as a fact one day will be refuted the next. For example, beta blockers were once contraindicated in heart failure and now they are almost first-line treatment. Such changes further challenge the notion of certainty in medicine. In real world medicine, clinical decisions are constantly required and, despite the primacy of patient autonomy and importance of shared decision-making, legal responsibility for these decisions generally resides with the physician.

- The ultimate challenge is not merely to make a decision in the face of uncertainty, but to make an ethical decision that embraces different values, i.e. for the clinician to make a 'good enough' decision in a situation where it appears impossible, because of the patient's resistance to treatment, to make what a doctor might consider an optimal decision. As Goodman[69] states, 'the embracing of such a view rescues us from the extremes of decision incapacity or inertia on the one side, and winging it on the other'.

Application of core concepts to Case 57

- Whilst accepted guidance on the management of hypertension, such as that coming from NICE, may be clear, Mr Warren is a capacitous patient who is reluctant to take what appears to be indicated and much needed medication for his hypertension. His blood pressure (BP) is very high and any clinician will seek to do the best for him. Therefore a passive acceptance of his capacitous, apparently informed decision may not be adequate, particularly given that he mentions that his father had died soon after starting treatment for hypertension.

- Simply telling Mr. Warren that treating his BP is likely to reduce his risk of stroke or heart attack is insufficient. Here is a patient who has strong beliefs about the value or otherwise of 'evidence'. And, given that every patient is different, and there is disagreement between hypertension treatment guidelines, he is, to some extent, correct to be sceptical about the validity of guideline-informed prescribing and treatments. This scenario exemplifies the ways in which medicine is practised in a social context. Whether Mr Warren perceives there to be a choice or decision to be made at all is a social and value-laden personalized process.

- This case also illustrates the complexity of ethical decision-making in an apparently straightforward case. It may seem obvious that there is a 'right way' to proceed: citing guidelines may be as much about seeking certainty and resolution as providing optimal care. Might the quest for certainty in treating Mr Warren conflict with the ethical principle of autonomy?

- Mr Warren is correct to note that in medicine the sands do also shift. This should be acknowledged rather than becoming defensive about Mr Warren's apparent challenge to 'best practice' or clinical evidence.

- Respecting Mr Warren's autonomy means that the skilful clinician will seek to negotiate understandings, foster an informed perspective thereby empowering, supporting, and enabling him to make a meaningful choice. Despite wanting to promote his well-being and health, a physician's belief system about managing hypertension is likely to be at variance with that of Mr Warren.

- There is much that can be done to inform Mr Warren and to maximize his autonomy to ensure that his choice is credible. However, explicit acknowledgement of his values and careful reflection on the conflict between biomedical values and his beliefs is needed.

- The mention by Mr Warren of his father is key—such statements are rarely, if ever, incidental. This is not a standard consultation where a blood pressure measurement requires unquestioning implementation of guidelines but a sensitive interaction which will determine future care. With that in mind, it is the time for patient exploration of Mr Warren's history, experiences, and perceptions.

- It may not be possible to implement the 'best practice' guidance on initial meeting, but it is possible to develop a trusting relationship with Mr Warren which maximizes the chances that he will return to the clinic and remain open to effective treatment in future. This consultation encapsulates what might be described as the ethics of complexity in which the real world clinical and social contexts combine with deontological principles through the moral sensitivity of the physician who must be alert to the uncertainty, tensions, and unpredictability of their work even in apparently 'routine' encounters.

- This may be a frustrating encounter, but with careful communication, it could be the beginning of an effective therapeutic relationship. It is only by exploring Mr Warren's beliefs, concerns, and fears, that trust can be established. To dismiss, or seek to 'correct' Mr Warren's perception is likely to compromise rather than enhance care. Quite simply, Mr Warren cannot be forced to take medication and the best prospect of change depends on calm, empathic professionalism. This is a situation in which the journey to informed and authentic consent is far longer than merely producing a form to be signed or a prescription to be dispensed.

Further information

- In the clinical setting, belief systems influence decisions and ultimately all decision-making is value laden. Evidence-based medicine, so Sackett et al.[70] say, is 'the integration of best research evidence with clinical expertise and patient values'. However, this begs the question of what one means by, and who defines, 'best research evidence' and 'clinical expertise' as well as the 'patient values' already discussed. Sackett and colleagues' definition has been used by governments on both sides of the Atlantic to further the implementation of national guidelines.

- So what are the values that should inform evidence based medicine? Sackett et al. define them as 'the unique preferences, concerns and expectations each patient brings to a clinical encounter and which must be integrated into clinical decisions if they are to serve the patient.' This seems laudable, if ambitious, but does highlight the fact that patients may have a different mindset to doctors struggling to balance their scientific training with the reality of clinical uncertainty.

- At an individual level, the clinician bears a responsibility to the patient to facilitate optimal health and uses a combination of unwritten and written rules or guidance to achieve this end. Clinical guidelines are one such aid, but that is all: they are an aid to a process of moral sensitivity in which the doctor recognizes differential values and belief systems must be shared, embraced, and acknowledged if optimal health is to be achieved. Guidelines may be seen as instructions for action and apply equally to social interaction as medical intervention. Clinical guidelines would be straightforward if simple research showed unambiguously which treatment worked, how low blood pressure should really be, what the best level of cholesterol is. But the world isn't simple and is not predictable. Likewise, ethical behaviour is not always straightforward. So if science and ethical behaviour are uncertain, and evidence constantly changing, how can clinical and ethical decisions be made and what of the role of guidelines?

- Guidelines, in short, must have credibility. Merely describing something as a guideline does not lend it magical and unquestionable superior status. In addition to summarizing the best evidence for health professionals, guidelines may address, with varying degrees of transparency, the vexed issue of resource and seek to incorporate diverse and competing agendas. Furthermore, the ethical aims of guidelines differ and may conflict: e.g. to endorse patient autonomy and maximize patient choice whilst simultaneously fulfilling obligations to use resources well and maximize public health. Guidelines are multilayered and have many different purposes.

- What is the legal position in respect of an individual clinician who chooses not to follow guidelines in his practice? The test remains that is used in all claims of negligence against doctors. Namely, the claimant will have to demonstrate that the doctor's engagement or lack thereof with guidelines fell short of, or differed from, those of a body of reasonable practitioners. Therefore, if an expert witness stated that a doctor's choice not to follow guidelines was that of a reasonable practitioner and the choice withstands logical analysis, it is most unlikely that he would be found liable for negligence. In the high-profile case of Anthony Bland,[71] the guidelines produced by the BMA Medical Ethics Committee were praised by the House of Lords,[72] and it was suggested that legal protection was afforded to clinicians who followed the guidelines. This does not however mean that the converse position for a doctor who deviates from guidelines is that he is legally unprotected. Indeed, notwithstanding the comments about the legal acceptability of the guidelines in the *Bland* case, the House of Lords still ruled (albeit implicitly) that reliance on guidelines alone was not acceptable, by declaring that all such cases should be brought before a court for approval. Moreover, if the court is convinced by expert evidence that guidelines are unreasonable or flawed then they will not be applied by the court at all in its determination of whether or not a doctor was negligent. Essentially, the court will seek to assess whether the guideline is *established*. Do the guidelines contain recognized, relevant, and well-developed practice? The answer to this question is likely to come from an expert witness (or several) giving evidence. It is also important to remember that guidelines can sometimes follow, rather than lead, effective medical practice.[73] Notwithstanding the rise of evidence-based medicine, the courts have traditionally been quick to recognize that medicine is an art and not a science.[74]

- It is common for clinicians to speculate on the implications that increasing numbers of guidelines and protocols may have on clinical freedom. However, as yet, there is no legal authority to assume that deviation from guidelines will be considered indicative of negligent practice.[75] It remains the position that the court will examine whether the clinician's actions were reasonable with reference to whether or not the defendant's actions were acceptable to a reasonable body of practitioners (who need not necessarily form the majority opinion) *in the particular circumstances of the* case.[76] Perhaps the best advice one can offer to a clinician concerned about deviating from guidelines is that, as in any area of medical practice, actions and decisions must be justifiable for, should there ever be a court case, that clinician will surely be asked why a decision not to follow guidelines was taken[77].

Case 58 ◆ Responding to refusal of consent by a competent patient (indicated ECG)

Mr Hassid, aged 53, attends A&E about 6 a.m. with his wife who, he says, 'made him come because she is making something out of nothing'. Mr Hassid had an episode of what he describes as 'indigestion' following a heavy meal the previous evening but his wife insists the episode was 'not just indigestion'. Mr Hassid is alert to give the history. His wife is also present. He says that he was unable to sleep because he was in such discomfort. He took some 'Gaviscon' tablets about 2.30 a.m. Although Mr Hassid thinks the pain is wearing off, he remains a bit 'uncomfortable'. When asked, he indicates the centre of his chest as the site of the pain and 'does not think' it is radiating. Mr Hassid is a 'moderate' smoker. His BMI is 29 and, his BP is 130/85mmHg. He is not short of breath. His temperature is 36.9 and pulse is

72bpm. When it is explained that an ECG and further investigations are indicated to exclude a myocardial infarction, Mr Hassid says that he 'has had enough of all this nonsense. It was just a nasty bout of indigestion'. On discussion, it becomes clear that Mr Hassid is keen to leave the hospital to go to work where he is tendering for a new contract in an important presentation.

Core concepts

- A capacitous patient has the freedom to choose to accept or reject medical treatment even where that choice appears to be unwise or frustratingly ill-advised.
- Ultimately therefore, patients who have capacity can self-discharge against medical advice.
- However, there are important points to remember when a patient is wishing to self-discharge, namely:
  - A patient's actual understanding of risks and potential consequences should be checked. Merely because something has been said, understanding cannot be assumed to follow.
  - Compromise may be possible, but if not, explore the options for the patient should the symptoms worsen and the scope for follow-up in primary care, e.g. informing the patient's GP of the hospital visit and subsequent concerns.
  - Enable patients to return should they change their mind or the situation worsens. Patients who do not feel judged or reprimanded are more likely to be able to return to the hospital should they reconsider or become sicker. Encourage the patient to return should he deteriorate or simply change his mind. Remind the patient that there are a number of ways of accessing care should he become unwell quickly, e.g. ambulance service, A&E, etc.
  - Inform the patient in a non-judgemental way that when patients choose to leave without receiving the recommended care, the hospital asks that the patient signs a form to confirm that he understands that he is choosing to leave even though the clinical team would like him to stay.
  - Document all discussion in the notes comprehensively and clearly, and cross-refer to the self-discharge form.
  - Inform the consultant in charge immediately.

Application of core concepts to Case 58

- Although Mr Hassid may appear to be making a decision that seems clinically unwise or foolish, candidates must strike the balance between explaining why it would be advisable to remain in hospital and acknowledging that the choice is ultimately Mr Hassid's to make.
- Building a rapport with Mr Hassid is essential. He has apparently come to the hospital reluctantly and his concerned wife remains present. Candidates need to remember that they know nothing of the couple's relationship. Candidates should therefore ask neutrally whether Mr Hassid would prefer to talk alone or with his wife present.
- The scenario requires candidates to demonstrate two core communication skills, namely (a) checking and (b) explaining whilst developing and maintaining an effective therapeutic relationship.
- Explore what Mr Hassid understands about his experience so far. Is he aware that there are some significant unanswered questions regarding his heart? What does he understand about myocardial infarctions, if anything? Explanations should be clear and avoid jargon or technical language.

- Mr Hassid can be presumed to be a capacitous adult. There is nothing in the presentation to suggest his capacity could be impaired (compare this situation with, for example, a patient presenting with diabetic ketoacidosis where capacity may need to be assessed). It is therefore his choice to refuse treatment even if his refusal seems bizarre or could result in his death.

- In order to make a meaningfully autonomous decision, Mr Hassid does need to know the risks and potential consequences of his choice. Explaining in a patient, honest way why you are concerned about his heart and why the investigations are indicated are key to ensuring that Mr Hassid is fully informed and his decision ethico-legally valid.

- Although Mr Hassid has identified an important presentation at work as the reason he wishes to discharge himself, it may be that he is afraid, in denial, or simply unaware that he is potentially at risk. Being alert to the verbal and non-verbal cues from Mr Hassid is likely to lead to a better understanding of his wish to leave the hospital.

- The possibility of his chest pain being cardiac has to be explained to Mr Hassid, but not confront him in a bullying, frightening, or alarmist way. Likewise, whilst candidates should seek to persuade Mr Hassid to stay, chiding, agitating, or overbearing dogmatism are to be avoided. Empathic acknowledgement of the inconvenience of his symptoms at such an important time in his working life, exploring whether there are other solutions and demonstrating a willingness to listen are crucial.

- If Mr Hassid insists that he wishes to leave the hospital, candidates should follow the procedure for self-discharge against advice and ensure that there is safety netting, e.g. encouraging Mr Hassid to return should he change his mind, advising him of changes in symptoms that warrant urgent attention, suggesting alternative sources of care, and communicating with his GP.

- If Mr Hassid wishes to leave hospital against medical advice, it is usual for a counter-signed note to be made in the medical records and/or for him to sign a self-discharge form. Documentation is very important in these circumstances.

- Seek to maintain an organized, calm, and non-judgemental approach throughout the consultation.

Case 59 ◆ Jehovah's Witness patient refusal of consent for blood transfusion

Miss Keane, aged 23, is brought to A&E following a road accident. She has acute heavy blood loss (c: 40%) as a result of her injuries. Miss Keane is conscious and tells staff that she is a Jehovah's Witness and 'must not receive blood products under any circumstances'. Miss Keane tells a nurse that she will find a card in her purse which she carries at all times to ensure, even if she were to be found unconscious, that no one would give her blood products. The nurse asks you what to do.

Core concepts

- Although Jehovah's Witnesses are often discussed separately in the ethico-legal literature, the correct analysis of this scenario is based on first principles.

- Remember that capacity is a decision-specific concept and can vary. The criteria are described in detail above.
- Irrespective of the reasons for refusal, if the patient has capacity, he or she is entitled to refuse treatment.
- Patients who have particular beliefs that may affect medical treatment in an emergency will sometimes carry some sort of documentation to express and confirm their wishes. Such documentation should be considered as an advance statement or decision and therefore assessed in accordance with the criteria for validity set out in the Mental Capacity Act 2005 (discussed above).
- Cultural and religious sensitivity is required and it is essential not to make assumptions. For example, there is a range of views, as occurs in other religious groups, amongst Jehovah's Witnesses regarding the acceptability of blood products.[78] It may be acceptable to some people who are Jehovah's Witnesses to receive minor processed blood fractions or certain components.[79]
- In many areas, a local 'hospital liaison committee' will exist to facilitate greater understanding between the Jehovah's Witness community and clinicians. Such committees provide contact details of doctors experienced in working with Jehovah's Witnesses, reviews of alternatives to blood products and they may be a valuable resource in difficult cases, time and circumstance permitting.

Application of core concepts to Case 59

- Miss Keane is an adult who is refusing indicated medical treatment. Therefore the first question is whether she is capacitous.
- As an adult Miss Keane should be presumed to have capacity, although depending on her injuries and their effects, there may be a case for assessing her capacity formally.
- If her capacity is assessed, the question will be whether Miss Keane can understand, retain, and weigh up information about her circumstances and then communicate her decision. If so, she has the capacity to choose and refuse treatment like any other adult.
- The card Miss Keane is carrying is equivalent to an advance statement and is not unusual amongst Jehovah's Witnesses. The criteria for validity therefore turn on whether it was made at a time when she had capacity, with adequate information, and is specific to the current situation. If those criteria are met, it is a valid, written advance statement and, within the terms of the Mental Capacity Act 2005, must be respected as such. The only caveat is that as Miss Keane is refusing treatment that may be life-saving, her advance statement should have been witnessed and signed.[80] However, given that she is conscious and confirming her wishes verbally and in real time, the advance statement is not determinative.
- Miss Keane needs the same level of information that would be given to any patient. Candidates should beware of making assumptions because she has disclosed that she is a Jehovah's Witness. The need and probable urgency for blood transfusion following extensive blood loss should be clearly and accurately explained to her without exaggeration or over-playing the risks—it has been noted that Jehovah's Witnesses often have better outcomes than would be expected given the refusal of blood products.[81]
- Ultimately, it is Miss Keane's decision whether or not she receives blood products. She has expressed her wishes both verbally and in writing. Such a decision may be shocking, incomprehensible, or distressing to staff, but it is Miss Keane's decision to make. The clinical team has done its job ethically by ensuring she makes a capacitous and informed choice: it is meaningful respect for Miss Keane's autonomy and the provision of care that is responsive to the patient's values and beliefs.
- By maintaining an open, non-judgemental and professional approach to Miss Keane throughout, the therapeutic relationship remains intact and allows for the possibility of

dialogue, perhaps even enabling Miss Keane to change her mind. Although it is unlikely that she will change her mind given her strongly expressed resistance to blood products, it is possible and because the nature of capacity is that it is decision-specific, Miss Keane is free to alter her views albeit within a limited time scale.

- Candidates may wish to explore the involvement of a local liaison committee depending on whether such a group exists and whether time allows.

- It is best practice to ensure, wherever possible, that consultants are involved in such cases and that the decision process is clearly and accurately documented. The documentation should ideally be signed, counter-signed, and witnessed.

Further information

- The law on consent and refusal of treatment has been thrown into sharp relief by a number of cases involving patients who are Jehovah's Witnesses with young lives being lost as a result of clinicians respecting a patient's refusal of blood products. It can, understandably, be immensely difficult for clinical teams to stand by and watch patients making choices that may lead to an avoidable death, but the law is clear: no one can override a capacitous patient's informed refusal of treatment.

Confidentiality and Information Sharing

Confidentiality and Healthcare Information: Clinical Cases

Case 60 ◆ Public interest limits to confidentiality—serious risk presented by patient with epilepsy who continues to drive

You are a junior doctor working in the neurology outpatient clinic. Mr Parsons is a 42-year old man diagnosed with grand mal epilepsy a year ago, for which he has been taking medication. However, despite several changes in treatment, his epilepsy remains poorly controlled. Mr Parsons has continued to have fits, mostly at night, but his notes record that he has had one recent fit during the day at the bank where he works. You are aware that the consultant has advised Mr Parsons to cease driving and informed the DVLA of his diagnosis. The consultant has explained to Mr Parsons that he should stop driving and that the DVLA must be informed of his diagnosis of epilepsy. You recognize Mr Parsons immediately as the same man who parked his car next to yours in the hospital car park this morning. You recall with certainty that he was alone and was driving when he pulled into the space in the car park. Mr Parsons has come in for a routine clinic appointment today.

Please acknowledge that you have seen Mr Parsons driving and discuss with him the implications of continuing to drive whilst he has poorly controlled epilepsy.

Core concepts

- Driving may present particular risks when patients have diagnoses or symptoms that potentially compromise their awareness and control of the vehicle. Driving when unsafe to do so is a significant issue. Nearly half the instances of unconsciousness at the wheel of a vehicle are epileptic in origin and the condition is often undisclosed.
- The Driver Vehicle and Licensing Agency (DVLA) has a specialized unit, the Drivers' Medical Group, which is responsible for establishing whether people are fit and safe to drive. The DVLA uses a system of expert panels to set standards (and those standards are reviewed every six months) and advise on the implications of driving with specific medical symptoms or conditions. The categories covered by the DVLA panels are shown in Box 9.

> **Box 9** Secretary of State's Honorary Medical Advisory Panels
>
> * Alcohol Drugs and Substance Misuse and Driving
> * Cardiovascular System and Driving
> * Diabetes Mellitus and Driving
> * Disorders of the Nervous System and Driving
> * Psychiatric Disorders and Driving
> * Visual Disorders and Driving

* Although it is a criminal offence for a person not to disclose a relevant medical condition to the DVLA, it is insufficient for doctors to rely entirely on patients to make the appropriate disclosure. Doctors have specific professional obligations in ensuring that the DVLA is aware of anyone with a medical condition that potentially impairs safety when driving. The assessment of how well candidates understand those professional obligations is the primary aim of this scenario.

Application of core concepts to Case 60

* This is a scenario that inevitably involves conveying information that Mr Parsons will not welcome. Talking about driving also reminds the patient of the reality and impact of his disease which is likely to be difficult and painful. It is therefore to be expected that the patient will become emotional, perhaps angry. Effective communication will be needed that conveys the essential message about the unacceptability of Mr Parsons continuing to drive whilst acknowledging the significant impact of ceasing to drive on the patient's life.
* The first task is to acknowledge to the patient that he has been observed driving. This should be addressed factually and neutrally once the initial introductions have been made. It is important to avoid being or appearing judgemental, or worse, confrontational.
* Candidates should explore what Mr Parsons has been told about driving and the risks of his continuing to drive with poorly-controlled epilepsy. Although there is a note recording that the consultant has discussed the issue with him, candidates should not make assumptions about how the information has been received. This means that initially, candidates will need to listen carefully to Mr Parsons because what follows should reflect what Mr Parsons does or does not know and believe to be the risks of him continuing to drive.
* The information about risk that has to be conveyed should be carefully explained in a calm and factual way. Alarmist, patronizing, or chiding approaches should be avoided. The risks to Mr Parsons and others should be neither under- nor over-stated. Candidates should contextualize the information by explaining that Mr Parsons potentially presents a risk to public safety.
* If Mr Parsons refuses to inform the DVLA, candidates should explain that where a patient presents a serious risk of physical harm to others, confidentiality can be breached. However, candidates should continue to encourage Mr Parsons to approach the DVLA himself and be explicit that it would be preferable for Mr Parsons to do so.
* The discussion with Mr Parsons should be documented accurately and completed.
* Throughout the consultation, candidates should remain non-judgemental, avoid 'scolding', acknowledge the impact of not being able to drive on Mr Parsons and remain calm.

Further information

* Confidentiality is considered a somewhat strange area medico-legally. It is clearly a highly valued area of medical practice, much emphasized by the professional codes of conduct and

governing bodies. However, the law has very little to say about breach of confidence, and case law on the subject is very thin on the ground. This is partly because there are few remedies for breach of confidence, and therefore it tends to be a matter for professional discipline rather than legal redress.

- It has been suggested that there should be a statutory offence of breach of confidence[82] that would extend to the doctor–patient relationship. The introduction of such a statutory offence would place the UK in a comparable position to that of many European countries.[83]

- Whilst acceptance of a duty of confidentiality is almost universal amongst doctors, the extent to which this duty is absolute or may be compromised is not necessarily a matter of agreement. There are several widely accepted common law justifications for breaking confidentiality which are discussed below. However, on closer examination, these can actually prove to be little more than very general labels which actually give the doctor very little substantive information about when she may be justified in breaking confidentiality. In addition, there are several statutory provisions that cover the disclosure of confidential information in certain specific circumstances.

- Other than the statutory requirements relating to information sharing, breach of confidence can usually only be justified in one of three principal ways, namely when:
  - (i)   the patient consents;
  - (ii) divulgence is in the patient's best interests, and it is neither desirable nor practicable to seek consent; or
  - (iii) divulgence is in the public interest.

- When one considers what these three justifications for breach of confidence actually mean in practice, it is clear that there is significant room for interpretation on the part of the practitioner. Therefore, a doctor needs to feel that a decision to breach confidence is an ethical decision, which can be justified both internally and externally.

Case 61 ◆ **Risk and confidentiality—drug abusing patient**

Mr Caan, aged 31, attends A&E in an intoxicated state. He is agitated and repeatedly requests opiates to **'calm him down'**. *In discussion, he reveals that he is a frequent and heavy user of drugs, taking crack, heroine, cocaine, marijuana, and alcohol on a regular basis and benzodiazepines occasionally. He asks if you are going* **'to tell anyone'** *about his drug misuse.*

Core concepts

- This scenario has been included because some clinicians, particularly those not working regularly with drug dependent patients, are confused about the duty of confidentiality in respect of misuse of drugs.
- There was previously a legal duty on doctors to notify the Home Office under the Misuse of Drugs Act 1971 of drug abusing patients. However, that duty no longer exists in England and Wales. Instead, prescribers of controlled drugs are expected to return forms

(either electronically or in hard copy) that contribute to the local or national drug misuse database.

- Otherwise, the duty of confidentiality to a drug abusing patient is the same as for any other patient, i.e. it can be qualified by (a) the patient's consent; (b) the patient's best interests where it is impracticable or impossible to seek consent; and (c) where there is a serious risk of physical harm to an identifiable person or persons.
- There will, of course, be local protocols regarding the storage, prescribing, and documenting of controlled drug provision.

Application of core concepts to Case 61

- A clear, calm, and professional consultation with Mr Caan is the aim, just as it would be with any other patient.
- Having introduced oneself and listened to Mr Caan's concerns, the task is to explain politely and without judgement what can and cannot be offered to him in an A&E department.
- His intoxication may render him confused and confusing. Such confusion does not mean that Mr Caan lacks capacity. Rather efforts should be made to maximize his capacity and, if there is no immediate risk to his health, waiting until he is sufficiently sober that he can make decisions about his care.
- If possible, candidates should explore why it is that Mr Caan is specifically requesting opiates. In the absence of any indication for the prescription of opiates, candidates have to explain to Mr Caan why such a prescription would be inappropriate. Furthermore, even if there is indication for opiates, it will not be possible to give Mr Caan such medication whilst he is intoxicated. Either way, the aim is to explain to Mr Caan that his request cannot be met and remain calm in the face of challenge.
- Mr Caan asks specifically about the effect of his disclosure on patient confidentiality. Candidates must respond by setting out the ways in which the disclosure he has made about his drug misuse will inform his care and be recorded.
- Candidates are not required to know about the specialist treatment of drug misuse, but are expected to treat Mr Caan with courtesy, showing an awareness of how his drug misuse will affect his health and identifying appropriate further sources of care and support.
- Mr Caan should be reassured that there is no statutory basis on which his information will be shared with external agencies and that details of his health will remain within the healthcare team who are responsible for his care.
- The only basis on which information about Mr Caan's drug and alcohol abuse could possibly be shared is where he presents a serious risk to an identifiable individual, e.g. if he were actively using drugs and alcohol whilst in a position of responsibility and the safety of others were likely to be compromised as a result.
- Addiction and drug dependency are complex and unlikely to be resolved in a busy A&E department. Unfortunately, Mr Caan may decide that he does not want to engage in any sort of specialist care and, ultimately, that is his choice to make.

Further information

- Patients who abuse drugs can be difficult and frustrating. However, the duty of care and right to general medical services are equivalent to any other person irrespective of the patient's willingness or capacity for ceasing his or her drug misuse. Professional bodies are unequivocal that doctors must not discriminate, judge, or act prejudicially with regard to people who are abusing drugs.

- Indeed, based on the legal standard of care test, it is reasonable to expect a doctor who does not specialize in drug dependency to discuss the options for further specialist care alongside providing general medical care. And general medical care should, of course, take account of the increased risks to drug abusing patients, e.g. blood borne viruses.

Case 62 ◆ Confidentiality and relatives— relatives seeking information about a patient's diagnosis (leukaemia)

You are an F2 doctor working in oncology outpatients. Muriel Howes has come alone and asked to see one of the doctors in the clinic. Her husband was diagnosed with acute myeloid leukaemia last week. You remember Mr Howes and were there when the consultant told him of the diagnosis and discussed treatment. You recall that he attended alone. Mrs Howes is visibly upset. She tells you that she is **'very concerned'** *about her husband. He is so pale and tired but is* **'secretive'** *about what the doctors said to him last week. She knows that Mr Howes had some* **'sort of blood tests'** *but nothing more. Mrs Howes tells you that she found the clinic's appointment card in her husband's jacket and decided to come to clinic today because she is* **'out of her mind with worry'**. *She asks you to tell her* **'what on earth is going on?'; 'What is wrong with my husband?'**

Core concepts

- Doctors working for the NHS do not have a contract with their patients; a duty to keep confidences is inferred at common law for all doctors.[84] Therefore, doctors have a legal obligation not to divulge voluntarily information that they obtain during the course of their medical relationship with a patient without that patient's express consent[85] even to a spouse, partner, or close relative.
- In the UK, in common with most Western bioethical traditions, the construct of the doctor– patient relationship is dyadic, which can present difficulties when a doctor has contact with relatives, be it formally or, as in this scenario, informally. Clinicians may become very used to seeing family members visiting a patient on a ward or accompanying a patient to clinic. Such familiarity does not alter the fundamental principles of confidentiality that apply to each and every patient independently of his or her family.
- It is essential to remember that the decision whether or not to share information with relatives and to involve third parties in care is the patient's alone (assuming he or she has capacity). It may seem surprising or even foolish of a patient to wish to keep information private, but it is his or her choice to make and should not be judged or compromised by well-meaning but misguided clinicians.

Application of core concepts to Case 62

- This scenario assesses not only whether candidates know that confidentiality cannot be breached without the patient's permission, but also how well candidates handle a difficult situation with an anxious and upset relative.

- In addition to the knowledge needed to explain to Mrs Howes why the team is unable to share information about her husband's care with her in the absence of Mr Howes's permission, the consultation has to be conducted in a way that acknowledges Mrs Howes's distress, explores options for facilitating a discussion with her husband, and ameliorates rather than exacerbates her emotional state.

- This is a challenging situation and the candidate's communication skills may either inflame or diffuse the situation depending on the extent to which Mrs Howes feels heard, understood, and supported. And it is possible to listen, empathize, and support Mrs Howes whilst not breaching the patient's confidentiality.

- First, the relationship of Mrs Howes to the patient, i.e. her husband, should be confirmed. Candidates should verify whether she is attending clinic alone and if her husband is aware of her visit.

- Mrs Howes is extremely worried—she is sufficiently anxious to have tracked down the details of the clinic, travelled to the hospital, and waited to see a doctor without an appointment. It is essential that her anxiety, fear, and concerns are heard and acknowledged.

- There is a fine line between exploring with Mrs Howes why her husband is apparently refusing to talk to her and making uninformed judgements or inadvertent but damaging comment on her marital relationship. Phrases such as *'Is everything alright in your marriage because it seems odd to me he won't talk to you'* or *'This is a situation which makes me think you ought to consider marriage guidance counselling'* should be avoided! Alternative ways of discussing her husband's reluctance to talk to her might include phrases such as *'You are obviously and understandably very worried. Does your husband know how concerned you are?'* or *'it sounds as though it is an even more frightening situation for you because your husband won't talk to you. Do you have any thoughts about why that might be?'*

- Candidates will have to tell Mrs Howes something that she does not want to hear, i.e. that confidentiality cannot be broken even though she is the patient's wife and in obvious distress. Mrs Howes may, perhaps even is likely to, respond with frustration and become more upset, possibly even angry. Allowing Mrs Howes to express her feelings whilst remaining calm is crucial.

- The scenario presented here is simple in terms of ethico-legal content if not in terms of the challenge it poses to candidates' communication skills. Without Mr Howes's permission, no information can be shared with his wife. The ethico-legal rationale being that the first criterion by which a duty of confidence is qualified is having the consent of the patient to talk to a third party. That consent has not been given by Mr Howes and therefore the task is to explain the position to Mrs Howes and its foundation in professional guidance, law, and ethical practice.

- Throughout this consultation, candidates may themselves feel frustrated and even upset—no one likes to be in a situation where they are unable to help, feel ineffective, or perhaps personally criticized. It is important that these feelings are not conveyed to Mrs Howes either verbally or non-verbally. Maintaining eye contact and an open body posture throughout is important.

- The unwelcome information that candidates have to tell Mrs Howes, namely that confidentiality precludes clinicians from sharing information without the patient's permission, may need to be repeated. The so-called 'broken record' technique is probably not required, but clear, calm, and, if necessary, a patiently repeated explanation that no one can give Mrs Howes details of her husband's care without his permission is essential.

- Candidates should explore whether there might be ways in which discussion between Mr Howes and his wife could be facilitated. Suggestions might include:
  - ◆ Mrs Howes returning with her husband for a joint consultation;
  - ◆ exploring with Mr Howes, at his next appointment, the impact of his diagnosis and treatment on his family life—and perhaps 'reality testing' and gently checking the sustainability of not wanting his wife to know anything about his care;
  - ◆ involving the family's GP and reminding Mrs Howes that the GP is available to support her through this difficult time;
  - ◆ asking sensitively whether Mrs Howes and her husband have friends or family who may be sources of support—is there someone whom Mr Howes trusts and who may be able to convey to Mr Howes how concerned his wife is without worsening the impasse?
- At the end of the consultation, candidates may want to reiterate regret that they have been unable to help Mrs Howes as she asked. However, an appropriate closure would be to summarize the possibilities for encouraging a discussion between her and her husband, reminding her of ways the clinical team may be able to contribute to supporting them as a couple through a painful time.

Case 63 ◆ Confidentiality on the telephone—a call to a patient enrolled in research

Ms B, who has Systemic Lupus Erythematosus (SLE), attended the gynaecology department for a termination of pregnancy. Whilst at the hospital, she had signed a form agreeing that her cases notes could be used as part of a research project into termination of pregnancy in patients with SLE. Six months later, Ms B returned home with her boyfriend and switched on the answer phone in the sitting room where they both heard the following message **'Good Afternoon this is Dr S at X hospital. I am a doctor working with the SLE research team on the termination of pregnancy study. I was wondering whether you could call me back and answer a couple of simple questions. Thank you and I look forward to hearing from you. Good bye'.**

Ms B's partner had not known she had been pregnant, still less about the termination. He ended their relationship. Ms B complained to the hospital and threatened legal action.

Core concepts

- Confidential information can be shared with a patient's consent. However, as this scenario demonstrates, a patient may happily consent to information being shared amongst medical professionals under particular circumstances, but this does not necessarily mean that he or she is consenting to all potential uses of the information.
- When calling patients, careful regard should be had to confidentiality. Even though a patient may have supplied a telephone number, there can be pitfalls for the unwary medical caller.

- It is good practice when asking for a telephone number to check with the patient (a) if this is a personal line; (b) if there is a time when the patient is more likely to be able to talk freely; and (c) whether it is acceptable to leave a message if the patient is not available. Unfortunately, best practice may not be possible, particularly in the monolithic systems of the NHS where the recording of telephone numbers if part of routine administration that does not allow for these three simple enquiries.

- In all situations, doctors should be extremely circumspect in giving information over the phone. The scenario demonstrates that even calling 'with consent' can result in indefensible breaches of patient confidentiality.

Application of core concepts to Case 63

- If, as is common, a doctor has to call a patient on the phone without knowing whether the number is one on which the patient will be available and able talk privately, it is sensible to be cautious.

- Ask the name of the person to whom you are speaking before identifying yourself. If you have not reached the patient, politely saying that you will call back is the best option.

- Should you reach an answer-phone or voice mail service, it is preferable not to leave a message. Occasionally, it may be very important to make contact with the patient as soon as possible, in which case, a neutral message asking for the person concerned to call you and leaving a telephone number is probably the most pragmatic solution as the potential breach of confidentiality is weighed proportionately against the urgency and need to contact the patient. In the scenario presented here, it was not sufficiently urgent to justify leaving a message for the patient on an insecure answering machine.

- Ms B has a legitimate complaint. Her confidentiality has been breached, albeit inadvertently, and the consequences for her are considerable, i.e. the end of her relationship and loss of privacy. A response should conform to the process requirements of local complaints policies and must represent an honest and sincere apology for a serious error.

- Many patients who complain cite the wish to inform and improve future practice as their motive rather than the pursuit of money. Indeed, a truthful, open, and timely response is likely to prevent future dispute and legal action. Any response should explain the ways in which Ms B's experience will be used to enhance practice and prevent recurrence.

Further information

- It should be emphasized that in UK law, partners, spouses, and putative 'fathers' do not have any right or entitlement to be informed of a woman's decision either to proceed with, or terminate, a pregnancy. As such, a man can neither prevent a woman from having a termination of pregnancy nor can he oblige her to have a termination. The decision is, at law, entirely the woman's choice and as such, the fundamental principles of confidentiality mean that medical information about either a termination or antenatal care can only be shared with a male partner with her express consent.

Information Sharing: Clinical Cases

Case 64 ◆ **Patient calling to follow-up investigation results**

You are a Junior Doctor working in a sexual health clinic. Mr Franks, aged 36, presented for a 'check up', last week. A full sexual health screen was undertaken. The serology results are:

- *HBsAg*   **Positive**
- *Anti-HBc*   **Positive**
- *IgM anti-HBc* **Positive**
- *Anti-HBs*   **Negative**

Mr Franks calls the clinic reception and asks to be put through to you. He tells you that he is calling to **'find out the test results from last week'.**

Core concepts

- Many hospitals and clinical units will have rules about giving information over the telephone and it is common for 'confidentiality' to be cited as the rationale for such rules.
- The principal concerns about disclosing medical information over the telephone are twofold. First, there is the question of identity, i.e. how can the clinician establish that the person to whom they are speaking is the patient? In reality, the worry about caller identity seems a somewhat unnecessary preoccupation given that there are myriad ways in which financial and other organizations verify identity such as secret questions, checking personal details, asking for specific characters of passwords, etc.
- The second concern about discussing test results over the phone is that if the information is sensitive or in any way unwelcome news, patients should be seen in person to allow for a proper discussion which goes beyond merely giving the information to explore patient response and future management options. This second concern about the therapeutic vacuity of the telephone seems more valid than worries about identity.

Application of core concepts to Case 64

- Even if it is assumed that Mr Franks's identity is not in question, hepatitis is a complex disease and Mr Franks needs to be able to discuss the diagnosis rather than merely 'hear' it.
- The telephone is unlikely to be the best medium for conveying significant news and giving Mr Franks the opportunity to consider the effect of a diagnosis of hepatitis on his life. Therefore, Mr Franks needs to be invited in to meet a clinician to discuss his test results.
- The content of the telephone discussion therefore needs to be honest and simple conveying to Mr Franks that you would like to discuss the tests he had in person and you can arrange a priority appointment for him.

- Candidates should be prepared to answer Mr Franks's questions and must not mislead him. Remember when speaking on the phone it is harder to gauge a person's emotional state and you cannot see non-verbal cues, so listen carefully and adapt your communication skills accordingly.
- The conversation should conclude with a clear confirmation of how and when Mr Franks will hear about his promised priority appointment and when he is likely to be able to come into the clinic to discuss his test results.

Further information

- This scenario takes place in a sexual health context and it is noteworthy that sexual health has been one of the most progressive areas of medicine in its use of technology to communicate with patients[86] leading one sexual health team to establish an innovative clinical service conducted entirely online.[87] Research suggests that the two main preferences for receiving sexual health test results are either during a face to face consultation or over the telephone.

Case 65 ◆ Patient requesting access to medical records (neurology outpatient)

Mrs Hinks has been a patient of the neurology team for 2 years following referral for investigation and management of her headaches. She attends the outpatient clinic one morning and tells you that she would like to see her medical records. She asks you to share her notes with her and talk her through their contents during the appointment.

Core concepts

- The most important piece of law with which to be familiar is the Data Protection Act 1998 in relation to the sharing of healthcare records. The Data Protection Act 1998 (DPA) largely superseded the Access to Health Records Act 1990.[88] The DPA 1998 is an immensely complex piece of legislation and only the basic principles of the statute are discussed here.
- The data protection legislation should also be read in conjunction with the Freedom of Information Act 2000 which has less direct application to healthcare records but, in some circumstances, may be relevant.
- A useful starting point for specific queries is the Information Commission Office's website which can be found at http://www.ico.gov.uk/. Local NHS Trusts will also have policies describing the application of the statutory framework to patient requests[89] to see healthcare records.
- The DPA 1998 is essentially based on eight principles of data protection. The definition of 'data' within the 1998 Act includes information being *recorded as part of a relevant filing system* and forming *part of an accessible record* (DPA 1998, s 1(1)). Note that no distinction is drawn between manual and electronic data, i.e. written and electronic healthcare records and notes are treated identically for the purposes of the law.

- It does not matter when the information was recorded in considering the request for information. The emphasis is on the thematic 'setting' or structuring of information rather than the physical filing, chronology, or other organizational systems used.
- 'Personal data' comprise that information in which an individual can be identified and includes statements of opinion (as well as fact) and indications of any intentions of the data controller in respect of the named individual.
- Data should be accurate and the onus is on the data controller to take all reasonable steps to verify the accuracy of the data, rather than simply rely on the word of third parties. This may be particularly relevant when considering information recorded about incompetent patients.[90]
- Individuals are entitled to be told by data controllers whether data is being processed about them by or on behalf of an organization, e.g. as part of the NHS or, strictly speaking, on behalf of the Secretary of State for Health. If data are being so processed, individuals can seek a description of (a) the data held; (b) the purposes for which data are being processed; and (c) persons/third parties to whom data may be disclosed.
- Patients who have capacity can ask for a copy of the data (which must be in an accessible and intelligible form which may raise particular challenges in the context of complex medical information and, as a less serious aside, doctors' handwriting!).
- Requests can be made informally and there is no provision in law that explicitly prohibits doctors from showing patients their records but many Trusts prefer that a formal request is made in writing and a fee may be charged.
- There are circumstances under which a request to see healthcare records can be refused, namely:
  - if the records identify a third person, other than a fellow healthcare professional who has also been involved in treating the patient; and
  - if it disclosure is likely to adversely affect the patient's mental and/or physical health.
- Different rules apply in relation to requests to see the records of a deceased patient which, although broadly congruent with the principles of the DPA 1998, are sufficiently complex to warrant seeking immediate advice from the relevant department in the hospital or PCT.

Application of core concepts to Case 65

- Mrs Hinks has made a request that is increasingly common. She has not given a reason for her wish to see her medical records, nor does she have to do so. As a patient with capacity, she is entitled to see her healthcare records and any other information that is held about her.
- A sensitive exploration of Mrs Hinks's request may be useful in case she has become particularly concerned about something. However, care must be taken to avoid interrogating Mrs Hinks and the emphasis should be on establishing whether there is something specific with which you may be able to help or whether she wishes to see her entire records. It may be that Mrs Hinks is motivated by a potential legal or insurance claim, a desire for greater information about her health or simple curiosity, but she does not need to explain herself to anyone.
- The response to Mrs Hinks request will be informed both by the law on sharing information and by local policy on disclosure of medical records.
- It is important to check the local policy on sharing healthcare information when considering how to respond to Mrs Hinks. It is likely that the hospital will require a formal request in writing from Mrs Hinks and an administrative fee before records are disclosed. This should be explained to Mrs Hinks and she should be clearly advised how to proceed, e.g. to whom should she write, what is the likely timescale, why is there a fee, etc?

- Whilst it would not be unlawful to do as Mrs Hinks has asked and discuss her notes with her during the consultation, it is likely to be contrary to local practice and possibly infringe employment terms by breaching institutional policy.
- On a purely practical level, the time such immediate disclosure and concomitant discussion would take in a busy neurological outpatient clinic is likely to preclude instant accession to Mrs Hinks' request.

Further information

- The DPA 1998 significantly broadened the definition of data 'processing' to incorporate the obtaining, holding, and disclosing of information about living people. Data controllers should seek consent from those about whom they are holding data to share information. In general, the more ambiguous and implied the consent on which the data controller relies, the more likely the Information Commission Office may be to question its validity.
- More generally, the importance of comprehensive, contemporaneous records in clinical care cannot be overstated. Notes and records have been said to be the single most important piece of evidence in any complaint or even legal action. Some experts will actually discuss the notes and medical records under a distinct heading in their medico-legal reports: a trend that is increasingly being encouraged by those with responsibility for advising on the compilation of such reports.[91]
- Moreover, given the delay that commonly occurs between a cause of action occurring and any ensuing proceedings, good notes are vital not only as formal evidence but as a means of recalling the events accurately and consistently should the defendant be subjected to cross-examination.
- So, what constitutes 'good' record keeping for medico-legal purposes? An article in the Medical Defence Union Journal[92] made the following recommendations:
  - notes should be legible;
  - the date and time of the consultation must always be included (when this is corroborated with an appointment book this can prove particularly significant in court proceedings);
  - all notes should be signed by name, and ideally a signature should be accompanied by a printed name;
  - only approved and unambiguous abbreviations should be used;
  - an entry should never be altered nor an addition disguised;[93]
  - if computer records are used there should ideally be an 'audit trail' which gives assurance that the records have not been altered;
  - insulting, humorous, or personal comments should be avoided as they 'lower the overall tone' of the records and make it harder for the defence to construct a case based around them;[94]
  - if notes/letters are dictated and typed up by someone else, the contents of the hard copy should be checked to ensure that it is an accurate representation of the dictated version;
  - reports should be seen, evaluated, and signed by a clinician before they are filed;
  - records should not be thrown away; and
  - access to records should be provided in accordance with the statutory provisions.

Case 66 ◆ Interactions with the police—requests for information about a patient with a blood disorder following an assault

You are working as an SHO in haemotology. The police visit the department and ask you to disclose the records of all your patients with sickle cell anaemia. There has been an assault in the area following a fight in a local bar. The police advise you that the forensic team has identified that the assailant was very likely to have sick cell disease.

Core concepts

- Requests from the police for medical information are common. And there are, of course, circumstances where doctors will work with the criminal justice system to provide care and services. In law, the police have no greater claim to automatic access to medical information than any other individual or organization.[95] However, there are certain statutory exceptions to this general rule, e.g. information following traffic accidents,[96] and information relating to terrorism.[97]

- Clearly, the lack of a general obligation to furnish the police with confidential information does not permit a doctor to act in such a way as to be considered an obstruction to police investigation. Whether or not a doctor is acting in a way that could be considered an 'obstruction' turns on the concept of 'lawful excuse',[98] i.e. if a doctor refuses to answer questions, and has a lawful excuse for such refusal, she is not being obstructive. The considered opinion appears to be that the obligation of confidence would constitute 'lawful excuse'.[99]

- It should be noted, that concealing information for gain is a crime,[100] whether or not the offender is a doctor!

- The default position is that, in the absence of a court order requiring disclosure, the consent of the patient should be sought before any personal or clinical details are disclosed to the police.

- Where requests are received from the police for clinical information or access to medical records, most NHS Trusts have protocols defining how such requests should be made and by whom they should be handled.

- Clearly, the question of whether one supplies the police with information that would otherwise be confidential is, to a significant extent, a matter of ethical deliberation for the individual doctor, given the limits of the legal provisions within this area. The BMA have issued guidance for doctors which covers cooperation with the police.[101] This advice suggests that a doctor should consider disclosing information only in the case of *serious* crimes whilst recognizing that the definition of severity is confusing.

- The core BMA guidance is derived from the concept of serious arrestable offences under the Police and Criminal Evidence Act 1984. A serious arrestable offence is defined as an offence that has caused or may cause:
  - serious harm to the security of the state or to public order;
  - serious interference with the administration of justice or with the investigation of an offence;

- ◆ serious injury;
- ◆ substantial financial gain or serious loss; or
- ◆ death.

- Therefore the BMA guidance suggests that confidentiality may be breached where crimes such as murder, manslaughter, rape, treason, kidnapping, and abuse of children or other vulnerable people have been committed.
- Furthermore, the BMA guidance proposes that serious harm to the security of the state or to public order and serious fraud will also fall into the category of crimes where information may be shared with the police.
- In contrast, the BMA notes, in cases of theft, minor fraud or damage to property where loss or damage is less substantial, a breach of confidence would not generally be justifiable.
- Sometimes the police will seek, and be granted, a court order under the Police and Criminal Evidence Act 1984 permitting access to healthcare records as part of the investigation of a crime. It is good practice to ask the police if they have obtained a court order enabling them to access medical information and, if a court order has not been sought, to wait until a decision has been made before granting access to medical information without consent. It is by no means certain that a circuit judge will always look favourably on police applications for access to healthcare records.
- Finally, in addition to the statutory frameworks and professional guidance within which disclosure of information to the police should be considered, the common law provides that a doctor is entitled (note not required) to share information where it is in the public interest as defined by the case of *W* v *Egdell*,[102] i.e. where there is a serious risk of physical harm to an identifiable individual or individuals.

Application of core concepts to Case 66

- On the assumption that it is in accordance with local protocol and policy to respond directly to the police, this scenario presents a situation where the severity of any risk and the value of the clinical information requested are debatable.
- First, the police should be asked whether they have a court order sanctioning the provision of healthcare information.
- If there is no court order, it would be best practice to advise the police to seek such an order. Given the extent of the information that is requested and that the confidentiality of many patients, rather than a single individual patient, would be compromised by supplying such information, it is not certain that a court order would be granted.
- Clearly, if the police either have a court order already or are granted such an order after a formal request, the information requested should be provided in accordance with the terms of the order and local protocols on sharing healthcare information with the police.
- If an order is not granted, the information requested by the police should not be shared. If a judge has not been persuaded by the seriousness of the risk and the value of the information to a criminal inquiry, doctors should conclude that there is no legitimate basis on which to share confidential information.

Further information

- Ethicists have further suggested that regard should be given to the potential usefulness or otherwise of any confidential information that may be given to the police.[103] That is to say, when considering whether or not to share confidential information without a specific court order requiring it, doctors should consider how useful such information is likely to be in solving the crime. However, in practice, such a prospective utility test may be a frustrating and time-consuming exercise in second guessing and is probably better left to a judge to assess whilst deciding whether to grant a court order requiring medical information to be disclosed to the police.

Case 67 ♦ Firearms and a patient in A&E

Mr Monkton, aged 21, is brought to A&E by ambulance after being discovered collapsed in the street. He is bleeding from what appear to be two gun shot wounds. What obligations, if any, does the clinical team have to disclose information about Mr Monkton?

Core concepts

- Gun shot wounds have special status and form a distinct category in professional guidance on confidentiality.[104] Essentially, the advice from the GMC is that doctors should always notify the police where a patient, such as Mr Monkton in the scenario above, has a gun shot wound or wounds. The rationale being that patients who arrive with a wound from a gun pose a serious risk of harm to others, i.e. this is a situation that falls within the scope of the 'public interest' qualification to the duty of confidentiality.

- As with other cases where confidential information can justifiably be shared with a third party, the details disclosed should be limited to that which is essential to avert risk and only given to the person or persons who need to know.[105]

Application of core concepts to Case 67

- In practical terms, the advice is that someone from the clinical team (and the task can be delegated by doctors) should advise the police as soon as possible after Mr Monkton's arrival at the hospital. The police are then responsible for assessing the extent of the risk posed to the 'public interest' and will commonly visit the department.

- Whilst the police are likely to wish to talk to Mr Monkton as a priority, his medical interests come first. Doctors are entitled to ensure that Mr Monkton is in a stable condition and fit to talk before the police are permitted to interview him.

- If Mr Monkton is, or becomes, unconscious, and therefore unable to talk to the police, the situation falls within the standard *W v Egdell* criteria for determining whether the public interest warrants disclosure without Mr Monkton's consent; there is a full discussion of the *W v Egdell* case and the relevant criteria for assessing the 'public interest' in relation to disclosure of confidential medical information above (see Case 66 Police Requests for Information).

Further information

- Following recent concern about the increase in knife attacks, particularly in cities, the government has proposed that doctors should routinely inform the police of serious injuries inflicted by knives.[106] At the time of writing, it is unclear whether the reporting of knife wounds is a recommendation to doctors, or a requirement. However, the standard criteria for 'public interest' disclosure are likely to apply in cases where serious injuries have been inflicted by knives. The common law 'public interest' justification for disclosure is in evidence in the interim guidance on knife wounds published by the GMC and the Department of Health.[107]

Case 68 ◆ Information sharing and a notifiable disease—patient with TB

Mr Ukhono, aged 37, presented in A&E because he had been **'coughing and sweating'** *for several weeks. Mr Ukhono lives temporarily at a local hostel and tells you that he was living on the streets until recently. Having taken a history and examined Mr Ukhono, TB is part of the differential diagnosis. Investigations and X-rays confirm that Mr Ukhono has TB. He is reluctant to be admitted to a ward. Mr Ukhono also pleads with you not to tell anyone at the hostel because he* **'will be kicked out'.**

Core concepts

- Many questions in public health are less philosophical and more political than in almost any other area of healthcare practice. The underlying ethos of public health is necessarily utilitarian (i.e. put simplistically, to provide the greatest good for the greatest number) and communitarian, but the application of the ethos must be pragmatic, constrained as it is by political agendas, resource constraints, socio-economic inequalities, and legal frameworks.

- The traditional model in medical ethics and law has been of an encounter between an individual clinician and patient. In such a model, all ethico-legal duties, rights, and dilemmas are understood as flowing from this dyadic (and often one-off) encounter. It is perhaps not surprising that this particular model of the medical encounter dominated the agenda for so long given the way in which medical training and the regulation of the medical profession by the GMC stress the role of the doctor as advocate for the individual patient. However, there is increasing attention being paid to the population perspective and the ethico-legal issues that arise thereof, e.g. the allocation of resources, screening programmes, epidemiological research, and immunization to name but a few.

- Article 5 of the Human Rights Act ('HRA') 1998, which articulates the right to liberty and security of the person, has obvious relevance when considering the management of patients with communicable diseases. For example, the controversial suggestion that patients with TB, who are non-adherent to treatment, could be forced to have treatment (in a way similar to that described in New York in the late 1990s) is likely to be unlawful when considered in the context of this article of the HRA 1998.

- Likewise, article 8[108] which provides for the right to respect for private and family life also has implications for a range of public health activity including the notification of appropriate authorities about communicable diseases.

- The problems posed by communicable diseases are increasingly significant with several areas reporting local outbreaks of tuberculosis in the last five years. Internationally, the fight is even greater: the World Health Organization (WHO) has described failings in tuberculosis control as 'a global emergency'.[109]

- Adherence and concordance on the part of patients who are diagnosed with tuberculosis are vital if relapse and the development of drug resistant disease are to be avoided.

- What powers do and should doctors have in respect of patients who are smear-positive and are, at best, erratic about complying with treatment regimes? Should practitioners have the power to detain compulsorily such patients? The moral rationale for compulsory detention is generally said to be the utilitarian argument that the effect on individual autonomy of compulsory detention is a smaller loss than the potential damage such an individual can cause to society if he is not detained. However, given that patients with TB are frequently (but not necessarily) 'marginalized' within society, it has been suggested that such measures are indicative of discrimination (which is of course, explicitly prohibited under the HRA 1998). Coker[110] has argued that ethical practice demands that clinically informed assessment of risk and the exploration of less restrictive alternative approaches to adherence must precede any move towards compulsion.

- The Public Health (Control of Disease) Act 1984 and specifically sections 37 and 38 which, on the authority of a Magistrate (Justice of the Peace), permitted the removal and detention of patients to prevent infection, have been the subject of both academic debate and an extensive consultation on reform.[111]

- The consultation led to the Health and Social Care Act 2008 which received Royal Assent in July 2008. The specific powers provided by the 2008 Act, which amends the Public Health (Control of Disease) Act 1984 enable a Justice of the Peace to make an order where a person poses a risk of infection and that order may require a person to:

  - have a medical examination;
  - be removed to a hospital or other suitable establishment;
  - be detained in a hospital or other suitable establishment;
  - remain in isolation or quarantine;
  - be disinfected or decontaminated;
  - wear protective clothing;
  - provide information or answer questions about his or her health or other circumstances;
  - cooperate in the monitoring of his or her health and the reporting of the results of that monitoring;
  - attend training or advice sessions on how to reduce the risk of infecting or contaminating others;
  - be subject to restrictions on moving around or interacting with others;
  - abstain from working or trading.

- However, at the time of writing, the Health and Social Care Act 2008 is yet to come fully into force and the existing provisions relating to the removal and detention of patients with TB as set out by the Public Health (Control of Disease) Act 1984, sections 37 and 38 continue to apply to Mr Ukhono. A commencement order (the term for delegated or secondary legislation which brings primary legislation into force, often at different times and on specific dates) will follow in due course.

- Notification should be made in the correct form to the consultant in communicable disease control because TB[112] is a notifiable disease. Indeed, it is not widely known, but for a doctor to fail to advise the consultant in communicable disease control promptly of a patient with a notifiable disease, is actually a criminal offence.

- National guidance is available to provide clinicians with ready access to best practice in the management of TB[113] and covers the important issues of notification, monitoring, contact tracing, and treatment adherence.

- Unfortunately, misunderstandings about transmission and stigma, which may be culturally specific, persist. Local authorities in urban areas have begun working effectively across the social care, health (with particular attention to the primary and secondary care interface) and education sectors to ensure that those who may already be disadvantaged are not further marginalized by a diagnosis of TB.

Application of core concepts to Case 68

- For the purposes of discussing process with Mr Ukhono, it is important first to ensure that he is aware of his diagnosis and receives optimal treatment. Therefore, communication should optimize the prospect of a trusting therapeutic relationship and patient courtesy is likely to go further than cajoling, admonishing, or even threatening him with compulsory powers.

- You should explain to Mr Ukhono what the role of the consultant in communicable disease control is, why you are informing him or her and what is likely to happen next especially with regard to contact tracing.

- Most NHS Trusts will have local guidance on how to involve the infectious disease unit or team within the organization when a patient is suspected to have, or diagnosed as having, a communicable disease. And it is important to inform the relevant staff of Mr Ukhono's presence in the hospital, and to seek advice on managing and treating him.

- Once the required notification and proper treatment has been instigated, the importance of preventing further transmission should be explained to Mr Ukhono. His legitimate concerns about his housing must not be ignored and the discussion should be informed by resources that describe the support available to people who are at risk of unlawful eviction.

- Services may be available that will ease the burden of treatment for Mr Ukhono, particularly costs relating to transport, temporary housing, and prescription charges. Demonstrating both an understanding of stigma, empathy for Mr Ukhono's fear regarding his hostel place, and knowledge of the resources available to minimize the impact of diagnosis and treatment make it more likely that Mr Ukhono will understand rather than fear the notification and contact tracing process. Emphasizing that information will only be shared on a 'need to know' basis as part of a well-established and legally regulated process is also important.

- In conclusion, the complexities of compulsion should not dominate the discussion with Mr Ukhono. The aim is to respond as required by law to notify the appropriate people that there is a case of TB in the hospital whilst developing a relationship of trust with a vulnerable man who is frightened that he will be further marginalized. Such a relationship is likely to be the foundation for an effective treatment programme and protect both Mr Ukhono's individual interests and those of the wider community.

Further information

- The incorporation of the European Convention of Human Rights into English law in the form of the HRA 1998 provides further questions and dilemmas for practitioners working in public health. The HRA 1998 contains broad provisions that lay down rights in very general terms. It must be remembered that all statutory law needs to be interpreted by the courts and the degree of interpretation and guidance available on the effect of the HRA 1998 is presently quite limited. Box 10 sets out the provisions of the HRA 1998.

> **Box 10** European Convention on Human Rights and its relationship to the Human Rights Act 1998
>
> - Art 1—Obligation to respect human rights[*]
> - Art 2—Right to life
> - Art 3—Prohibition of torture
> - Art 4—Prohibition of slavery and forced labour
> - Art 5—Right to liberty and security
> - Art 6—Right to a fair trial
> - Art 7—No punishment without law
> - Art 8—Right to respect for private and family life
> - Art 9— Freedom of thought, conscience and religion
> - Art 10—Freedom of expression
> - Art 11—Freedom of assemble and association
> - Art 12—Right to marry and found a family
> - Art 13—Right to an effective remedy[*]
> - Art 14—Prohibition of discrimination
>
> [*] Articles 1 and 13 are not formally incorporated into the Human Rights Act 1998 because the government believed that rights are protected through the domestic courts and therefore these two provisions are automatically ensured.

- The provisions of the HRA 1998 apply only to public bodies (although this includes individuals acting on behalf of public bodies, e.g. doctors working on behalf of a health authority or NHS Trust).
- It is important to note that different articles within the HRA have different status. Thus, articles 3 (Prohibition of torture, inhuman or degrading treatment or punishment), 4 (Prohibition of slavery and forced labour), and 7 (No punishment without law) are absolute rights from which no derogation is permitted (although the rights contained within these articles must be interpreted). In contrast, articles 8–12 are qualified rights where derogation is permitted but any action must be (a) based in law; (b) meet Convention aims; (c) non-discriminatory; (d) necessary in a democratic society; and (e) proportionate.
- Thus, for all but the absolute rights, the HRA is to be interpreted in the context of existing legislation. If existing legislation is found to prevent a public body acting in accordance with the HRA 1998, the court has the power to declare the legislation to be 'incompatible' with the Act (but not to repeal or otherwise to set aside the offending statutory provision).
- The sections of the HRA most likely to be of interest and relevance to clinicians are the rights contained in Articles 2 (Life), 5 (Liberty and security of the person), 8 (Respect for private and family life), and 14 (Non-discrimination in the protection of rights provided for by the HRA 1998).
- The BMA advises that the practice of doctors seeking to comply with the HRA must adapt to a new model in which two questions are asked of every decision, namely (a) are someone's human rights affected or potentially affected by the decision; and (b) is it legitimate to interfere with them? Medical decision-making both at an individual and a population level will be increasingly challengeable and the process of reaching the decision is as important as the substance of the decision itself.

Professionalism, Probity, and Accountability

Professionalism, Probity, and Accountability: Clinical Cases

Case 69 ◆ **Professional boundaries—the flirtatious patient**

Miss Martina Holland is 22 years old. You admitted her to the ward, via A&E, following a severe asthma attack. Once she was stablized in A&E, she made several comments about her **'luck'** *in* **'meeting such a gorgeous doctor'** *and made a note of your name from your ID badge. When you visit her on the ward the following morning, Miss Holland is overtly flirtatious. She says she has* **'put on her makeup and best underwear'** *ready for your examination. You feel very uncomfortable.*

Core concepts[†]

- Although this scenario concerns a female patient, flirtation and sexual innuendo can occur during any doctor–patient combination of both sexes.
- Boundaries are commonly considered with reference to sexual transgressions. Whilst sexual boundary violations do, regrettably, occur in healthcare,[114] the broader issue of maintaining healthy professional boundaries is an integral part of professionalism. Boundaries are essential because of the stubbornly constant power that resides in healthcare professionals' daily work. For however much knowledge is accessible, and shared rather than rarefied, there is an unavoidable power imbalance. The patient has a problem and needs the clinician's advice, opinion, or skills. The patient is dependent in a way that the clinician is not in the encounter. The trick then is not to seek to eliminate power, but to recognize it as inevitable and facilitate mutual trust and respect.
- Sexual boundary violations are usually preceded by slips in boundaries spanning time, and many healthcare professionals will never transgress sexually but do have difficulty maintaining boundaries in their relationships with others.
- The first and crucial stage in maintaining a healthy awareness of boundaries is to establish a shared working definition of what boundaries are in practice. The concept has been variously described but all interpretations commonly encapsulate the notion of the limits that exist (physical, behavioural, and emotional) to ensure a safe and effective therapeutic or working relationship. Boundaries are the fence within which a secure, clearly delineated professional space is created and maintained.

[†] The discussion and guidance notes in this scenario are adapted from an earlier paper; see Bowman D Guidelines on Gynaecological Examinations: Ethico-legal Perspectives and Challenges. Current Obstetrics and Gynaecology 2005; 15(5):348–52.

- The concept of boundaries is more complex and subtle than its common reduction to the issue of sexual transgression would suggest. Self-disclosure, differential availability, attention or allocation of resource, mixing personal and professional contact, gifts,[115] emotional involvement, financial transactions, time, 'rule-bending', and 'making exceptions' can all indicate that boundaries are becoming blurred. Moreover, boundary pushing, crossing, and violating can come from any direction, i.e. the patient may try to push the boundary with the clinician or the student with the clinical teacher. However, the onus is on the healthcare professional to maintain boundaries.

- A useful distinction drawn by Coe and Hiltz,[116] is between boundary crossings (in which harm may not necessarily occur) and boundary violations (in which harm does occur).[117] What then makes a professional more or less likely to push or cross boundaries? Research has demonstrated that the following variables make a clinician more susceptible to crossing or violating boundaries:

  ◆ poor setting of limits;
  ◆ a personal crisis, particularly in relationships;
  ◆ idealization of, or identification with,[118] a 'special' patient;
  ◆ illness, isolation, or other personal vulnerability;
  ◆ lack of awareness or denial of the importance of boundaries;
  ◆ excessive self-disclosure to patients;
  ◆ confidential 'off the record' conversations;
  ◆ extended/additional appointments or rescheduling to the end of the day;
  ◆ contact outside appointments.

- The importance and integrity of the human body is reflected in two dominant principles in contemporary healthcare ethics and law, namely the pre-eminence of autonomy and its legal translation in the concept of informed consent. Chaperoning policies and other professional guidance provide explicit direction for clinicians as to how to protect and prioritize autonomy and the integrity of the human body.

- Guidance on performing so-called 'intimate examinations' (although the term 'intimate' is controversial[119]) is available from the GMC.[120] However, the mere existence of guidelines does not act as an ethico-legal panacea and challenges remain for clinicians, particularly with regard to the place of professional judgement. Clinicians may be required to rely on judgement (paradoxically), both to set aside, and embrace more comprehensively, the guidelines.

- Advice on chaperones and dignity is often admirably rigorous, reflective, and practical. Particularly commendable are guidelines where there is recognition of the value of chaperones irrespective of the gender of the clinician, thereby avoiding presumptions about sexuality, and consideration of the relative benefits and limitations of using different groups as chaperones. However, questions remain about the extent to which chaperoning is *offered* (in the way any investigation or treatment is offered), or *required* as a routine part of examinations.

- Perhaps one of the reasons that these questions remain is because the function of the chaperone is ambiguous. The use of chaperones is not merely protective to, and therefore presumably in the interests of, the patient, but has an important function in protecting doctors too. Therefore, if a patient refuses a chaperone, what is the position of the doctor who wishes to have a chaperone present?

- Ethically, the principle of patient autonomy in Western ethics is core. All competent patients have the right of self-determination and their choices should be respected. Does this ethical model in which autonomy is the predominant principle translate into unfettered choice in all healthcare encounters? It is argued that this is not the case because such a conclusion depends on a simplistic misinterpretation of, and response to, the concept of autonomy, both personal and professional. The way in which the ethical question or 'problem' is understood and phrased is integral to the ensuing analysis and eventual conclusions. Therefore, careful attention should be paid to the 'naming' of an ethical problem. In this situation, it is not whether a patient's autonomy takes priority over a doctor's professional autonomy that is the question, but how autonomy can be facilitated, developed, maximized, and shared by the parties.

- As such, 'autonomy' (personal or professional) is not something to be fought over, but a common aim of clinician and patient in which sharing contrasting, or even conflicting, perspectives allows for and demands dialogue, discussion, and decision-making based on mutual respect and increased understanding. The fostering of, and respect for, patient autonomy is integral to ethical practice and clinicians should be sensitive to the inherent power imbalance; perhaps this imbalance of power is even more acute when considering patients who may feel both vulnerable and embarrassed.

- Given the relative positions of clinician and patient in the consultation, what does it mean to foster patient autonomy? Perhaps it means rejecting notions of autonomy that are constructed in an artificially binary way, as 'all or nothing' choices. Meaningful choices cannot be made in a moral and social vacuum. Just as cultural relativism recognizes and explores the social, temporal, and geographical determinants that result in varied constructions of moral principles, so too ethicists who argue for the pre-eminence of patient autonomy should reflect on the social and cultural context in which autonomy is not only constructed, but can be developed and respected. Frequently, in healthcare, this is an imperceptible daily negotiation in which compromise is possible, but occasionally a patient's choice is in direct opposition to a doctor's choice. In such circumstances, it is unhelpful and possibly unethical for the conflict between doctor and patient preference to become a battle: such an approach is likely to result in dissatisfaction for both parties. Rather, this is the time to explore why there is an apparent irreconcilable difference between patient and doctor perspectives and return to perhaps the primary duty of the clinician: to serve the patient's interests in a professional, altruistic, and disinterested way.

- In order to do this, an exchange of information about why there is a difference between the doctor's and the patient's perceptions of whether and how a chaperone and appropriate professional boundaries contribute to the common goal of 'best interests' is required. Reasons both for a doctor's insistence on maintaining a neutral, professional demeanour and the need for a chaperone, and a patient's refusal of the chaperone, are varied. A doctor may feel that a chaperone is essential because of local employment policy, or based on the advice of her defence organization or simply because of an intuition that the presence of a chaperone would be wise.

- Although allegations of impropriety and sexual assault are rare, does the comparative infrequency of serious allegations sufficient justify doctors acting in a way that is contrary to their professional judgement and places patient autonomy above all else?

- In contrast, a patient may feel that the presence of a third party is intrusive or adds to the embarrassment she feels about the examination, she may be disconcerted by what she perceives as the reframing of her relationship with a clinician whom she trusts and with whom she is flirting only to conceal her discomfort. To represent the complexity of variables that influence both professional and patient responses to chaperones as a competition between doctor and patient choice is simplistic, unhelpful, and ultimately counter-therapeutic.

- The GMC has adopted a pragmatic response to this ethical dilemma; a response which has an eye on the medico-legal implications of conflicting patient and practitioner preference with regard to chaperoning. The advice for the doctor whose offer of a chaperone is refused is to acquiesce, but also to document that a chaperone was refused by the patient. This response is practical and has much to commend it to a busy clinician who has little time to ponder the tensions between the philosophical constructions of professional and patient autonomy, but it doesn't address the ethical question; a question that has implications for all of medical practice.

- The notion that professional autonomy is subservient to patient autonomy on every occasion is to render clinicians to the status of patient-directed technicians and diminishes the knowledge, skills, and therapeutic value of medical training (although it might equally be argued that requiring absolute adherence to formalized professional guidelines likewise diminishes professional expertise). Patient autonomy does not mean that a patient is able to determine absolutely what she would like without reference to professional judgement. For example, few clinicians would accede to a request for a beta blocker from a nervous but seriously asthmatic patient about to take her driving test or an examination. Of course, it does not follow that if patient autonomy, if not respected absolutely, is inevitably sacrificed at the altar of paternalistic medical authority. Rather it reflects that autonomy is less about a competition in which patient and professional preferences jostle for philosophical priority, but depends on an ethos of respect, equality, trust, and shared enterprise in which conflicting interests are balanced, and yet neither completely dominant nor eliminated entirely.

- Once autonomy is reinterpreted for both doctor and patient as a common process in which information is equitably exchanged with the shared aim of improving health, the issue of which party's preference should 'trump' the other party's preference in the consultation becomes redundant. Thus in the beta blocker example above, the ethical issue is not whether a patient can demand treatment that is likely to have adverse consequences, but whether the clinician can create a non-judgemental atmosphere in which the patient feels she can explain her preference, and the clinician can enhance her autonomy by explaining why her preference is ill-advised. It is not about either party 'defending' their position but exploring, and explaining, the differences in their respective perspectives. To do so is to create, perpetuate, and respect autonomy in a far more meaningful and ethically sustainable way than to merely accede to, or refuse, patient 'demands'.

- To return to the chaperoning example when a flirtatious patient is behaving in a way that is discomforting, what should a clinician do when a patient refuses a chaperone? The practical advice of the GMC is a good starting point, but on what ethical basis can this course of action be explained? First, it implies that the doctor and patient will have a discussion about the nature of their relationship and the presence of a chaperone. The doctor will be able to explain that he or she is seeking to follow 'best practice', and clarify the role of the chaperone in the examination. In return, the patient has an opportunity to explain why she does not wish a chaperone to be present allowing the doctor to understand her perspective and to ask questions.

- From the sharing of information comes awareness and challenging of assumptions and the 'problem' can be reframed: no longer is it a question of frustration at conflicting professional and personal wishes, but a process of understanding that the 'wishes' of both doctor and patient are socially, psychologically, and culturally located.

- The exchange of information is, it is argued, the ultimate ethical tool, and without it, discussions of autonomy are meaningless. Of course, even after exploring patient and professional preference, difference may still remain. However, the scene has been set for negotiation, compromise, and reconciliation. This may mean that the doctor decides to proceed without a chaperone: however, it is likely that he or she will do so feeling more comfortable with their decision having heard why it is that the patient is so reluctant to have a chaperone present. Conversely, the doctor may ultimately decide that he or she will not examine the patient without a chaperone, and request that the patient sees a colleague (perhaps of another sex), but the patient is more likely to understand why this is suggested rather than feeling that the doctor has exercised his or her authority and is expressing disapproval of the patient's 'non-compliance'.

Application of core concepts to Case 69

* Miss Holland is apparently pushing professional boundaries. There may be many reasons for her behaviour: she might be using flirtation as a defensive mechanism against insecurity, fear, embarrassment, or vulnerability. It may be transference which is not confined to psychiatric and mental health services. Whatever the 'motive' or 'explanation' however, a professional response is required that is not defensive, hostile, or even similarly flirtatious.

* Intuition is a powerful tool in medicine and it is important to use the discomfort of encountering Miss Holland to take positive action. Candidates should be confident to be explicit about the boundaries of the doctor–patient relationship and explain honestly that they are going to ask a chaperone to be present whilst examining Miss Holland. To do so is not to thwart her autonomy but to treat both the patient and professional with respect and dignity.

* Maintaining a neutral, but polite, approach throughout and simply stating that a chaperone would be a good idea is an effective and non-confrontational way to ensure that professional boundaries are maintained and both parties are protected.

Further information

* Whilst, the predominant focus of most discussions of boundaries is the relationship between clinician and patient, boundaries can be pushed or violated within any relationship, e.g. between colleagues (especially where there is a hierarchical or power imbalance), or between clinical teachers and students.

* Notwithstanding the importance of boundaries in protecting clinicians and patients, education and training about boundaries is variable and the subject is frequently limited, if not completely absent from many curricula. As such, working on the basis that an explicit statement of standards is essential if a culture of professionalism is to exist, attention should be given to the issue of boundaries in both codes of conduct and staff development programmes. There are a number of established training organizations offering well-received training and staff development in the field of boundaries, notably Jonathan Coe's organization, WITNESS.[121]

* For further guidance on professional boundaries in clinical practice, the 'Clear Boundaries' project conducted by the Council for Healthcare Regulatory Excellence is an excellent resource.[122]

Case 70 ♦ **Conflict and anger management — patient and relatives perceiving poor treatment in A&E following musculo-skeletal presentation**

Marcus Matthews, a 15 year old boy, attended A&E with his mother after his leg 'froze' in mid-air whilst he was playing football. The F2 doctor in A&E elicited a history of pain down the right thigh which worsened on movement. Marcus could not recall any injury. On examination, Marcus was found to have a pronounced limp with pain on external and internal rotation of the hip. The F2 doctor diagnosed a groin strain and advised Marcus and his mother that he should return if the symptoms persisted. Four days later, the boy returned to A&E with both his parents. This time, Marcus was seen by another F2 doctor who confirmed the previous findings. The second doctor prescribed Norgesic tablets for Marcus and, once again, advised him to return if the symptoms persisted. Two days later, Marcus fell at school and was unable to stand on his right hip. He was brought back to hospital in a teacher's car and joined by his parents. You are working in A&E and see Marcus. Radiography reveals a slipped upper femoral epiphysis. Marcus's parents are very angry about the suboptimal care they believe their son received in A&E on his first two visits to the department. They ask how their son's diagnosis could have been missed and want to make a formal complaint. How should you respond?

Core concepts

- Complaints, and ensuing litigation, often occur when patients feel aggrieved because of something quite separate from the clinical care that has been received. It is an old and untraceable adage that 'a doctor who is nice to his patients can get away with murder' but the spirit of this saying may be true. Such a statement is not intended to be trite or facetious—there is much a clinician can do to manage anger and dissatisfaction which influences both whether a complaint is pursued and, more importantly, how patients and families feel about the clinical care that has been received.

- It is important to be familiar with, and able to explain, the ways in which complaints are handled both in your local NHS Trust and nationally. In April 2009, the complaints proce- dure changed and a national scheme comprised of two stages was introduced.[123] The first stage is local resolution and requires institutions to respond to individual complaints. The second stage enables patients or their representatives to refer the matter to the Parliamen- tary and Health Service Ombudsman.

- Without exception, NHS Trusts will have dedicated departments to handle complaints. It is the role of that department to meet statutorily defined timescales, arrange meetings, and lead investigations—it not the role of individual doctors. However, front-line clinicians are effectively the gatekeepers to, and public face of, the hospital as far as patients and their relatives are concerned. As such it is essential to know how to respond immediately and to whom patients should be referred.

- Figure 70.1 shows in simplified form the ways in which disputes in the NHS can progress.

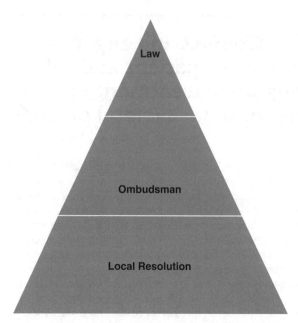

Figure 70.1 The progression of disputes in the NHS.

- Where a dispute has not become formalized, it may still require discussion and resolution. Third parties and external groups may be useful in this context. These might include clinical ethics committees, clinical governance meetings, mediators, conciliators, senior clinicians, managers, and faith group leaders. These are ad hoc systems that tend to be organic, in that they evolve according to perceived need and are usually without statutory force.

- The process of complaints is important and, to proceed, the stages shown in Figure 70.1 need to be pursued in order. If legal proceedings are initiated, i.e. negligence claims, the complaints process ceases. Note that the 'law' at the top of the complaints' process diagram refers only to judicial review of the process of making a complaint. In addition to negligence actions, patients or their representatives may, in some circumstances, wish to make a complaint to the professional regulatory body, e.g. the GMC, about an individual practitioner. Complaints to the regulatory body about a clinician can co-exist with a complaint made under the NHS complaints procedure.

- A complaint should be made within twelve months of the incident. A complaints' manager has discretion to extend the time limit if the circumstances show that the complaint could not have been made earlier, and if it is still possible to investigate the complaint.

- Patients should receive an acknowledgement of their complaint within three working days and be kept informed about its investigation. The purpose of local resolution is to provide an opportunity for the complainant and the organization (or individual), to attempt a rapid and fair resolution of the problem. The process should be open, fair, flexible, and conciliatory, and should facilitate communication on all sides. The procedure introduced in April 2009 places greater emphasis on face to face meetings.

- NHS Conciliation is one method of facilitating a dialogue to resolve an issue and the aim is that a third party will help the parties to reach a common understanding. 'Conciliation' is often used interchangeably with 'mediation' or confused with 'arbitration'. In the NHS, mediation is often associated with claims settlements, i.e. it is used to negotiate the terms of a settlement once a family or patient has initiated negligence proceedings at law. As the NHS complaints and claims systems are currently separate, it is not useful to use the term 'mediation' in relation to the complaints procedure. However, many conciliators will use mediation skills. Arbitration is very different to both conciliation and mediation in that it is often not voluntary and the arbitrator may make a judgement and impose a settlement. There are certain principles which must apply when conciliation is adopted, namely:

- ◆ conciliation encourages and maintains the voluntary participation of all parties;
- ◆ it is confidential;
- ◆ it is without prejudice, i.e. it will not influence potential or actual legal proceedings that might ensue;
- ◆ the conciliator is impartial, independent, and non-judgemental;
- ◆ it encourages the participation and self-determination of all the parties so that they retain responsibility for both the content of the conflict and the outcome of the conciliation;
- ◆ conciliation is a collaborative and not an adversarial process;
- ◆ it offers a structured and challenging approach to conflict resolution;
- ◆ it seeks to help parties identify their own and others feelings and interests rather than defend positions.

- The conciliator's report does not form part of the complaint file, but would usually note agreed action points or outcomes (e.g. an explanation or an apology), which with the agreement of both parties, can be shared. There are no judgements or recommendations.
- If local resolution is concluded and the complainant remains dissatisfied, he or she can refer the case to the Health Service Ombudsman. The Ombudsman considers complaints made by or on behalf of people who have suffered an injustice or hardship because of unsatisfactory treatment or service by the NHS or by private health providers who have provided NHS funded treatment to the individual. The Ombudsman can consider complaints about:
  - ◆ unsatisfactory care or treatment, including the exercise of clinical judgement;
  - ◆ failure to provide a service that ought to have been provided; and
  - ◆ poor administration, which might include poor complaint handling, rudeness, misleading advice, refusal to provide information to which an individual is entitled, or clerical error.
- Bodies or individuals under investigation must, in law, provide any evidence requested by the Ombudsman and must otherwise assist with her investigation in any way she requests. The appointment of a designated officer within NHS bodies responsible for each complaint is also expected to ensure effective liaison during the investigation—usually the designated officer will be located in the local NHS Trust complaints department.
- Upon completion of an investigation, the Ombudsman may uphold the complaint in full or in part or may not uphold the complaint at all. In any case, she will set out her findings and the reasons for those findings in her report. Where the complaint is at least partially upheld, she may make recommendations for appropriate redress, which might include an apology, an explanation, improvements to practices and systems, or, where appropriate, financial redress. She also has the power to refer individual clinicians to regulatory bodies, such as the GMC, in the interests of patient safety where she considers that this is appropriate. The Ombudsman will expect her recommendations to be implemented and will contact the relevant NHS provider to find out how her recommendations have been implemented.

- The final possible stage in the complaints procedure is judicial review. If a patient, or his representative, is unhappy with the Ombudsman's investigation and conclusion, it may be possible for the complainant to pursue a judicial review action. In brief, judicial review is a process whereby the decisions of public bodies or organizations are reviewed for procedural propriety, reasonableness of process and administrative fairness.

- Although handling anger and receiving complaints is stressful and not something any clinician welcomes, understanding that the ways in which one communicates and familiarity with the correct NHS complaints procedure can do much to diffuse a difficult situation can be reassuring. All the major defence organizations identify calm, clear, and accurate communication as the best protection against disputes escalating.

Application of core concepts to Case 70

- Marcus's family is angry. It may be that there is just cause for their anger, or it may be that the progression of their son's symptoms masked the true diagnosis to such an extent that the two doctors who had been consulted earlier were appropriate in their assessment. At this stage, it does not matter whether Marcus's parents are justified or not in their anger. The task now is to provide good clinical care to Marcus, to listen and acknowledge his parents' concerns, and to identify ways in which they can record their dissatisfaction formally.

- People who are angry need to feel heard. Inviting Marcus's parents to a quiet room where you will not be disturbed and creating an environment in which they can express themselves is essential. It is worth considering whether there are any staff in the A&E department with whom Marcus and his family established a relationship and, if so, inviting that person to accompany you.

- Once in a private area, allow Marcus's parents to speak. Be clear that there are defined processes for making a formal complaint and this meeting is not a substitute for proper procedure—it is your chance to hear their story and express personal regret for what they have experienced. It does not matter whether you believe their interpretation of events has merit, this is about relationship building: taking them seriously and really listening to people who are very unhappy.

- It is essential to remain calm, be informed about the steps Marcus's family have to take to make a formal complaint and demonstrate empathy. Avoid judging, being defensive, debating the 'facts' of their perceptions and interrupting. You should listen, offer information on their options with regards both to the future clinical management of Marcus's care and their dissatisfaction, and provide the contact details of those who will be able to support and guide them through hospital procedures. Although Marcus is the patient, his parents are entitled to make a complaint on his behalf as his representatives.

- You might also mention to Marcus's parents that the Patient Advocacy and Liaison Service (PALS) can be useful to some and the Independent Complaints Advocacy Service (ICAS) is an alternative, non-hospital affiliated, source of advice and support. ICAS services are sometimes, but not routinely, provided by the Citizens Advice Bureau (CAB).

- Listening and explaining, in simple and non-technical language, to Marcus's parents what has happened and what the options are for addressing their concerns should be the priority in this scenario. Appropriate apologies and honest explanations do not, contrary to popular misconception, render clinicians legally vulnerable but do much to obviate the risk of protracted disputes. Remember to record what you discuss in both the medical records and with the Complaints' Department. You should inform and involve your consultant at the earliest opportunity even if he or she was not available to meet the family. No one wants to hear of a dispute in their department via the hospital grapevine.

- It is also likely that there will be a need to communicate with the two F2 doctors who initially saw and treated Marcus—feedback to the junior staff involved is probably the responsibility of the consultant but to be effective will need to be informed and accurate so it depends on your management of the information you received both from the notes, treating Marcus and speaking to his family.
- Attentive listening, patient understanding, and empathic responses will go a long way to diffusing the anger felt by Marcus's parents. It is not an easy consultation, but it is a vital consultation with the potential to reduce conflict, repair relationships, and build trust.

Further information

- If and when a dispute proceeds to being a formal legal action, all other procedures described above cease. Traditionally, clinical negligence has been an adversarial process that could result in either pre-trial settlement or proceed to a hearing (usually in the High Court). However, in recent years there has been increasing interest in mediation as a means of resolving clinical negligence disputes. Indeed, both the NHS Litigation Authority and the Legal Services Commission encourage greater use of mediation.
- Legal action is governed by a procedure known as the 'pre-action protocol'. The protocol recommends a timed sequence of steps for patients and healthcare providers, and their advisers, to follow when a dispute arises with the aim of facilitating and speeding up the exchange of relevant information. The protocol aims to maximize the chances that a dispute can be resolved without resort to a full legal hearing. Only once the protocol has been followed should an action proceed to court where the legal rules of negligence will apply, namely:
  - ◆ duty of care;
  - ◆ standard of care;
  - ◆ causation; and
  - ◆ proximity of loss.

Case 71 ◆ **Adverse event/critical incident reporting procedures**

Ms Felicity Hughes attended A&E following a fall during a club hockey match at the weekend. She complained of pain in her left wrist and hand. On examination, the area is slightly swollen and Ms Hughes is mildly tender over the anatomical snuff box but does not appear to feel pain on palpation. Imaging appears not to show any fracture and Ms Hughes is discharged with analgesia. At the X-ray review meeting, a senior doctor identifies a small scaphoid fracture.

Core concepts

- Missed scaphoid fractures are common. In addition to ensuring that Ms Hughes receives appropriate treatment and complications prevented by calling her back as soon as possible and explaining why such fractures are commonly missed, this episode constitutes a critical incident or adverse event which should be recorded and used to inform learning.

- For critical incident reporting to be meaningful, it must be more than a paper-based exercise in administrative rule observance. Most NHS Trusts will have a prescribed system and form for recording details of the incident. Forms may vary but thought should be given both to the data recorded and the ways in which those data are likely to be most useful in influencing learning and future practice at a systemic level.
- The basic information that should be recorded is:
  - the date, time and location of the incident;
  - the names, addresses, and status of the people involved including cross references to patient numbers, staff identifiers, departmental locations and relationships of third parties;
  - a brief factual account of the incident;
  - the action taken to resolve the incident;
  - the names of all additional people with actual or potential professional responsibility and interests;
  - observation/reflection on the situation/context in which the incident occurred;
  - any injury or damage that occurred;
  - any additional comments that seem relevant either to what happened or to learning from what happened.
- In addition to merely completing the paperwork, it is good practice to talk to senior staff, e.g. the consultant(s) overseeing the departments (in this case A&E, radiology, and possibly orthopaedics), senior nursing and therapies clinical leads whose staff have been involved (or should have been involved) in the incident, any third parties with responsibility for the patient, etc. Such conversations are likely to enhance the way in which the form is completed and ensure that it is a valuable learning exercise rather than a tick box procedure.
- Although the scenario described here is a straightforward, if common, clinical error, critical incident reporting is wide-ranging and episodes of violence, aggression, health and safety concerns, near misses, interpersonal conflict, miscommunication, and leadership failures should also be included in systemic reporting.
- Information should be recorded in as much factual detail as possible. Reflection on the incident is invaluable but impressionistic generalization should not substitute for accurate, honest, and comprehensive description. Consideration or analysis of the impact or significance of an incident should be located in examples and the details of what occurred. Cultural norms, values, and attitudes can be usefully illuminated in critical incident reporting, but must be grounded in examples or patterns of behaviour. Those reviewing critical incidents should have to 'read between the lines' as little as possible.
- Ideally, the premise for critical incident reporting is that it is a positive way to achieve systemic improvement in practice and not a managerial tool for individual blame. However, without effective leadership and individual cooperation at all levels, critical incident reporting can be variably effective. It is as much a professional duty to ensure that incidents are properly reported whilst members of staff are appropriately supported as it is to be competent in biomedical knowledge and clinical skills.

Application of core concepts to Case 71

- Ms Hughes should be contacted straight away, probably by telephone (being alert to the challenges of communicating by phone as discussed in Case 63 Confidentiality and the Telephone) and asked to come back to the hospital as a priority.

- She should be told honestly what has happened, i.e. *'At our X-ray review meeting, we picked up a fracture that should be treated called a scaphoid fracture. I am sorry to have to ask you to come back to the hospital.'* Although it is acceptable to explain that such fractures are easy to miss, care should be taken to avoid sounding defensive, complacent, or indifferent.

- If Ms Hughes has questions about why the fracture was missed, the effects of missing the injury and the purpose of the X-ray review meeting, these should be answered truthfully, openly, and without defensiveness.

- Once Ms Hughes has been seen and treated appropriately with arrangements in place for follow-up, the critical incident process should be considered. Has a form been submitted and by the appropriate person? In addition to the 'paper-based' review, is it important to talk to other staff who may not have attended the review meeting but have a stake in the patient's experience?

- Discussions should take place in an environment of support, honesty, and learning—the aim is not to humiliate, belittle, or criticize individuals.

Further information

- Although the analysis of critical incident forms may be beyond the remit of many MRCP candidates, it is useful to have an idea of what constitutes appropriate analysis of critical incidents and how reporting is used to develop clinical practice. Although systems of analysis will differ, the core principles are common, namely:

  ◆ to review practice to identify patterns, recurring themes, and areas for attention;

  ◆ to assist with the above in classifying incidents according to severity and frequency;

  ◆ to maintain a central record of cross-specialty practice that is inter-professional, inclusive, and non-hierarchical; and

  ◆ to use best practice guidance to facilitate root cause analysis of critical incidents and inform improvements in practice and learning.

Case 72 ◆ Medical error in medication administration—penicillin to known allergic patient

Mrs Newman was admitted to the ward via her general practitioner. On admission she informed the on-take team that she was allergic to penicillin and her referral letter from the GP also noted the allergy. On admission, a note of her allergy was duly recorded in the medical record. The following morning, a locum doctor on your team prescribed penicillin for Mrs Newman. As soon as Mrs Newman received the penicillin she began to have a serious anaphylactic reaction. The nurse who administered the penicillin to Mrs Newman put out an emergency call and Mrs Newman responded well to immediate treatment with epinephrine and corticosteroids.

(i)   *How should the clinical team respond to this error?*

(ii) *Would Mrs Newman be able to bring an action for negligence?*

Core concepts

- Before turning to the specific scenario, it is worth spending a little time explaining how to distinguish between medical error and medical negligence. Whilst most claims of negligence will involve errors, not all errors constitute negligence.

- The first component of a negligence claim is to establish that the defendant owed a duty of care to the claimant. Usually, this is not terribly difficult in cases of medical negligence, as all doctors are considered, at common law, to owe a duty of care to their patients. Indeed, in an emergency, this duty may extend beyond the patients on a doctor's list to anyone whom one may encounter depending on the circumstances.

- The technical difficulties lie in the next two stages of establishing negligence, namely:

  - proving that the duty of care was breached in such a way as to fall below the standard of care that could reasonably be expected of a medical practitioner in similar circumstances; and

  - establishing that it was this breach of duty by the medical practitioner that actually *caused* (both in law and in fact) the damage suffered by the patient.

- The judgment in *Bolam* v *Friern Management Committee* has long been the source from which professional standards are derived and against which a clinician's actions are assessed in a negligence action. The essence of the test is to examine whether or not a practitioner's actions fall short of, or differ from, those of a body of reasonable practitioners. Therefore, on the application of the *Bolam* test, if an expert witness stated that a doctor's actions were those of a reasonable practitioner, it was most unlikely that he would be found liable for negligence.

- However, in November 1997, during the case of *Bolitho* v *City and Hackney Health Authority* the 'reasonable practitioner' standard of care test was amended. The House of Lords held that the court was not bound to accept that a clinician was not negligent merely because an expert (or number of experts) could be found to affirm that a defendant's actions were reasonable. In addition, there was a requirement that, in order to be judged 'reasonable', a defendant's actions (and the expert's opinion of those actions) should be capable of 'withstanding logical analysis' by the court.

- The decision was greeted with much excitement in the medico-legal press and interpreted as marking the demise of the traditionally accepted power of the medical profession to determine an appropriate standard of care. However, in practice, it is likely that only a negligible number of cases will produce expert opinions that are so unreasonable that they do not withstand logical analysis.

- It would seem that, although in theory the perceived protection afforded to the medical profession by the *Bolam* test has been modified by the judgment in *Bolitho*, in practice the effect of such a modification is likely to be highly limited if not undetectable. Furthermore, as McHale[124] points out, 'their Lordships were, in fact, quite circumspect in their approach'. It would seem that although in theory the perceived protection afforded to the medical profession by the *Bolam* test has been modified by the judgment in *Bolitho*, in practice the effect of such a modification is likely to be limited and perhaps the real power of the decision is, as McHale goes on to suggest, in sending out a signal for future clinical litigation.

- It is the issue of causation on which many medical negligence cases turn and this can be an extremely complex and technical area (and usually occupies most of the expert witnesses' time). In situations where patients have been unwell over a significant period of time, it can be extremely difficult to say when the damage occurred, and at what point a doctor was negligent. Thus many cases will fail on the basis of causation. For example, where steroid eye drops are prescribed and continue to be prescribed for a longer period than is indicated, appropriate, or safe, a potential negligence action will depend on the point at which the prescription became inappropriate and whether this coincided with the damage caused to the patient from the continued prescription. The legal significance of causation is further illustrated by litigation relating to the prescription of benzodiazepines. In many of these cases, the initial decision to prescribe a tranquillizing drug was appropriate but the continued prescription of the drug without review when, the claimants allege, information was available to show that these were a group of drugs perhaps even more addictive than heroine or cocaine was inappropriate. Therefore, the claimant has to establish, on the balance of probabilities, exactly when he became addicted to the drug, and whether this coincided with inappropriate prescribing based, of course, on the information available at the time of the prescription. Only if the point at which the patient became addicted, the inappropriate prescribing and awareness by the doctor of the risk of addiction coincide to cause damage to the patient, could any action succeed.

- The courts are neither concerned with best practice nor with unfeasibly high standards of care. It is not expected that doctors are 'super doctors' who always make perfect decisions, accurately identify rare conditions, and never make a mistake. What is expected is that doctors behave in a way that accords with the practice of a reasonable doctor—and the reasonable doctor is not perfect.

- There is much that clinicians can do to prevent formal complaints and litigation. Openness is a valuable asset in clinical practice generally and, particularly when something has gone wrong. The question of whether or not to apologise when something has gone wrong used to be a particularly confusing area for many doctors. However, the current advice from defence organizations is that a prompt apology is an appropriate response to an adverse incident, as is an accurate account of the facts. Indeed, the GMC goes further and states that all doctors have a moral obligation to apologise and explain when medical errors and accidents occur. As a doctor, you are not compromising your position by apologising. On the contrary, you may be preventing further complaints, and/or future legal action by a courteous and appropriate apology.

- Finally, the equation of competence and negligence is, it is suggested, to be avoided. Given the fallibility of human endeavour, any doctor may make an error that constitutes negligence. However, this does not render that doctor incompetent. It is generally accepted that inherent in the definition of incompetence is time, i.e. *patterns* of error or *repeated* failure to learn from error. In short, many doctors who have been held to be negligent are competent and many incompetent doctors will never have been, nor will be, held to be negligent.

Application of core concepts to Case 72

- It is significant that this scenario involves how Mrs Newman's allergy to penicillin was recorded and communicated. Contrary to popular belief, many negligence actions in medical practice emanate from errors in communication and administration, rather than from clinical and diagnostic errors. The legal implications of this are numerous and all too easily overlooked as the failure of the simplest processes can break the chain of delivery of service and expose patients to harm.[125]

- In the case of Mrs Newman, the criteria for a negligence claim do appear to be satisfied. Clearly the clinical team, including locum staff, owes Mrs Newman a duty of care. The receiving on-take team recorded Mrs Newman's allergy in the records and therefore to prescribe penicillin was to fall below the standard that could be expected of a reasonable body of medical practitioners and does not withstand logical analysis. The ensuing anaphylactic reaction was causally related to the negligent prescription of penicillin and the proximate damage was reasonably foreseeable. If Mrs Newman were to bring an action it would, by virtue of the Crown Indemnity scheme, be against the hospital rather than named members of the team. Given the circumstances it is likely that the Trust would settle the claim as there is little to defend given the nature of the errors.

- However, merely because Mrs Newman can bring a negligence action, it does follow that she will do so. A prompt apology for the error and the willingness to discuss what has happened may go a long way to vitiating any intention to litigate. More prosaically, to bring an action would require money, energy, and investment of time: Mrs Newman may well, in common with many patients who experience avoidable error during care, decide that she is prepared to forgive fallibility and never go near a lawyer's door.

Further information

- Aside from the interpretative character of the standard of care tests used in court, there are further limits to using the law of negligence as a definitive source for defining the competent practitioner.

- First, case law is a partial and skewed corpus of material: many of the most catastrophic cases of clinical negligence never reach the court and are therefore never subject to, nor contribute to the evolution of, the legal standard of care because they are settled out of court (i.e. a payment is made on behalf of the defendant doctor or health authority to the claimant before the case is heard in court).

- Secondly, for a claim of negligence to be instigated, not only must the patient have suffered damage, but he or she must have sufficient insight to question whether the care provided by the doctor may have fallen below the appropriate standard of care. This is no mean feat for a non-expert. One of the reasons that *Bolam* remained the accepted test of the standard of care in clinical negligence for so long was because the courts necessarily relied on medical expertise because the ability of non-clinicians to understand, still less assess, the quality of medical care provided is often limited. If the powerful and disinterested legal system struggles to evaluate medical care, it is even more difficult for a patient.

Case 73 ◆ **Recognizing and admitting limits of own competence**

Louise is a newly qualified nurse working on a medical ward. You are covering that ward as a second year Foundation doctor. A patient has been admitted to a ward who is taking three types of medication, Aluminium Hydroxide suspension 4% 5–10mls four times a day, Ranitidine 150mg twice daily and 'Drug X' 2mg twice daily. Louise is responsible for the patient's care and has asked you to 'refresh her memory' about the purpose and actions of the patient's three medications because 'the patient has been asking all day'. You are familiar with Aluminium Hydroxide and Ranitidine, but you have never heard of 'drug X'. There is no British National Formulary to hand and you are in a hurry.

Core concepts

- The aim of this scenario is to admit uncertainty honestly and offer Louise options for finding out more and accurate information before she tells the patient anything of which you are both unsure. It is the explanation of the third drug, 'drug X', that provides the core of the assessment. It has been chosen and left unnamed because the purpose is to pose a scenario to candidates where their capacity to be honest about the limits of their knowledge and admit uncertainty are assessed. In practice, it is likely that the third drug, investigation, or intervention will be named but chosen for its obscurity.

Application of core concepts to Case 73

- The principal function of this scenario is to assess a candidate's willingness to acknowledge the limits of his or her competence and his or her readiness to admit uncertainty. Although candidates are expected to discuss the purpose and action of drugs, this is *not* the primary aim of this assessment.
- The first task is to establish what Louise already knows about the patient's medication. Candidates will be familiar with the first two drugs and should explain in simple and clear terms the purpose and action of Aluminium Hydroxide and Ranitidine, namely, e.g., saying something like *'Aluminium Hydroxide is symptomatic treatment for dyspepsia and works by neutralising gastric acid'* and *'Ranitidine treats conditions like peptic ulcers and gastro-oesophageal reflux disease by blocking histamine H2 receptors, which reduces acid secretion'*.
- As regards the third medication, 'drug X' and assuming it is unfamiliar, at all costs avoid guessing, dissembling, or confabulating. The most that can be offered are sensible ways of finding out what the drug is and its significance to the patient, i.e. via a British National Formulary (BNF) or Medline.
- Candidates should ask the nurse whether she has understood what has been explained and whether she has any remaining questions. It probably goes without saying that a cooperative manner that avoids condescension is required throughout.

Further information

- Renee Fox[126] has argued that uncertainty is inevitable and falls into two categories. The first refers to the limitations of an individual practitioner's knowledge; the second (and more significant) describes the intrinsically limited nature of healthcare knowledge itself. Biomedicine is incomplete, controversial, and contested, and there remains an infinite amount of unanswered, and perhaps, unanswerable questions. It is, posits Fox, the conflation of these two types of uncertainty with which every healthcare professional must learn to cope in practice.

Case 74 ◆ **Reference request from former medical student whose consultant refused to 'sign her off' following a clinical attachment**

Katia was a medical student on the firm on which you are a specialist trainee. She was not an asset to the team and was regularly absent. When Katia did attend, she was flippant and sometimes rude to staff, appeared to have limited knowledge, was overconfident and demonstrated poor clinical skills. Indeed, so limited was Katia's contribution to the clinical team that your consultant refused to 'sign her off' and she had to repeat the attachment during her elective period with another firm. You worked a lot with Katia and found her frustrating but tried to be supportive throughout her time on the firm. You have not heard from Katia since she left the firm last year until you receive, out of the blue, an email from her asking you to be her referee in support of her applications for Foundation year training jobs. Katia says that she is asking you because **'you were always so nice to me'** *and goes on to say that as a* **'younger doctor, you'll know we all make mistakes as students and should be given a second chance'.** *How should you respond to Katia's request?*

Core concepts

- Reference requests are commonplace in the NHS, and it is easy to forget the importance of such requests in a busy working life.

- Medical students may struggle to distinguish themselves or be memorable to their seniors, but Katia has, unfortunately, become memorable for undesirable reasons. Her task therefore is to take responsibility for poor performance as a medical student, not to seek to 'cover it up' by obtaining a reference from a junior doctor whom she may perceive to be a 'soft touch'.

- The reference is not merely a document that goes into the application ether. It is a statement on which employers, colleagues and Deaneries rely. Katia's future patients, the receiving clinical team(s) of which she will be a member and the Deanery that is responsible for her training are depending on a full and accurate account of her knowledge, skills, and professionalism.

Application of core concepts to Case 74

- Katia is asking something that has significant implications for her, for you as the potential referee, for the profession, and for patients.

- Taking each of the parties affected by this reference request in turn, let us consider Katia first. Katia is about to begin her career in medicine and is seeking her very first position. She is at the bottom of the medical hierarchy and the early experiences of training are likely to shape her perception of medicine and possibly her future. Although the process of applying for Foundation jobs can appear like an extension of medical school, Katia is about to become an employee for the first time. She may have given varying degrees of consideration to her choices for foundation positions but, at the very least, she should not begin her career with dishonesty or misrepresentation.

- The implications of Katia's request for you are considerable. An honest reference will be of limited value, and indeed may be damaging, to Katia. Therefore, it seems likely that she is expecting a misleading reference that omits or distorts the facts about your working relationship.

- Indeed, her statement about your relative youth and understanding suggests that she is expecting you to produce a reference that does not reflect the true nature of her performance on the firm. To do so is to lie: you will be placing the interests of a fellow, albeit nascent, member of the profession above the interests of those of patients and her NHS employers and may enable her, in the language of the criminal law, to obtain a pecuniary advantage by deception.

- In short, to attest to Katia's suitability for the profession in a reference is to call into question the referee's own suitability for the profession.

- In response to Katia's email, an expression of surprise at being asked to act as a referee given the less than ideal way in which you met and worked together would seem the most appropriate reaction. That expression of surprise may yet be sufficient to enable Katia to realise that she has misjudged you and should not have asked you to act as a referee for her.
- It may be telling that she has sought out a junior member of a firm on which she was not signed off rather than her repeated placement or indeed other attachments from her final year. If Katia remains obtuse about the inappropriateness of her reference request, a clear statement explaining why you would not be able to say anything positive about her work supported by examples of her poor performance during the attachment is required, perhaps with an accompanying comment on the assumptions she appears to have made about the support you offered her during her time on the firm and the relative seriousness with which she seems to believe younger doctors treat reference requests.

Case 75 ◆ A colleague who causes concern—possible alcohol abuse

Dr Peters is a consultant in your Trust. He has been a consultant for ten years and is well liked and respected by both colleagues and patients. For several weeks now, however, you have noticed that Dr Peters seems to smell of alcohol at odd times of the day and, on a couple of occasions, he has appeared not to be completely sober at team meetings. One day as a patient is leaving the outpatient clinic, she remarks that **'I don't see Dr Peters these days because he's getting a bit too fond of the drink isn't he doctor?'**

What would you do in this situation? Why?

Core concepts‡

- Clinical accountability has become a much-debated issue in the last decade. Media sensationalism, the public perception of a sometimes 'closed shop' approach, clinicians' (sometimes justified) frustration at the avaricious and mercenary lawyer swooping on human errors, and the long-held belief that to criticize one's colleagues publicly is simply not appropriate, have all contributed to a situation where the various parties have taken up sometimes intractable and often poorly-reasoned positions in the debate. In the wake of high profile public inquiries,[127] and the well-publicized responses from the Chief Medical Officer on behalf of the Department of Health,[128] there has a significant move towards open and accountable practice. Doctors are required to reflect on their practice and demonstrate their competence throughout their careers. Furthermore, there is a responsibility on all healthcare professionals to be alert to their colleagues' competence.

---

‡ The discussion and guidance notes pertaining to this scenario are adapted from an earlier publication; see Bowman D Fallible, Unlucky or Incompetent? Ethico-legal Perspectives on Competence in Primary Care. In Bowman D and Spicer J, Primary Care Ethics. Oxford: Radcliffe Medical Press; 2007.

- In relation to the work of healthcare professionals, section 18(1) of the Health Act 1999 imposes a duty of quality on all those working in the NHS. It is this provision that underpins the principles of clinical governance: the formalization of a professional duty to scrutinize practice with the aim of maintaining and improving standards in the broadest sense. Clinicians have a collective responsibility, therefore, not only to reflect on their own practice but also to be aware of and, if necessary, respond to the practice of colleagues even in the absence of formal line-management responsibilities.

- Another statute that may be relevant to those concerned with a doctor's performance is the Public Interest Disclosure Act 1998, which provides protection for those who express formal concern about a colleague's performance. Essentially the statute is an amending Act and states that it is a breach of employment legislation to penalize or dismiss an employee who makes a 'qualifying disclosure'[129] under the statute (and information regarding the health and safety of persons is explicitly included within the list of qualifying disclosures under s 1).

- As well as constituting a 'qualifying disclosure', concerns must be expressed using appropriate procedures and be made in good faith. While the law clearly seeks to support those who make the difficult decision to blow the whistle, its effect in practice may be limited. Although 'disadvantage' and 'dismissal' are prohibited by the Act, it cannot prevent intense discomfort, isolation, and subtle expressions of hostility.

- It is, of course, the GMC that defines standards of professional practice and has ultimate responsibility for investigating when a doctor's standard of practice is questioned. Professional bodies, such as the GMC, BMA, and the Royal Colleges have diverse but often overlapping roles in developing, defining, and revising standards for doctors. It is worth examining the specific guidance provided by the GMC in greater detail, specifically in relation to the issues of competence and underperformance. The principal publications in which the GMC sets out standards and obligations could all be said to contribute to defining the competent doctor, but three requirements are of particular relevance, namely that a doctor must:
  - Keep his or her professional knowledge and skills up to date.
  - Recognize the limits of his or her professional competence.
  - Act quickly to protect patients from risk where he or she has good reason to believe that a colleague may not be fit to practise.

- The work of the GMC in regulating the profession does not reach the majority of practising doctors. Even though there have been suggestions recently that the GMC is being over-zealous in pursuing doctors about whom there are concerns, it remains likely that expressions of concern will be shared, initially and perhaps exclusively, with other clinicians and possibly managers. The discretion of first-line responders is considerable and the ways in which those initially approached choose to interpret the problem and subsequently respond carries considerable moral and professional responsibility.

- If concern is expressed about a doctor, the first ethical duty of his colleagues is to explore the diverse perspectives of those involved and negotiate the naming of the problem. It is only by this process that an appropriate response can be provided—values, interpretations, perceptions, and opinions are not irritants to be neutralized in the pursuit of an illusory objective process, but integral to providing a fair and transparent process.

- For those who are concerned about a doctor's performance, there will be conflicts of interest. Ethically, conflicts of interests are important because they influence and sometimes determine the ways in which we perceive and respond to a problem. Traditionally, in the ethico-legal literature, conflicts of interest have been characterized as denoting personal or professional gain, often in a financial sense. However, there are more subtle ways in which conflicts of interest can and should be considered. Consulting styles, prescribing choices and preferences for particular consultants are all likely to influence practice. If a fellow clinician doesn't share one's preferences, how might this affect a judgement of competence? It is relatively easy to recognize a financial or political conflict of interest, but it is more difficult to recognize these subtle, yet potentially powerful, influences on how one constructs medical practice and therefore the competent practitioner.

- A rigorous and ethical response to performance problems in healthcare demands that the participants engage in the important stages of:
  - naming the problem and exploring how others name the problem;
  - identifying conflicts of interest (interpreted broadly) that may influence responses to the problem;
  - locating the duties owed to patients in ethical theory;
  - learning from, and sharing, the experience.
- The law, professional guidance, and policy provide an unequivocal starting point: inaction in the face of justifiable concerns about a colleague's performance is not an option. However, to travel ethically and defensibly from this unequivocal starting point remains challenging—clear and factual expressions of concern, documented meetings, timescales for change, and ultimately prioritizing the patient are always essential, but rarely easy.

Application of core concepts to Case 75

- In the case of Dr Peters, potential conflicts of interest abound. First, one is likely to feel loyalty towards Dr Peters as a colleague, and perhaps even a friend. The longer one works with colleagues, the stronger the bonds of loyalty may be. It has been argued that those who raise concerns about clinical performance are most likely to be new to existing organizations and systems.[130]
- In addition to the personal loyalty to Dr Peters as a colleague, there may be other conflicts of interest. Clinical teams are rarely over-staffed and the impact of disruption is potentially considerable. In addition to the inconvenience and cost of losing Dr Peter's services either temporarily or permanently, there may be less quantifiable effects on the reputation of the team, the relationship of the department with external parties who may have an interest in Dr Peters' performance, the ways in which Dr Peters' difficulties reflect on those who appointed him and staff workload.
- Given that significant numbers of doctors don't register with a GP, self-medicate and/or find seeking help difficult,[131] it is important to establish whether Dr Peters has access to advice and support outside the Trust occupational health service, for example, a GP and/or support organization specifically aimed at doctors.
- Having argued that naming the problem and considering conflicts of interest broadly are the first two stages in responding ethically to concerns about Dr Peters, in what ways might the core ethical concepts of duty and consequences further inform the analysis?
- In the case of Dr Peters, one might ask whether there are principles or obligations that are relevant to the case, for example, with regard to truth-telling, putting patients first above all other groups, or respect for persons.
- Consequentialism, in contrast, seeks to explore problems with reference to the likely consequences: in the case of Dr Peters, one might ask what the consequences of possible actions or inactions might be. For example, are there circumstances in which truth is likely to have adverse consequences for Dr Peters himself or patients? What would the net gains and losses be if the Trust suspends or even dismisses Dr Peters? How would decisions affect Dr Peters' career and well-being?

- Although there is a clear difference between deontology and consequentialism, it may be misleading to imply that a theoretical choice has to be made. The development of moral obligations and rules is often informed by likely consequences. It is also possible simultaneously to make deontological and consequentialist points to support a moral position.
- Dr Peters' colleagues may feel that they owe duties to two parties, namely patients and Dr Peters himself. Using Ronald Dworkin's[132] terminology, the duty to patients is clear, 'trumps' the duties to Dr Peters and the profession, and is reinforced by the GMC, which states unequivocally *'you must make the care of the patient your first concern'* and:

  you must protect patients from risk of harm posed by another doctor's… conduct, performance or health… the safety of patients must come first at all times. Where there are serious concerns about a colleague's performance, health or conduct, it is essential that steps are taken without delay to investigate the concerns to establish whether they are well-founded, and to protect patients[133]

- These ethical imperatives could be said to be based on the principle of respect for persons. Patients are not a means to an income, professional security, or self-worth, but are ends in themselves. Patients are dependent upon doctors for care and they do not come to the relationship with equal status or knowledge. Put simply, most patients trust their doctors: they believe they are competent. Thus Dr Peters' colleagues have a duty to investigate the concerns. The only way in which the ethical imperative to place patients first can be fulfilled is to address the concerns about Dr Peters' performance.
- If there is reason to be concerned about Dr Peters' competence, it is likely that someone senior will want to talk to Dr Peters directly. In the course of this conversation, it is possible for a senior colleague to have regard to the secondary duty of care to Dr Peters himself by offering advice and support, provided that the senior colleague does not lose sight of his primary duty—to protect patients.

  If there is, as I have argued, an ethical obligation to tackle the question of Dr Peters' performance once the concerns are found to be warranted, is there any place for a consequentialist analysis of the problem? Reviewing the source of the principle that demands action by staff and the broader literature on performance and accountability in medicine, it is evident that consequences are very important. The GMC invokes the concept of risk repeatedly in its statements that doctors must act in the event of poor performance. Clearly medicine is a risky enterprise, but the moral acceptability of risk is connected to competence. Thus most would accept that a surgeon conducting an operation may have a 70% mortality rate, provided he has done all he can to ensure he is proficient at performing the operation, that he performs it to the best of his ability, and that he reviews his practice to ensure that he remains acceptably proficient; but not if the same surgeon has a 70% mortality rate for an operation for which he is inadequately trained, that he conducts with a hangover or other impairment and that he chalks up to experience. Doctors must put themselves in the best position to be competent notwithstanding the inherent risks of medicine: the moral difference is between avoidable and unavoidable mistakes.
- If Dr Peters accepts that there are problems with his performance, it may be possible to negotiate actions that will ameliorate the situation, particularly if careful and close attention is played to naming the problem and matching the response. For instance, is the problem a knowledge deficit (educational remediation, mentoring, and perhaps supervised practice may be appropriate), is it a health or stress-related problem (access to independent support, advice, and treatment are indicated), or are there systems problems (attention to the surgery and its ways of working would be warranted)?
- If, as is perhaps more likely, Dr Peters does not accept there is a problem with his performance, how should his colleagues proceed? Again, the GMC is clear:

you must give an honest explanation of your concerns to an appropriate person from the employing authority... . If there are no appropriate local systems, or local systems cannot resolve the problem, and you remain concerned about the safety of patients, you should inform the relevant regulatory body.

• It is likely that the next stage for senior colleagues would be to contact the service centre director or medical director. Another source of advice is the National Clinical Assessment Service (formerly the National Clinical Assessment Authority), which draws on its national and international expertise in performance problems while emphasizing local resolution.

• Implicit in the emphasis on consequences is harm, which prompts the question of whether poor performance matters independent of consequences. It is submitted that poor performance matters very much whether or not harm is likely or ensues: patients come to doctors expecting a basic level of competence and care, and the relationship depends on trust. A hospital makes representations to patients that foster and maintain trust. Representations that a doctor is someone in whom a patient should place his trust inform the whole process of seeking care. If Dr Peters continues to practise while there are serious concerns about his performance, this is ethically unacceptable, irrespective of the risk of harm, because it indicates collective misrepresentation and dishonesty by the NHS.

Further information

• Given the range of sources available to those seeking external guidance on competence and performance in medicine, why do performance problems remain among the most challenging of all ethical dilemmas? The clue may be the word 'ethical'. Pellegrino and Thomasma[134] argue that the inherent humanity of the doctor and the patient endows the clinical encounter with a moral force that is more powerful than basic legal rules, guidelines, and codes of conduct. Jacob,[135] commenting on Thomasma and Pelligrino also accepts that ethics have regulatory function. Jacob frames regulation as something to which the medical profession reacts.

• However, given the determination with which the profession has fought (and may continue to fight) to protect the principle of self-regulation, it could equally be argued that the profession is proactive not reactive and shapes the nature of its own regulation. Regulation may be necessary but it will rarely be sufficient. As such, the place of ethical analysis is integral to the identification and management of a performance problem—and ethical analysis is difficult.

• The naming of a problem is not a neutral process. Implicit in the identification, interpretation and presentation of a problem are values, preferences, and choices, which may reflect deeper philosophical and political allegiances. For example, what a patient values may be quite different from what the doctor values and this difference may result in disparity in how each party defines competence. The place of values is particularly evident when reviewing the ways in which clinical competence has been considered by academics and professionals, even without taking into account patient perceptions.

• It is perhaps unsurprising that it can be very difficult to determine 'competence' in medicine. There has been significant research on this topic by, among others, Marilyn Rosenthal[136] and she suggests several reasons for this difficulty, namely:-

  ◆ As in any other profession, very few doctors (if any) get through their careers without making a mistake (or several). This cannot and should not mean that they are labelled incompetent.

  ◆ Continuum and consistency in performance appear to be vital when doctors are asked to judge their peers. Thus it is only after a certain number of mistakes that questions begin to be asked about competence. However, the judgement about competence is made more difficult by the fact that it is extremely hard to draw the boundary between the 'avoidable' and the 'unavoidable' mistake in a discipline as uncertain as medicine.

- ◆ Doctors are trained to be aware of the fallibility of the human being and are perhaps more forgiving and 'loyal' than other professions when it comes to judging the actions of their colleagues. There is, Rosenthal suggests, a norm of non-criticism.

- The literature on clinical competence has focused variously on systems, individual responsibility and personal experience, the taxonomy and classification of error, intention and the moral aims of doctors and medicine, quantitative measures of performance and statistical analyses of outcomes, stress, ill-health, psychology and other influences on competence, professional identity, power and collective culture, and responses to errors or poor performance. These differences are important. They are not just indicative of vital academic debate, but demonstrate first, how difficult it is merely to name the problem with which one is dealing when reflecting on clinical performance, and second, how the ways in which one eventually elects to name the problem determines ensuing analysis and decisions.

- Finally, is there an ethical way in which to move on from performance problems? The literature suggests that there is a moral imperative to learn, both individually and collectively from medical error if not poor performance. In a fascinating review of error reporting in the nascent specialty of neurosurgery between 1890 and 1930, Pinkus demonstrates how the focus on positive results in medicine was not always the preferred model.[137] Indeed, just as medical research shapes and limits not only the knowledge base but also the culture and identity of medicine, so too does professional and academic publishing. Could it be that there is an ethical imperative, if not to publish, at least to share experiences of assessing and responding to performance problems? May we yet see the day when *The International Journal of Medical Errors, Poor Performance and Negative Findings* takes pride of place on journal subscription lists?

- Certainly, there has been a long-held view that there is an imperative to learn from error, if not more generalized patterns of poor performance. Charles Bosk's seminal and groundbreaking work[138] described how young surgeons are expected to respond to their errors by remembering and learning. The value and desirability of learning is evident in the importance attributed to significant event and critical incident analyses where participation is now a professional obligation. If there is a moral obligation to learn from discrete events and individual clinical cases, could this be part of a wider imperative to review how one assesses and responds not only to one's own performance, but also to that of colleagues?

- The issues of competence and accountability within the medical profession will continue to prompt loud and often passionate debate from all quarters of society (many, of course, with perceived or actual vested interests). However, there are no easy answers to the questions of competence and accountability. A 'whistle-blower' can be a heroic paragon of courageous conviction willing to fight for truth and justice in the face of hostile and aggressive opposition from his colleagues and at the expense of his own career prospects. However, he may equally well be a vexatious, jealous, and spiteful under-achiever motivated solely by the base desire to undermine and perhaps even destroy the reputation of a fellow doctor. How reliably can the distinction be drawn between these two extremes? It seems certain that the somewhat populist broad-brush stroke of the recent legislation does nothing to answer this most crucial of questions. Equally, whilst clinical governance, performance assessment and revalidation procedures may highlight 'poor performers', such measures will not *per se* offer the appropriate support and help that such 'poor performers' need and deserve.

References for cases 41–75

1. Harris D, Davis R. An Audit of 'Do Not Attempt Resuscitation' Orders in Two District General Hospitals: Do Current Guidelines Need Changing? Postgraduate Medical Journal. 2007; 83:137–40.

2. Current guidance appears in a document produced jointly by the Resuscitation Council, the British Medical Association (Medical Ethics Department) and the Royal College of Nursing and can be found at www.resus.org.uk.

3. Ebrahim S. Do Not Resuscitate Decisions: Flogging Dead Horses or A Dignified Death? BMJ. 2000; 320:1155–6.

4. Hakim R et al. Factors Associated with Do Not Resuscitate Orders: Patients' Preferences, Prognosis and Physicians' Judgements. Annals of International Medicine. 1996; 125:285–93. Cherniack E. Increasing Use of DNR Orders in the Elderly Worldwide: Whose Choice Is It? Journal of Medical Ethics. 2002; 28:303–7.

5. Age Concern. Turning Your Back on Us: Older People and the NHS. London: Age Concern, 2000.

6. A label that has been adapted from a philosophical school formally known as 'Futilitarianism' which proposes that all human endeavour is ultimately futile.

7. Bowker L, Stewart K, Hayes S, Gill M. Do General Practitioners Know When Living Wills are Legal? J R Coll Physicians. 1998; 32:351–3.

8. Zaman S. and Battock T. Doctors Need to Know More About Advance Directives. BMJ. 1998; 317:146.

9. R (Lesley Burke) v General Medical Council [2004] EWHC 1879.

10. Re T (Adult: Refusal of Treatment) [1992] WLR 6, 782–6.

11. The role of the Lasting Power of Attorney replaces the Enduring Power of Attorney that was largely confined to acting for those lacking capacity in financial and property decisions.

12. For guidance and further information on the role of Lasting Power of Attorney, see the Office of the Public Guardian website—www.publicguardian.gov.uk

13. The Court of Protection has the power to remove someone from the role of Lasting Power of Attorney if it is satisfied that the attorney is not acting in the best interests of the incapacitous person.

14. Schneiderman LJ, Jecker NS, Jonsen AR. Medical Futility: Its Meaning and Ethical Implications. Ann Internal Medicine. 1990; 112:949–54. Truog RD, Brett AS, Frader J. The Problem with Futility. N Engl J Med. 1992; 326:1560–4. Weijer C, Elliott C. Pulling the Plug on Medical Futility. BMJ. 1995; 310:683–4. Weijer C. Why I Am Not A Futilitarian. CMAJ. 1999; 869–70. Weijer C. Cardiopulmonary Resuscitation for Patients in a Persistent Vegetative State: Futile or Acceptable? CMAJ. 1998; 491–3.

15. For a clear and accessible summary of the IMCA service and its work, see Making Decisions: The Independent Medical Capacity Advocacy (IMCA) Service. London: Department of Health; 2007.

16. Redley M et al. Evaluation of the Pilot Independent Mental Capacity Advocate Service. London: Department of Health; 2006.

17. Waller BN, Repko RA. Informed Consent: Good Medicine, Dangerous Side Effects. Cambridge Quarterly of Healthcare Ethics 2008; 17: 66–74.

18. Chester v Afshar [2004] 4 All ER 587, HL.

19. Mason K, Laurie G. Reproductive Counselling and Negligence. In Mason and McCall Smith's Law and Medical Ethics. 7th ed. Oxford: Oxford University Press, 2006. p. 184 ff.

20. See http://www.cancerscreening.nhs.uk/bowel for further information on the national screening programme.

21. For a summary of the literature on genetics and bowel cancer, see http://info.cancerresearchuk.org/cancerstats/types/bowel/molecularbiologyandgenetics [Accessed 3 June 1008].

22. Cochrane Database of Systemic Reviews. Screening for Colorectal Cancer using the Faecal Occult Blood Test: An Update. 2006.

23. See http://www.cancerscreening.nhs.uk/bowel.

24. Rance v Mid-Downs AHA [1991] 1 All ER 801.

25. *R v Cambridge HA, ex parte B* [1995] 1 WLR 898, CA and *R v Cambridge HA, ex parte B (No 2)* [1996] 1 FLR 375.

26. Per Lord Bingham.

27. Estimated at between 10 and 20%; see The Provision of Hospital Care. In Kennedy I, Grubb A, editors. Principles of Medical Law. Oxford: Oxford University Press.

28. See Rawls J. A Theory of Justice. Cambridge MA: Harvard University Press; 1971.

29. Horton R. Herceptin and Early Breast Cancer: A Moment for Caution. Lancet. 2005; 366:1673.

30. Romond EH, Perez EA, Bryant J, et al. Trastuzumab plus Adjuvant Chemotherapy for Operable HER2-positive Breast Cancer. N Engl J Med. 2005; 353:1673–84. Piccart-Gebhart MJ, Procter M, Leyland-Jones B, et al. Trastuzumab after Adjuvant Chemotherapy in HER2-positive Breast Cancer. N Engl J Med. 2005; 353:1659–72.

31. Richards C, Dingwall R, Watson A. Should NHS Patients be Allowed to Contribute Extra Money to their NHS Care? BMJ. 2001; 323:563–5.

32. See Muncie, J. Criminological Perspectives. Oxford: Oxford University Press; 1997; Homer AC, Gilleard C. Abuse of Elderly People by their Carers. BMJ. 1990; 301:1359. Ogg J, Bennett G. Elder Abuse in Britain. (BMJ. 1992; 305:998.

33. Harris D, Davis R. An Audit of 'Do Not Attempt Resuscitation' Orders in Two District General Hospitals: Do Current Guidelines Need Changing? Postgraduate Medical Journal 2007; 83:137–40.REP

34. Current guidance appears in a document produced jointly by the Resuscitation Council, the British Medical Association (Medical Ethics Department) and the Royal College of Nursing and can be found at www.resus.org.uk.

35. Bouchner H, Vinci R, Warning C. Pediatric Procedures: Do Parents Want to Watch? *Pediatrics* 1989; 84: 907–9.

36. Ardley C. Should Relatives be Denied Access to the Resuscitation Room? Intensive Crit Care Nurs. 2003; 19:1–10. Azoulay E, Sprung CL. Family–Physician Interactions in the Intensive Care Unit. Crit Care Med. 2004; 32:2323–8. Baskett PJF, Steen PA, Bossaert L. European Resuscitation Council Guidelines for Resuscitation: The Ethics of Resuscitation. Resuscitation. 2005; 6751:5171–80.

37. Compton S, Magdy A, Goldstein M. et al. Emergency Medical Service Providers' Experience with Family Presence during Cardiopulmonary Resuscitation. Resuscitation. 2006; 70:223–8. Ong ME, Chung WL, Mei JS. Comparing the Attitudes of the Public and Medical Staff towards Witness Resuscitation in an Asian Population. Resuscitation. 2007; 73:103–8.

38. Most of these cases have involved people travelling to the 'Dignitas' clinic in Switzerland.

39. In July 2009.

40. See the *Assisted Dying for the Terminally Ill*, a bill proposed by Lord Joffe but which did not complete its passage through Parliament.

41. The concept was first described by a judge named Devlin (later Lord Devlin) in his summing up to the jury in a murder trial in 1957; see *R v Adams* [1957] Crim LR 365.

42. *Airedale NHS Trust v Bland* [1993] AC 789.

43. See for example Helme J, Padfield A. Safeguarding Euthanasia, NLJ. 1992; 142:1335 in which the authors declared the decision to prosecute Dr Cox 'disproportionate' to any wrong committed by the defendant.

44. British HIV Society, British Association for Sexual Health and HIV, British Infection Society. UK National Guidelines for HIV Testing 2008. Available at http://www.bhiva.org [Accessed 16 July 2009].

45. HIV Post-Exposure Prophylaxis: Guidance from the UK Chief Medical Officer's Expert Advisory Group on AIDS. London: Department of Health; September 2008.

46. Good Medical Practice. London: General Medical Council; 2006.

47. Christakis DA, Feudtner C. Ethics in a Short White Coat: The ethical dilemmas that medical students confront. Acad Med. 1993: 68(4):249–54. Caldicott Y, Pope C, Roberts C. The Ethics of Intimate Examination—Teaching Tomorrow's Doctors. BMJ. 2003; 826:97–9; Calton E, Essex J, Bowman D, Barrett C. Ethics Teaching for Clinical Practice: A Student Perspective. The Clinical Teacher. 2008; 5(4):222–6.

48. See the NHS Research Ethics Service, www.nres.npsa.nhs.uk, for the current regulatory framework within which clinical research must be conducted.

49. See www.nres.npsa.nhs.uk.

50. See Campbell A, et al. Research Ethics. In Campbell A, Charlesworth M, Gillett G, and Jones G. Medical Ethics.Oxford: Oxford University Press; 1997.

51. Risk should include not only physical risks, but also inconvenience, discomfort, embarrassment, and invasion of privacy.

52. See the 198. Revision of the Declaration of Helsinki.

53. Singer P. Animal Liberation. London: Random House; 1975.

54. Bentham J. An Introduction to the Principles of Morals and Legislation, section XVIII, IV (Dover Philosophical Classics). Mineola, NY: Dover Publications; 2007.

55. See 'The Use of Animals in Medical Research' in Campbell A, Charlesworth M, Gillett G, Jones G. Medical Ethics, 2nd ed. Oxford: Oxford University Press; 1997. p. 179.REP?

56. Fox MA Returning to Eden: Animal Rights and Human Obligations. London: Viking; 1980. p. 116.

57. Frey RG. Vivisection, Morals and Medicine. In Kuhse H, Singer P. editors. Bioethics: An Anthology. Oxford: Blackwell; 1999. pp. 471 ff.

58. Some commentators, notably Dr Stuart Derbyshire, have criticized the 3Rs suggesting that as the policy is motivated by animal welfare, the logical consequences of adopting such a perspective are bound to compromise the potential benefits of using animals in research.

59. British Medical Association. Survey of the Public's Attitudes to Presumed Consent. London: British Medical Association; 2008.

60. British Medical Association. Presumed Consent for Organ Donation. London: British Medical Association; 2007.

61. Department of Health. The Potential Impact of An Opt-Out System of Organ Donation in the United Kingdom: An Independent Report from the Organ Donation Taskforce. London: Department of Health; November 2008.

62. This scenario and the accompanying discussion are adapted from an earlier publication by the author; see Price J, Bowman D. Complexity, Guidelines and Ethics. In Bowman D, Spicer J. Primary Care Ethics. Oxford: Radcliffe Medical Press; 2007.

63. Grilli R, Lomas J. Evaluating the Message: Tthe relationship between compliance rate and the subject of a practice guideline. Med Care 1994; 32:202–13. Ellrodt AG et al. Measuring and Improving Physician Compliance with Clinical Practice Guidelines (a controlled interventional trial). Ann Intern Med. 1995; 122:277–82.

64. Atkinson P. Medical Work and Medical Talk. London: Sage; 1995.

65. Millman M. The Unkindest Cut: Life in the backrooms of medicine. New York: William Morrow; 1976. Cassell J. Expected Miracles: Surgeons at work. Philadelphia, PA: Temple University Press; 1991.

66. Mol A. The Body Multiple: Ontology in medical practice. Durham NC: Duke University Press; 2002.

67. Bosk CL. All God's Mistakes: Genetic counselling in a paediatric hospital. Chicago: University of Chicago Press; 1995.

68. Strong PM. The Ceremonial Order of the Clinic. London: Routledge; 1979.

69. Goodman K. Ethics and Evidence-based Medicine. Cambridge: Cambridge University Press; 2003. p.133.

70. Sackett DL, Strauss SE, Richardson WS, Rosenberg W, Haynes RB. Evidence-based Medicine: How to practise and teach EBM. Edinburgh: Churchill Livingstone; 2000.

71. *Airedale NHS Trust* v *Bland* [1993] 1 All ER 521.

72. 'if a doctor treating a PVS [persistent vegetative state] patient acts in accordance with (the guidelines)... he will be acting with the benefit of guidance from a responsible and competent body of professional opinion, as required by the Bolam test... I also feel that those who are... involved in a decision to withhold life support... would do well to study this paper.' (per Lord Goff in *Airedale NHS Trust* v *Bland* [1993] 1 All ER at 521).

73. For example, the practice of administering antenatal corticosteroids was well-established before the practice was included in guidelines issued by the Royal College of Obstetricians and Gynaecologists.

74. Indeed this was the principle underlying the formation of the *Bolam* test. The desire to protect clinical freedom has most recently been seen in the *Pfizer* case (*R* v *Secretary of State for Health, ex parte Pfizer* [1999] 2 CCLR 270) in which the court held that the actions of the Secretary of State for Health were unlawful because of the bald check on clinical judgement 'which is supreme'.

75. Although this has not prevented some interesting speculation on the future of guidelines in determining the standard of care: see Harpwood V. NHS Reform, Audit, Protocols and Standard of Care. Medical Law International. 2002; 1:241–59 in which it is suggested that deviation from guidelines should result in a reversal of the burden of proof (i.e. in the *defendant having to prove on the balance of probabilities* that he or she was not negligent in not adhering to the guidelines.).

76. See *Loveday* v *Renton and Wellcome Foundation Ltd* (1990) 1 Med LR 117.

77. This point reinforces the importance of good, accurate, and contemporaneous notes. For guidance on the appropriate standard of note-keeping, see Norwell N. The Ten Commandments of Record Keeping. The Journal of the MDU. 1997; 13(1):8–9.

78. See, for further information, Gillon R. Refusal of Potentially Life-Saving Blood Transfusions by Jehovah's Witnesses: Should Doctors Explain that not all JWs think it is Religiously Required? *J Med Ethics*. 2000; 26(5):299–301. Elder L. Why Some Jehovah's Witnesses Accept Blood and Conscientiously Reject Official Watch Tower Society Blood Policy. J Med Ethics. 2000; 26:375–80.

79. Management of Anaesthesia for Jehovah's Witnesses. 2nd edition. London: Association of Anaesthetists of Great Britain and Ireland; 2005.

80. The question of how much weight should be afforded to the so-called 'blood card' in emergencies where a patient is unconscious was controversial even before the Mental Capacity Act 2005 came into force. Following the passing into law of the Statute, it seems that changes may need to be made to the format of the card if it is to have the status of a valid advance statement.

81. Schiller H J Optimal Care for Patients who are Jehovah's Witnesses. Anesth Anal. 2007; 104:755–6.

82. The Law Commission. *Breach of Confidence* (1988) (Cmnd 8388), para 6.1, London.

83. In France and Belgium, confidentiality is protected by the criminal code. See the French Penal Code, art 378, and the Belgian Penal Code, art 458.

84. *Stephens* v *Avery* [1988] Ch 449 at 455.

85. *Hunter* v *Mann* [1990] 1 AC 109.

86. Dhar J, Leggat S, Bonas S. Texting—A Revolution in Sexual Health Communication. Int J STD AIDS. 2006; 17:375–7. Lim MS, et al. SMS STI: A Review of the Uses of Mobile Phone Text Messaging in Sexual Health. Int J STD AIDS. 2008; 19(5):287–90.

87. See www.drthom.com.

88. There remain a few circumstances in which the Access to Health Records Act 1990 applies, particularly in relation to deceased persons.

89. It is assumed in this discussion that the patient is an adult. Generally speaking, the healthcare records of minors who are not *Gillick* competent, and can therefore not consent to sharing information, should be disclosed only if such disclosure is in the child's best interests.

90. Where there is a valid lasting or enduring power of attorney, a request can be made from the person acting in that capacity provided that the information sought relates to an area covered by the power of attorney.

91. Ineson N. The Format of a Medico-Legal Report in The Medico-Legal Practitioner Series: General Practice. London: Cavendish Publishing; 1996.

92. Norwell N. The Ten Commandments of Record Keeping. The Journal of the MDU. 1997; 13(1):8–9.REP

93. If a request to change records is made by a patient, amendment should take the form of an addendum to the original inaccurate note—information should not be removed from the records.

94. For a case where the judge looked very harshly on a doctor who wrote 'usual list of neurotic symptoms—a waste of time', and 'same old sob story' in a plaintiff's notes, see *Rhodes* v *Spokes and Fairbridge* [1996] 7 Med LR 136 per Smith J. Note also her general remarks concerning the significance of poor notes: 'Any doctor who fails to keep an adequate note of a consultation lays himself open to a finding that his recollection is faulty and someone else's is correct'.

95. *Sykes* v *DPP* [1962] AC 528, per Lord Denning at 564.

96. Road Traffic Act 1988, s 172; *Hunter* v *Mann* [1974] QB 767.

97. Terrorism Act 2000.

98. *Rice* v *Connolly* [1966] 2 All ER 649.

99. Montgomery J. *Health Care Law*. Oxford: Oxford University Press; 1997. Ch. 11, p. 266.

100. Criminal Law Act 1967, s 5(1).

101. Confidentiality and Disclosure of Health Information Toolkit. BMA, July 2008.

102. [1990]. Ch 359; [1990] 1 All ER 835.

103. Draper H. Confidentiality. Med Def Union Journal. 1997; 13(2):28–30.

104. General Medical Council. Reporting Gunshot Wounds: Guidance for Doctors in Accident and Emergency Departments. General Medical Council, London; 2003.

105. Frampton A. Reporting of Gun Shot Wounds by Doctors in Emergency Departments: A Duty or A Right? Some Legal and Ethical Issues Surrounding Breaking Patient Confidentiality. Emerg Med J. 2005; 22(2):84–6.

106. Mulholland H. Doctors Told to Report Knife Wounds. The Guardian. 7 July 2008.

107. Reporting Knife Wounds: Interim Guidance from the General Medical Council and the Department of Health. London; August 2008.

108. This provision of the HRA must be read alongside the Data Protection Act 1998.

109. World Health Organisation. TB—A Global Emergency. Geneva 1994: World Health Organisation; 1994.

110. Coker R. Tuberculosis, Non-compliance and Detention for the Public Health. J Med Ethics. 2000; 26:157–9.

111. Department of Health. Review of Parts II, IV and VI of the Public Health (Control of Disease) Act 1984: Report on Consultation. London: Department of Health; November 2007.

112. Whether or not TB has been confirmed microbiologically; see Health Protection Agency UK Surveillance. http://www.hpa.org.uk/web/HPAweb&HPAwebStandard/HPAweb_C/1195733739390 [accessed July 2008].

113. Royal College of Physicians. Tuberculosis: Clinical Diagnosis and Management of Tuberculosis and Measures for its Prevention and Control. London: RCP; 2006.

114. Council for Healthcare Regulatory Excellence. Clear Boundaries Report. 2007. available at http://www.chre.org.uk/.

115. Bowman D. Probity and Presents: Ethical Perspectives on Gifts from Patients. Management in Practice. 2007; 10: September/October.

116. Coe J, Hiltz L. Handling Dilemmas and Lapses: Boundaries with Patients. Presentation at the NCAS National Conference, London; 2 March 2009.

117. See also Norris DM, Gutheil TG, Strasburger LH. This Couldn't Happen to Me: Boundary Problems and Misconduct in the Psychotherapy Relationship. Psychiatr Serv. 2003; 54:517–22.

118. Named after Michael Balint and his seminal work on the doctor–patient relationship, these groups provide a formal space in which to reflect on, and share, experiences and interactions between clinicians and patients.

119. Frayn EH. Mountains out of Molehills. Rapid Responses. 2003. bmj.com (http://bmj.bmjjournals.com/cgi/eletters/326/7380/97). Kaushik NC. What Examination is Not Intimate? Rapid Responses 2003. bmj.com (http://bmj.bmjjournals.com/cgi/eletters/326/7380/97). Ford S. Please Can We Avoid Dangerous Conflations? Rapid Responses. 2004. bmj.com (http://bmj.bmjjounrals.com/cgi/eletters/330/7485/234).

and MacKenzie GM. What Is an Intimate Examination? Rapid Responses. 2004. bmj.com (http://bmj. bmjjounrals.com/cgi/eletters/330/7485/234).

120. Intimate Examinations (2002) London: General Medical Council.

121. www.professionalboundaries.org.uk.

122. http://www.chre.org.uk/publications/#folder3 [Accessed 10 September 2008].

123. For further details of the NHS Complaints Procedure, see the regulations that accompany the new scheme—The Local Authority and National Health Service Complaints (England) Regulations 2009.

124. McHale J. Quality in healthcare: a role for the law? Qual Saf Health Care. 2002; 11(1):88.

125. Panting G. Continuity of Care. MPS Casebook. 1997: 9 Summer: 6 ff.

126. Fox R. (1957) Training for Uncertainty. in Merton R, Reader G, Kendall P. editors. The Student Physician. Cambridge, MA: Harvard University Press; 1957.

127. The Kennedy Inquiry is examining the events at the Bristol Royal Infirmary and has published an interim report; see www.bristolinquiry.org.uk. The Ritchie Inquiry examined the conduct of gynaecologist Rodney Ledward; see The Report and Inquiry into Quality and Practice within the NHS arising from the actions of Rodney Ledward.

128. See Department of Health. An Organisation with a Memory. London: TSO; 2000.

129. See s. 1 of the Public Interest Disclosure Act 1998.

130. Martin JP. Hospitals in Trouble. Oxford: Blackwell; 1985. Pilgrim D. Explaining Abuse and Inadequate Care. In Hunt G. editor. The Health Service: Accountability, law and professional practice. London: Edward Arnold; 1995.

131. Chambers R, Belcher J. Self-reported Healthcare over the Past Ten Years: A survey of general practitioners. BJGP. 1992; 42:153–6. Nuffield Provincial Hospitals Trust. The Provision of Medical Services to Sick Doctors: A conspiracy of friendliness? London: NPHT; 1994. Thompson WT et al. Challenge of Culture, Conscience and Contract to General Practitioners' Care of their Own Health: Qualitative study. BMJ. 2001; 323:728–31.

132. Although Dworkin uses the term 'trumping' in relation to rights; see Dworkin R. Taking Rights Seriously. London: Gerald Duckworth; 1977.

133. General Medical Council. Good Medical Pracitce, Section: 'Duties of a Doctor'. GMC; November 2006.

134. Pellegrino ED, Thomasma DC. The Virtues in Medical Practice. New York: Oxford University Press; 1993.

135. Jacob J. Doctors and Rules. London: Routledge; 1998.

136. See Rosenthal M. The Incompetent Doctor. Buckingham: Open University Press; 1996. Lloyd-Bostock S, Mulcahy L, Rosenthal M. Medical Mishaps: Pieces of the Puzzle. Buckingham: Open University Press; 1999.

137. Pinkus RL. Learning to Keep a Cautious Tongue: The reporting of mistakes in neurosurgery 1890–1930. In Rubin SB, Zoloth L. editors. Margin of Error: The Ethics of Mistakes in the Practice of Medicine. Hagerstown, MD: University Publishing Group; 2000.

138. Bosk C. Forgive and Remember: Managing medical failure. Chicago: University of Chicago Press; 1979.

INDEX